Respiratory Manifestations of Neuromuscular and Chest Wall Disorders

Editors

F. DENNIS MCCOOL
JOSHUA O. BENDITT

CLINICS IN CHEST MEDICINE

www.chestmed.theclinics.com

June 2018 • Volume 39 • Number 2

ELSEVIER

1600 John F. Kennedy Boulevard • Suite 1800 • Philadelphia, Pennsylvania, 19103-2899

http://www.theclinics.com

CLINICS IN CHEST MEDICINE Volume 39, Number 2
June 2018 ISSN 0272-5231, ISBN-13: 978-0-323-58392-3

Editor: Colleen Dietzler
Developmental Editor: Casey Potter

Clinics in Chest Medicine (ISSN 0272-5231) is published quarterly by Elsevier Inc., 360 Park Avenue South, New York, NY 10010-1710. Months of issue are March, June, September, and December. Periodicals postage paid at New York, NY and additional mailing offices. Subscription prices are $366.00 per year (domestic individuals), $691.00 per year (domestic institutions), $100.00 per year (domestic students/residents), $419.00 per year (Canadian individuals), $858.00 per year (Canadian institutions), $479.00 per year (international individuals), $858.00 per year (international institutions), and $230.00 per year (international and Canadian students/residents). International air speed delivery is included in all Clinics subscription prices. All prices are subject to change without notice. **POSTMASTER:** Send address changes to Clinics in Chest Medicine, Elsevier Health Sciences Division, Subscription Customer Service, 3251 Riverport Lane, Maryland Heights, MO 63043. **Customer Service: Telephone: 1-800-654-2452** (U.S. and Canada); **1-314-447-8871** (outside U.S. and Canada). **Fax: 1-314-447-8029. E-mail: journalscustomerservice-usa@elsevier.com (for print support); journalsonlinesupport-usa@elsevier.com (for online support).**

Reprints. For copies of 100 or more of articles in this publication, please contact the Commercial Reprints Department, Elsevier Inc., 360 Park Avenue South, New York, NY 10010-1710. Tel.: 212-633-3874; Fax: 212-633-3820; E-mail: reprints@elsevier.com.

Clinics in Chest Medicine is covered in *MEDLINE/PubMed (Index Medicus), Current Contents/Clinical Medicine, EMBASE/Excerpta Medica, Science Citation Index,* and *ISI/BIOMED.*

Printed in the United States of America.

Contributors

EDITORS

F. DENNIS McCOOL, MD
Professor of Medicine, Division of Pulmonary, Critical Care, and Sleep Medicine, The Warren Alpert Medical School of Brown University, Chief of Medicine, Memorial Hospital of Rhode Island, Pawtucket, Rhode Island, USA

JOSHUA O. BENDITT, MD, FCCP, RYT
Professor of Medicine, Director of Respiratory Care Services, University of Washington School of Medicine, Seattle, Washington, USA

AUTHORS

MAZEN O. AL-QADI, MD
Section of Pulmonary, Critical Care, and Sleep Medicine, Yale New Haven Hospital, Yale University School of Medicine, New Haven, Connecticut, USA

WILLIAM A. BAUMAN, MD
Professor of Medicine and Rehabilitation Medicine, Icahn School of Medicine at Mount Sinai, New York, New York, USA; Director, Rehabilitation Research & Development Center of Excellence for the Medical Consequences of Spinal Cord Injury, James J. Peters VA Medical Center, Bronx, New York, USA

JOSHUA O. BENDITT, MD, FCCP, RYT
Professor of Medicine, Director of Respiratory Care Services, University of Washington School of Medicine, Seattle, Washington, USA

DAVID J. BIRNKRANT, MD
Division of Pediatric Pulmonology, MetroHealth Medical Center, Professor of Pediatrics, Case Western Reserve University School of Medicine, Cleveland, Ohio, USA

ANDREW T. BRAUN, MD, MHS
Assistant Professor, Department of Medicine, Division of Pulmonary, Critical Care and Sleep Medicine, Johns Hopkins University School of Medicine, Baltimore, Maryland, USA; Division of Allergy, Pulmonary, and Critical Care, Department of Medicine, University of Wisconsin-Madison School of Medicine and Public Health, Madison, Wisconsin, USA

DEANNA BRITTON, PhD, CCC-SLP, BC-ANCDS
Assistant Professor, Department of Speech and Hearing Sciences, Portland State University (PSU), Department of Otolaryngology–Head and Neck Surgery, Oregon Health & Science University (OHSU), Northwest Clinic for Voice and Swallowing, Portland, Oregon, USA

CANDELARIA CABALLERO-ERASO, MD, PhD
Professor, Department of Medicine, Division of Pulmonary, Critical Care and Sleep Medicine, Johns Hopkins University School of Medicine, Baltimore, Maryland, USA; Medical-Surgical Unit of Respiratory Diseases, Institute of Biomedicine of Seville (IBiS), Centre for Biomedical Research in Respiratory Diseases Network (CIBERES), University Hospital Virgen del Rocío, University of Seville, Seville, Spain

JOHN C. CARTER, MD
Division of Pulmonary, Critical Care and Sleep Medicine, MetroHealth Medical Center, Assistant Professor of Medicine, Case Western Reserve University School of Medicine, Cleveland, Ohio, USA

ANTHONY F. DiMARCO, MD
Professor, Department of Physical Medicine and Rehabilitation, Case Western Reserve University, Research Scientist, MetroHealth Medical Center, Cleveland, Ohio, USA

ERIC J. GARTMAN, MD
Assistant Professor, Department of Medicine, Division of Pulmonary, Critical Care, and Sleep Medicine, The Warren Alpert Medical School of Brown University, Providence, Rhode Island, USA

DEAN R. HESS, PhD, RRT
Respiratory Care, Massachusetts General Hospital, Boston, Massachusetts, USA

JANET HILBERT, MD
Clinician, Department of Internal Medicine, Section of Pulmonary, Critical Care, and Sleep Medicine, Yale University, Yale University School of Medicine, New Haven, Connecticut, USA

IMRAN H. IFTIKHAR, MD, FACP, FCCP
Division of Pulmonary, Allergy, Critical Care and Sleep Medicine, Department of Medicine, Emory Sleep Center, Emory University School of Medicine, Atlanta, Georgia, USA

CHAFIC KARAM, MD
Assistant Professor, Department of Neurology, Oregon Health & Science University (OHSU), Portland, Oregon, USA

PATRICK KOO, MD, ScM
Department of Respiratory, Critical Care, and Sleep Medicine, University of Tennessee College of Medicine Chattanooga, Erlanger Health System, Chattanooga, Tennessee, USA

NOAH LECHTZIN, MD, MHS
Associate Professor, Department of Medicine, Division of Pulmonary, Critical Care and Sleep Medicine, Johns Hopkins University School of Medicine, Baltimore, Maryland, USA

KAMRAN MANZOOR, MD
Pulmonary Critical Care Attending, Assistant Professor of Medicine, Division of Pulmonary, Critical Care, and Sleep Medicine, The Warren Alpert Medical School of Brown University, Memorial Hospital of Rhode Island, Pawtucket, Rhode Island, USA

F. DENNIS McCOOL, MD
Professor of Medicine, Division of Pulmonary, Critical Care, and Sleep Medicine, The Warren Alpert Medical School of Brown University, Chief of Medicine, Memorial Hospital of Rhode Island, Pawtucket, Rhode Island, USA

TARO MINAMI, MD
Assistant Professor of Medicine, Division of Pulmonary, Critical Care, and Sleep Medicine, The Warren Alpert Medical School of Brown University, Director of the ICU, Memorial Hospital of Rhode Island, Pawtucket, Rhode Island, USA

ANDRE PROCHOROFF, MD
Division of Pediatric Neurology, MetroHealth Medical Center, Assistant Professor of Pediatrics, Case Western Reserve University School of Medicine, Cleveland, Ohio, USA

MIROSLAV RADULOVIC, MD
Assistant Professor of Medicine, Icahn School of Medicine at Mount Sinai, New York, New York, USA; Staff Physician, Internal Medicine, Co-Director, Pulmonary and Sleep Medicine Research Section, Rehabilitation Research & Development National Center of Excellence for the Medical Consequences of Spinal Cord Injury, The James J. Peters VA Medical Center, Bronx, New York, USA

JOSHUA ROLAND, MD
Emory Sleep Medicine Fellowship, Emory Sleep Center, Division of Pulmonary, Allergy, Critical Care and Sleep Medicine, Emory University School of Medicine, Atlanta, Georgia, USA

GREGORY J. SCHILERO, MD, FCCP, FAASM
Assistant Professor of Medicine, Icahn School of Medicine at Mount Sinai, New York, New York, USA; Director, Sleep Diagnostic and Treatment Center, Staff Physician, Pulmonary and Critical Care Medicine, Director, Pulmonary and Sleep Medicine Research Section, Rehabilitation Research & Development Center of Excellence for the Medical Consequences of Spinal Cord Injury, The James J. Peters VA Medical Center, Bronx, New York, USA

JOSHUA S. SCHINDLER, MD
Associate Professor, Department of
Otolaryngology–Head and Neck Surgery,
Oregon Health & Science University (OHSU),
Medical Director, Northwest Clinic for Voice
and Swallowing, Portland, Oregon, USA

JIGME M. SETHI, MD
Department of Respiratory, Critical Care, and
Sleep Medicine, University of Tennessee
College of Medicine Chattanooga, Erlanger
Health System, Chattanooga, Tennessee, USA

DANIEL W. SHEEHAN, PhD, MD
Division of Pediatric Pulmonology, John R.
Oishei Children's Hospital, Clinical Associate
Professor of Pediatrics and Associate Dean for
Medical Curriculum, University at Buffalo,
Buffalo, New York, USA

GEORGE E. TZELEPIS, MD
Professor of Medicine, Department
of Pathophysiology, University of
Athens Medical School, Athens,
Greece

Contributors

JOSHUA S. SCHINDLER, MD
Associate Professor, Department of
Otolaryngology-Head and Neck Surgery,
Oregon Health & Science University (OHSU),
Medical Director, Northwest Clinic for Voice
and Swallowing, Portland, Oregon, USA

ROME M. SETHI, MD
Department of Respiratory, Critical Care, and
Sleep Medicine, University of Tennessee
College of Medicine Chattanooga, Erlanger
Health System, Chattanooga, Tennessee, USA

DANIEL W. SHEEHAN, PhD, MD
Division of Pediatric Pulmonology, John R.
Oishei Children's Hospital, Clinical Associate
Professor of Pediatrics and Associate Dean for
Medical Curriculum, University at Buffalo,
Buffalo, New York, USA

GEORGE E. TZELEPIS, MD
Professor of Medicine, Department
of Pathophysiology, University of
Athens Medical School, Athens,
Greece

Contents

> The chest wall consists of various structures that function in an integrated fashion to ventilate the lungs. Disorders affecting the bony structures or soft tissues of the chest wall may impose elastic loads by stiffening the chest wall and decreasing respiratory system compliance. These alterations increase the work of breathing and lead to hypoventilation and hypercapnia. Respiratory failure may occur acutely or after a variable period. This article focuses on the pathophysiology of respiratory function in specific diseases and disorders of the chest wall and highlights pathogenic mechanisms of respiratory failure.

> Gas exchange between the atmosphere and the human body depends on the lungs and the function of the respiratory pump. The respiratory pump consists of the respiratory control center located in the brain, bony rib cage, diaphragm, and intercostal, accessory, and abdominal muscles. A variety of receptors and feedback pathways serve to fine-tune ventilation to metabolic demands. Appropriate evaluation and interventions can prevent respiratory complications and prolong life in individuals with neuromuscular diseases. This article discusses the normal function of the respiratory pump, general pathophysiologic issues, and abnormalities in more common neuromuscular diseases.

> Neuromuscular and chest wall diseases include a diverse group of conditions that share common risk factors for sleep-disordered breathing, including respiratory muscle weakness and/or thoracic restriction. Sleep-disordered breathing results from both the effects of normal sleep on ventilation and the additional challenges imposed by the underlying disorders. Patterns of sleep-disordered breathing vary with the specific diagnosis and stage of disease. Sleep hypoventilation precedes diurnal respiratory failure and may be difficult to recognize clinically because symptoms are nonspecific. Polysomnography has a role both in the diagnosis of sleep-disordered breathing and in the titration of effective noninvasive positive-pressure ventilation.

> Neuromuscular and chest wall disorders frequently compromise pulmonary function, and thorough respiratory evaluation often can assist in the diagnosis, risk assessment, and prognosis. Because many of these disorders can be progressive,

serial assessments are necessary to best define a trajectory of impairment (or improvement with therapy). This article covers the major respiratory testing modalities available in the evaluation of these patients, emphasizing both the benefits and shortcomings of each approach. Most parameters are available in a standard pulmonary laboratory (flow rates, volumes, static pressures), although referral to a specialized center may be necessary to conclusively evaluate a given patient.

Diaphragm dysfunction is defined as the partial or complete loss of diaphragm muscle contractility. However, because the diaphragm is one of only a few skeletal muscles that is not amenable to direct examination, the tools available for the clinician to assess diaphragm function have been limited. Traditionally, measures of lung volume, inspiratory muscle strength, and radiographic techniques such as fluoroscopy have provided the major method to assess diaphragm function. Measurement of transdiaphragmatic pressure provides the most direct means of evaluating the diaphragm, but this technique is not readily available to clinicians. Diaphragm ultrasonography is a new method that allows for direct examination of the diaphragm.

Section 2: Disorders

Pathologic processes that involve the central nervous system, phrenic nerve, neuromuscular junction, and skeletal muscle can impair diaphragm function. When these processes are of sufficient severity to cause diaphragm dysfunction, respiratory failure may be a consequence. This article reviews basic diaphragm anatomy and physiology and then discusses diagnostic and therapeutic approaches to disorders that result in unilateral or bilateral diaphragm dysfunction. This discussion provides a context in which disorders of the diaphragm and their implications on respiratory function can be better appreciated.

Chest wall disorders represent deformities and/or injuries that alter the rib cage geometry and result in pulmonary restriction, increased work of breathing, exercise limitations, and cosmetic concerns. These disorders are congenital or acquired and affect all ages. Disorders affecting the spine (kyphoscoliosis, ankylosing spondylitis), ribs (flail chest), and sternum (pectus excavatum) are discussed in this article, with emphasis on clinical presentations, pulmonary function abnormalities, diagnosis, and treatment.

Muscular dystrophies represent a complex, varied, and important subset of neuromuscular disorders likely to require the care of a pulmonologist. The spectrum of conditions encapsulated by this subset ranges from severe and fatal congenital muscular dystrophies with onset in infancy to mild forms of limb and girdle weakness with onset in adulthood and minimal respiratory compromise. The list and classification of muscular dystrophies are undergoing near-constant revision, based largely on new insights from genetics and molecular medicine. The authors present an overview of the muscular dystrophies, including their basic features, common clinical phenotypes, and important facets of management.

Amyotrophic lateral sclerosis (ALS) is a progressive neurodegenerative disorder that always affects the respiratory muscles. It is characterized by degeneration of motor neurons in the brain and spinal cord. Respiratory complications are the most common causes of death in ALS and typically occur within 3 to 5 years of diagnosis. Because ALS affects both upper and lower motor neurons, it causes hyperreflexia, spasticity, muscle fasciculations, muscle atrophy, and weakness. It ultimately progresses to functional quadriplegia. ALS most commonly begins in the limbs, but in about one-third of cases it begins in the bulbar muscles responsible for speech and swallowing.

Metabolic myopathies are a heterogeneous group of disorders characterized by inherited defects of enzymatic pathways involved in muscle cellular energetics and adenosine triphosphate synthesis. Skeletal and respiratory muscles are the most affected. There are multiple mechanisms of disease. The age of onset and prognosis vary. Metabolic myopathies cause exercise intolerance, myalgia, and an increase in muscle breakdown products during exercise. Some affect smooth muscle such as the diaphragm and cause respiratory failure. The pathophysiology is complex, and the evidence in the literature to guide diagnosis and management is sparse. Treatment is limited. This article discusses the pathophysiology and diagnostic evaluation of these disorders.

In the United States, approximately 17,500 cases of traumatic spinal cord injury (SCI) occur each year, with an estimated 245,000 to 345,000 individuals living with chronic SCI. Short-term management of respiratory dysfunction has resulted in improvement in early survival, but life expectancy remains less than that of the general population, and pulmonary complications are a leading cause of mortality. The global changes in pulmonary function, underlying pathophysiology, and the management options to improve respiratory muscle weakness and pulmonary clearance in persons with SCI are discussed. Given the high prevalence of sleep-disordered breathing among subjects with cervical SCI, this condition is also discussed.

Obesity hypoventilation syndrome has been noted for centuries, yet we still are trying to uncover the exact mechanisms behind the disease and best treatment modalities for patients afflicted by the condition. The syndrome, which results in symptoms based on a diverse spectrum of interactions between obesity, ventilatory drive, and sleep's impact on respiration, has been shown to worsen morbidity and mortality far beyond that of more typical sleep-disordered breathing. In this article, the authors discuss current knowledge and research about the epidemiology, patho-physiology, and clinical features, along with treatment considerations of obesity hypoventilation syndrome.

Section 3: Treatment

PROGRAM OBJECTIVE

The goal of the *Clinics in Chest Medicine* is to provide provide practitioners with state-of-the-art information that is clinically useful, concise, well referenced, and comprehensive.

TARGET AUDIENCE

All practicing physicians and healthcare professionals who provide patient care utilizing findings from *Chest Medicine Clinics of North America*.

LEARNING OBJECTIVES

Upon completion of this activity, participants will be able to:

1. Review disorders of the diaphragm and chest wall including the pathophysiology of chest wall and neuromuscular respiratory diseases.
2. Discuss swallowing and secretion management in and non-invasive ventilation for neuromuscular disease
3. Recognize pulmonary and diaphragm function testing, as well as sleep-disordered breathing in chest wall and neuromuscular diseases.

ACCREDITATION

The Elsevier Office of Continuing Medical Education (EOCME) is accredited by the Accreditation Council for Continuing Medical Education (ACCME) to provide continuing medical education for physicians.

The EOCME designates this enduring material for a maximum of 15 *AMA PRA Category 1 Credit*(s)™. Physicians should claim only the credit commensurate with the extent of their participation in the activity.

All other health care professionals requesting continuing education credit for this enduring material will be issued a certificate of participation.

DISCLOSURE OF CONFLICTS OF INTEREST

The EOCME assesses conflict of interest with its instructors, faculty, planners, and other individuals who are in a position to control the content of CME activities. All relevant conflicts of interest that are identified are thoroughly vetted by EOCME for fair balance, scientific objectivity, and patient care recommendations. EOCME is committed to providing its learners with CME activities that promote improvements or quality in healthcare and not a specific proprietary business or a commercial interest.

The planning committee, staff, authors and editors listed below have identified no financial relationships or relationships to products or devices they or their spouse/life partner have with commercial interest related to the content of this CME activity:

Mazen O. Al-Qadi, MD; William A. Bauman, MD; Joshua O. Benditt, MD, FCCP, RYT; David J. Birnkrant, MD; Andrew T. Braun, MD, MHS; Candelaria Caballero-Eraso, MD, PhD; John C. Carter, MD; Anthony F. DiMarco, MD; Colleen Dietzler; Eric J. Gartman, MD; Janet Hilbert, MD; Imran H. Iftikhar, MD, FACP, FCCP; Chafic Karam, MD; Alison Kemp; Patrick Koo, MD, ScM; Noah Lechtzin, MD, MHS; Kamran Manzoor, MD; Rajkumar Mayakrishnan; F. Dennis McCool, MD; Taro Minami, MD; Miroslav Radulovic, MD; Joshua Roland, MD; Gregory J. Schilero, MD, FCCP, FAASM; Gregory J. Schilero, MD; Joshua S. Schindler, MD; Jigme M. Sethi, MD; Daniel W. Sheehan, PhD, MD; George E. Tzelepis, MD.

The planning committee, staff, authors and editors listed below have identified financial relationships or relationships to products or devices they or their spouse/life partner have with commercial interest related to the content of this CME activity:

Deanna Britton, PhD, CCC-SLP, BC-ANCDS: receives royalties for prior publications and on-line presentations from Plural Publishing, Pro-Ed, Inc., and Medbridge Education.
Dean R. Hess, PhD, RRT: has served as a consultant/advisor for American Board of Internal Medicine, Philips Respironics, Inc. and Ventec Life Systems; he receives royalties and/or holds patents from Jones and Bartlett Learning Company, McGraw-Hill Education, and UpToDate; and has been employed by Daedalus Enterprises, Inc.
Andre Prochoroff, MD: has served as a consultant for PTC Therapeutics, Inc and Sarepta Therapeutics, Inc.

UNAPPROVED/OFF-LABEL USE DISCLOSURE

The EOCME requires CME faculty to disclose to the participants:

1. When products or procedures being discussed are off-label, unlabelled, experimental, and/or investigational (not US Food and Drug Administration [FDA] approved); and
2. Any limitations on the information presented, such as data that are preliminary or that represent ongoing research, interim analyses, and/or unsupported opinions. Faculty may discuss information about pharmaceutical agents that is outside of FDA-approved labelling. This information is intended solely for CME and is not intended to promote off-label use of these medications. If you have any questions, contact the medical affairs department of the manufacturer for the most recent prescribing information.

TO ENROLL

To enroll in the *Chest Medicine Clinics* Continuing Medical Education program, call customer service at 1-800-654-2452 or sign up online at http://www.theclinics.com/home/cme. The CME program is available to subscribers for an additional annual fee of USD $225.

METHOD OF PARTICIPATION

In order to claim credit, participants must complete the following:
1. Complete enrolment as indicated above.
2. Read the activity.
3. Complete the CME Test and Evaluation. Participants must achieve a score of 70% on the test. All CME Tests and Evaluations must be completed online.

CME INQUIRIES/SPECIAL NEEDS

For all CME inquiries or special needs, please contact elsevierCME@elsevier.com.

CLINICS IN CHEST MEDICINE

THE CLINICS ARE AVAILABLE ONLINE!
Access your subscription at:
www.theclinics.com

CLINICS IN CHEST MEDICINE

FORTHCOMING ISSUES

September 2018
Pulmonary Embolism
Peter Marshall and Wassim Fares, Editors

December 2018
Pneumonia
Michael S. Niederman, Editor

March 2019
Asthma
Serpil Erzurum and Sumita Khatri, Editors

RECENT ISSUES

March 2018
Interventional Pulmonology
Ali I. Musani, Editor

December 2017
Pulmonary Considerations in Solid Organ and Hematopoietic Stem Cell Transplantation
Vivek N. Ahya and Joshua Diamond, Editors

September 2017
Diagnosis and Treatment of Fungal Chest Infection
Eva M. Carmona and Andrew H. Limper, Editors

ISSUES OF RELATED INTEREST

Thoracic Surgery Clinics, Volume 27, Issue 2 (May 2017)
Disorders of the Chest Wall
Henning A. Gaissert, Editor

Preface

Progress in the Treatment of Patients with Neuromuscular and Nonmuscular Chest Wall Diseases

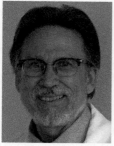 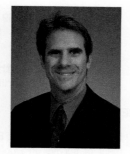

F. Dennis McCool, MD   Joshua O. Benditt, MD

Editors

Chronic neuromuscular and chest wall disorders that affect the respiratory system are comprised of congenital, genetic, and acquired diseases. These varied disorders range from processes that involve the bony structures of the chest wall, such as kyphoscoliosis, to diseases that directly impair skeletal muscle function, such as the muscular dystrophies. These disparate diseases all share the common thread of adversely affecting respiratory function without directly involving lung parenchyma. As a group, these disorders comprise a significant fraction of the patient population that the respiratory or ICU health care provider encounters and pose challenges to the clinician, which can be as daunting as challenges encountered in patients with diseases that directly affect lung parenchyma.

The leading causes of death and disability in patients with neuromuscular or nonmuscular diseases of the respiratory system are pneumonia and respiratory failure, both of which are eminently treatable as described in this issue of *Clinics in Chest Medicine*. In the past 2 to 3 decades, remarkable progress has been made in the treatment of respiratory complications of neuromuscular diseases. For example, in a retrospective

cohort study looking at survival in Duchenne muscular dystrophy, the authors showed that at the age of 20, the survival rate was 23.3% in individuals born in the 1960s, 54% in those born in the 1970s, and 59.8% in those born in the 1980s.[1] The authors concluded that the major factor responsible for this near tripling of survival to age 20 and beyond in this disorder was the use of noninvasive ventilation. This treatment modality also has proven to be beneficial in reducing morbidity and mortality for patients with nonmuscular disorders of the chest wall, especially those with severe kyphoscoliosis.

This issue of the *Clinics in Chest Medicine* details many of the important therapeutic and diagnostic developments. We start by looking at the pathophysiology of chest wall and neuromuscular disorders and then review the major specific disorders that the respiratory clinician is likely to see. Diagnostic evaluation is discussed, including a review of specialized pulmonary function testing and an update on methods used to assess diaphragm function. The issue is completed by articles assessing sleep-disordered breathing in this population, obesity hypoventilation, metabolic myopathies, and chronic spinal cord injury. The article by

Clin Chest Med 39 (2018) xv–xvi
https://doi.org/10.1016/j.ccm.2018.03.001
0272-5231/18/© 2018 Published by Elsevier Inc.

Hess reviews different types of devices for noninvasive ventilator support as well as their application. Other articles review the data supporting the use of noninvasive ventilation in specific diseases as well as discuss when invasive (tracheostomy) ventilation, or diaphragm pacing, should be considered.

A dramatic improvement in the understanding of the genetics and mechanism of many neuromuscular disorders has occurred of late. This has led to development of a number of drug interventions that are very promising but only treat a few of the disorders. Undoubtedly, much greater progress will be made in the coming years, which could help maintain muscle strength and reduce the burden of respiratory failure and pneumonia in these patients. Unfortunately, that day has not yet arrived. We hope that this issue of *Clinics in Chest Medicine* will be useful to respiratory clinicians, whose efforts are still needed in treating and improving the quality and length of life in patients with chest wall and neuromuscular respiratory disease.

F. Dennis McCool, MD
The Warren Alpert Medical School
of Brown University
Memorial Hospital of Rhode Island
111 Brewster Street
Pawtucket, RI 02860, USA

Joshua O. Benditt, MD
University of Washington
School of Medicine
UWMC, Box 356522
1959 Northeast Pacific Street
Seattle, WA 98195, USA

E-mail addresses:
F_McCool@brown.edu (F.D. McCool)
benditt@uw.edu (J.O. Benditt)

REFERENCE

1. Passamano L, Taglia A, Palladino A, et al. Improvement of survival in Duchenne muscular dystrophy: retrospective analysis of 835 patients. Acta Myol 2012;31(2):121–5.

Section 1: Basics

Chest Wall Diseases
Respiratory Pathophysiology

George E. Tzelepis, MD

KEYWORDS

- Chest wall • Respiratory failure • Kyphoscoliosis • Flail chest • Ankylosing spondylitis
- Hypoventilation

KEY POINTS

- Chest wall diseases produce restrictive pathophysiology with decreased lung volumes and reduced respiratory compliance, primarily owing to decreased distensibility of the chest wall.
- Patients with kyphoscoliosis may have significantly reduced chest wall compliance, whereas individuals with pectus excavatum or ankylosing spondylitis may have normal chest wall compliance.
- In obese individuals, the decreased respiratory compliance is largely due to a reduction in lung compliance.
- Respiratory failure may develop acutely as in flail chest or after a variable period, depending on the magnitude of the imposed elastic loads on the respiratory muscles.
- Sleep breathing abnormalities, age-related decreases in chest wall compliance, and associated lung dysfunction may also contribute to the development of respiratory failure.

INTRODUCTION

The chest wall is an essential part of the human ventilatory pump. It consists of the rib cage, abdomen, the spine and its joints, and the respiratory muscles with their nerves. The inspiratory muscles (diaphragm and intercostal inspiratory muscles) act to expand the chest wall and displace the abdomen outward. The increase in rib cage and the abdomen dimensions, alone or in combination, during inspiration are able to accommodate changes in lung volume. At all lung volumes, the elastic components of the lung promote passive inward recoil. Similar to the lung, the elastic components of the chest wall promote passive inward recoil at high lung volumes, 75% of vital capacity (VC) to total lung capacity (TLC). Unlike the lung, the elastic components of the chest wall promote passive outward recoil at low lung volumes, residual volume (RV) to 75% of the VC. Thus, at high lung volumes, chest wall expansion is due to contraction of the inspiratory muscles and not passive chest wall recoil.

In its normal state, the elastic components of the chest wall are easily stretched. Consequently, the chest wall has a relatively high compliance, equal to that of lung. Accordingly, the work of breathing is negligible when the respiratory muscles expand a healthy chest wall. However, the work of breathing may increase significantly when disorders stiffen the chest wall and decrease its compliance. These diverse disorders can affect the rib cage (kyphoscoliosis [KS], thoracoplasty, pectus excavatum, or flail chest), abdomen (obesity), spine (ankylosing spondylitis), and even skin (scleroderma, extensive burn scaring, massive subcutaneous emphysema). The common denominator

Disclosure Statement: The authors has no affiliations with or involvement in any organization or entity with any financial interest (such as honoraria; educational grants; participation in speakers' bureaus; membership, employment, consultancies, stock ownership, or other equity interest; and expert testimony or patent licensing arrangements), or nonfinancial interest (such as personal or professional relationships, affiliations, knowledge or beliefs) in the subject matter or materials discussed in this article.
Department of Pathophysiology, University of Athens Medical School, 75 M. Asias Street, Athens 11527, Greece
E-mail address: gtzelep@med.uoa.gr

Clin Chest Med 39 (2018) 281–296
https://doi.org/10.1016/j.ccm.2018.01.002
0272-5231/18/© 2018 Elsevier Inc. All rights reserved.

is decreased chest wall compliance, leading to an increased work of breathing. In this review, we focus on the pathophysiologic characteristics and factors involved in the pathogenesis of respiratory failure in these disorders.

KYPHOSCOLIOSIS

KS refers to a group of spinal diseases characterized by excessive spinal curvature in the lateral plane (scoliosis) and sagittal plane (kyphosis) as well as by spinal axis rotation. It is categorized as idiopathic (affecting adolescents, mostly females) or secondary or paralytic (associated with neuromuscular disease).[1] The severity of the spinal deformity is assessed by measuring the Cobb angle on a radiograph of the spine.[2] This angle is formed by the intersection of 2 lines, one parallel to the top and the other parallel to the bottom vertebrae of the scoliotic or kyphotic curve (**Fig. 1**). The greater the Cobb angle, the more severe the deformity; angles of greater than 100° are associated with respiratory symptoms, and angles of greater than 120° with respiratory failure.[3–6]

Respiratory Mechanics

The pathophysiologic hallmark of KS is severe restrictive respiratory impairment related to reduced distensibility of the chest wall, especially when the Cobb angle is greater than 90°.[7–9] In this setting, TLC (**Fig. 2**) and VC may be reduced to 30% of predicted.[4,8,10]

Respiratory system compliance is reduced, primarily owing to a decrease in chest wall

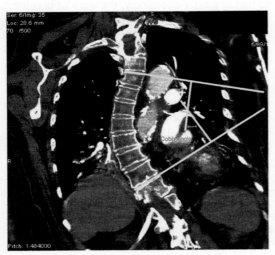

Fig. 1. Chest computed tomography scan (coronal view) of a patient with kyphoscoliosis. The angle formed from the 2 yellow lines drawn parallel to the vertebrae of the scoliotic curve is the Cobb angle.

compliance and, to a lesser degree, a decrease in lung compliance resulting from microatelectasis.[11–13] The volume–pressure relationship of the respiratory system curve is shifted to the right, thus, requiring greater than normal pressures to inflate the lungs (**Fig. 3**). In addition, the straight portion of the pressure–volume curve where compliance is relatively constant in the normal individual, is diminished.[12] This truncated section of the curve is largely the result of a significantly decreased TLC. The stiff chest wall reduces the resting position of the respiratory system (functional residual capacity [FRC]) and tidal breathing occurs on a flatter portion of the respiratory system volume–pressure curve.[12] This factor leads to greater inspiratory effort for relatively small tidal breaths, which increases the work of breathing.[12] The increase in the oxygen cost of breathing may reach values 3 to 5 times greater than those measured in healthy individuals[7,9,14] and, thus, place patients at risk for respiratory muscle fatigue.[15]

The decrease in chest wall compliance promotes breathing with shallow tidal breaths, and the decrease in FRC leads to breathing at low lung volumes, both of which predispose to the development of atelectasis.[7,10,16,17] Although lung compliance may be diminished, it is not as severely decreased as the chest wall compliance.[11,14,18] Because chest wall compliance decreases with age,[19] respiratory mechanics invariably deteriorate with age, even in the absence of worsening of the spinal deformity. Changes in respiratory system compliance primarily reflect decreases in chest wall, not lung compliance. Cobb angles of up to 50° have a minimal effect on respiratory system compliance as opposed to those greater than 100° (**Fig. 4**), which may decrease compliance to levels seen in acute respiratory distress syndrome.[20]

Concurrent respiratory muscle weakness considerably increases the severity of restriction. In the paralytic type of KS, the degree of lung restriction is determined primarily by the degree of the respiratory muscle weakness rather than by the degree of the spinal curvature.[21,22] Generally in these patients, the resulting lung abnormalities lead to a greater loss in VC for a given degree of spinal deformity than seen in patients with the idiopathic form of KS.[21,22]

Gas Exchange and Exercise Capacity

Hypoxemia is commonly found in patients with KS and correlates directly with VC and inversely with the angle of scoliosis. It is primarily due to ventilation–perfusion mismatch, and less often to

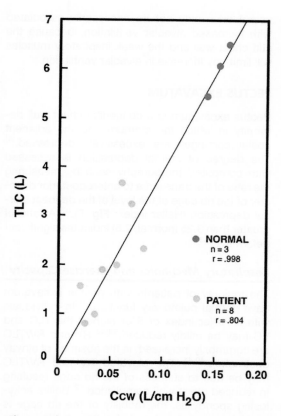

Fig. 2. Relationship between total lung capacity (TLC) and chest wall compliance (Cwc) in patients with kyphoscoliosis (*yellow circles*) and normal individuals (*blue circles*). (*Adapted from* Ting EY, Lyons HA. The relation of pressure and volume of the total respiratory system and its components in kyphoscoliosis. Am Rev Respir Dis 1964;89:384; with permission.)

intrapulmonary shunting from atelectasis.[8,10,12,23] In severe KS, oxyhemoglobin desaturation can occur with minimal activity.[12] Chronic hypoventilation may also contribute to hypoxemia. Hypercapnia initially occurs only during sleep or with exercise; as the disease progresses, it may occur at rest while awake.[5,24] Nocturnal hypoxemia typically predates the onset of respiratory failure in patients with KS. Hypoventilation during sleep is the most common abnormality and is related to a decreased neural drive to the inspiratory muscles during REM sleep.[25,26] Because these patients depend exclusively on the diaphragm to maintain alveolar ventilation during sleep, they are at risk to develop hypoxemia and hypercapnia.[27] However, the degree of nocturnal oxyhemoglobin desaturation may not correlate with the angle of spinal deformity.

Obstructive sleep apnea occurs with prevalence similar to that of general population and further aggravates hypoxemia and hypercapnia.[28] Tracheal distortion may predispose individuals with severe KS to obstructive sleep apnea. Chronic nocturnal desaturation and hypercapnia may further weaken the respiratory muscles, exaggerate hypoxemia, and lead to pulmonary hypertension and, ultimately, cor pulmonale.[12,24]

Exercise capacity may be severely limited in KS, especially with Cobb angles of greater than 60°. Decreased respiratory system compliance, increased work of breathing, and respiratory muscle weakness contribute to poor exercise capacity.[29-31] Maximal oxygen consumption is typically reduced to 60% to 80% of predicted, the heart rate is higher per workload, and the ratio of tidal

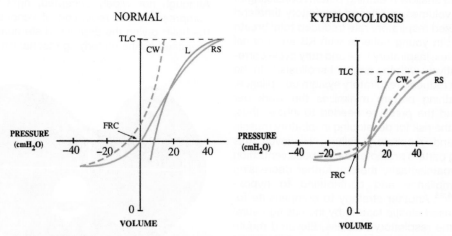

Fig. 3. Volume–pressure curves of a normal individual and of a patient with kyphoscoliosis (KS). Note that in KS the chest wall is less compliant, leading to a reduction in functional residual capacity (FRC), and positioning of tidal breathing on a flatter portion of the respiratory system volume-pressure curve. CW, chest wall; L, lung; RS, respiratory system; TLC, total lung capacity.

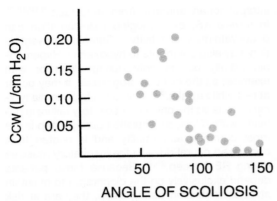

Fig. 4. Relationship between chest wall compliance (CCW) and angle of scoliosis in kyphoscoliosis. Note the negative correlation between angle of scoliosis and chest wall compliance. (*Adapted from* Kafer ER. Idiopathic scoliosis. Mechanical properties of the respiratory system and the ventilatory response to carbon dioxide. J Clin Invest 1975;55:1158; with permission.)

volume to VC is greater than 0.5. Because ventilatory reserve is reduced in severe KS, the ratio of maximum exercise ventilation to maximum voluntary ventilation can reach levels of greater than 0.7. In individuals with KS with Cobb angles of 20° to 45°, poor exercise tolerance with reductions in Vo_{2max} is usually due to limb muscle deconditioning rather than to ventilatory constraints.[32]

Control of Breathing

Patients with KS compensate for the increased elastic loads on the inspiratory muscles by adopting a rapid shallow breathing pattern consisting of low tidal volumes, shortened inspiratory time and an increased respiratory rate (reduced total breath time).[16,33] In young patients with KS and normal blood gases, inspiratory time and duty cycle correlate negatively with the angle of scoliosis.[33] In the setting of reduced respiratory system compliance, this breathing pattern minimizes the work per breath and the pressure needed to inhale, thus, lowering the risk for developing inspiratory muscle fatigue and respiratory failure. However, this breathing pattern promotes dead space ventilation and microatelectasis, thereby further decreasing lung compliance and contributing to hypoxemia.[15,34,35] Another strategy to compensate for the increased elastic load is by increasing neural drive to the respiratory muscles. Elevated mouth occlusion pressure at 100 msec, seen during quiet breathing, exercise, or breathing stimulated by hypercapnia in KS patients, correlates positively with the angle of deformity.[33] However, the increased

neural drive may not be necessarily associated with increased alveolar ventilation, because the stiff chest wall and the weak inspiratory muscles will limit any increase in alveolar ventilation.

PECTUS EXCAVATUM

Pectus excavatum is a congenital chest wall deformity in which the sternum and the adjacent costal cartilages are excessively depressed.[36] The degree of sternal depression is assessed with computed tomography scan by measuring the ratio of the transverse to anteroposterior diameter of the rib cage at the level of the deepest sternal depression (Haller index; **Fig. 5**).[37] A ratio of greater than 3.25 (normal, 2.5) indicates significant deformity.[36,38]

Respiratory Mechanics and Exercise Capacity

The majority of patients with pectus excavatum have normal pulmonary function.[39] In individuals with a Haller index of 5 or higher, the TLC and VC may be mildly reduced.[39,40] RV and RV/TLC are commonly increased, in the absence of airway obstruction.[40,41] The elevated RV and RV/TLC may be due to stiffness of the rib cage resulting in reduced chest wall compliance.[42] Unlike ankylosing spondylitis, the mobility of the rib cage is not decreased at rest or during exercise in pectus excavatum.[43,44]

Cardiopulmonary exercise testing is usually normal in pectus excavatum.[45,46] In individuals with severe deformities, mild decreases in the maximal work rate and oxygen consumption may occur, and often are out of proportion to the restrictive defect measured in these patients.[47–49] Although not widely accepted, right ventricular compression and reduction of venous return to the heart owing the depressed sternum has been proposed as the underlying mechanism.[49,50]

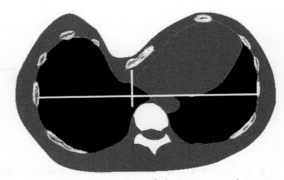

Fig. 5. Schematic drawing of chest computed tomography scan in pectus excavatum. The lines constructed are used to calculate the Haller index.

THORACOPLASTY

Thoracoplasty is a surgical procedure that consists of rib removal, rib fracture, phrenic nerve resection, lung compression, and filling the chest cavity with foreign material (ie, Lucite balls). It was frequently used to treat tuberculosis in the preantibiotic era (**Fig. 6**).[51] Although infrequent, it is still performed after complicated empyema operations, resection of chest wall tumors, management of chest wall trauma, and in patients with scoliosis.[52,53] Thoracoplasty is associated with a severe restrictive defect, which is comparable with that of KS.[54] These patients have impaired gas exchange, limited exercise tolerance, increased oxygen cost of breathing, and may eventually develop respiratory failure and cor pulmonale.[54]

FLAIL CHEST

Flail chest refers to a condition in which fractures of adjacent ribs produce a segment of the rib cage that deforms markedly during breathing. Double fractures of 3 or more adjacent ribs or combined sternal and rib fractures are required to produce a flail chest and lead to respiratory failure.[55,56] Multiple single rib fractures in a single plane can also lead to respiratory failure, a condition referred to as "nonintegrated chest wall" rather than flail chest.[57] The unstable segment of the chest wall moves paradoxically, inward with inspiration and outward with expiration (**Fig. 7**). The most common cause of flail chest in adults

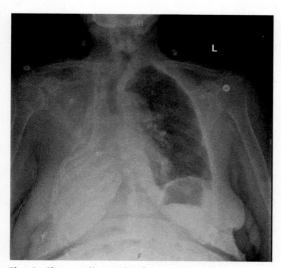

Fig. 6. Chest radiograph of a patient with hypercapnic respiratory failure, 60 years after thoracoplasty and right pneumonectomy for *Mycobacterium tuberculosis* lung infection.

is blunt chest trauma, especially with trauma after automobile accidents or falls.[58–60]

Respiratory Mechanics

Flail chest disrupts the anatomic integrity of the chest wall and renders the motion of the flail segment entirely dependent on intrapleural pressure changes. Thus, with inspiration and the decrease in intrapleural pressure, the flail segment moves inward, and during expiration, with positive pleural pressure, it moves outward.[61] Normally, rib cage expansion is accomplished through a coordinated action of the diaphragm and intercostal muscles, increases in intraabdominal pressure in the zone of apposition of the diaphragm to the rib cage, as well as through the passive outward recoil of the rib cage at low lung volumes. The contracting diaphragm exerts an inflationary action on the lower rib cage, and the inspiratory intercostal muscles exert an inflationary action on the upper rib cage. During inspiration, pleural pressure becomes subatmospheric, which is inflationary to the lung but deflationary to the rib cage. Multiple rib fractures can uncouple a segment of the rib cage from the rest of the chest wall. This uncoupled rib cage segment is subject to the deflationary effect of subatmospheric pleural pressure, but no longer subject to the forces promoting rib cage expansion. Thus, the uncoupled segment "flails" inward (instead of outward) during inspiration. During expiration, pleural pressure becomes more positive and the flail segment moves outward. This paradoxic motion of the flail segment is more pronounced when the swings in pleural pressure are amplified by a decrease in lung compliance related to pulmonary contusion and/or atelectasis, or increases in airway resistance related to bronchial secretions and/or bronchospasm.[61]

The location of the flail segment may influence the extent of paradoxic chest wall motion. Lateral flail chest, which is the most common, is associated with greater chest wall distortion. Posterior flail chest is associated with less severe clinical derangement owing to splinting provided by the back muscles. However, the pattern of chest wall distortion is not characteristic of a given location of the flail segment, and the same anatomic location may be associated with different patterns of distortion.[61] Paradoxic chest wall motion may occur within the rib cage itself (ie, between the upper and lower rib cage), or between the rib cage and the abdomen (ie, lower rib cage and anterior abdominal wall). These diverse patterns include (1) inward displacement of the lateral rib cage as the lower anterior rib cage and abdomen are

INSPIRATION   EXPIRATION

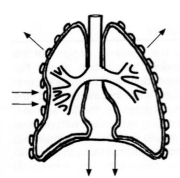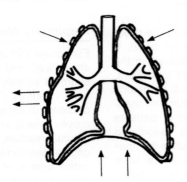

Fig. 7. The paradoxic motion of a rib cage segment in flail chest.

expanding, (2) inward displacement of the anterior lower rib cage and abdomen as the lateral rib cage is expanding, and (3) inward displacement of the anterior lower rib cage as the lateral rib cage and abdomen are expanding.[61]

Alterations in the pattern of respiratory muscle recruitment owing to severe chest pain are another factor contributing to different patterns of motion of the flail segment. Supporting evidence for this is the observation that electromyographic activity of the external intercostal muscles increases more than 3-fold in the flail region.[62–64] Clinical observations suggest that the change in the recruitment pattern of the respiratory muscles that follows traumatic flail chest may explain why some cases of flail chest remain unstable after prolonged mechanical ventilation, and why lateral flail segments have a greater propensity for dislocation after surgical fixation.[65,66]

VC and FRC can be reduced to as much as 50% of predicted in patients with flail chest.[67] In addition to an unstable rib cage, pulmonary contusion also contributes to the reduction in VC.[68] In patients with surgically corrected flail chest, VC usually returns to normal range in about 3 months. VC and FRC may remain reduced for years after flail chest, if lung fibrosis develops in regions of lung contusion.[67,69–71]

Respiratory Failure

The pathogenesis of respiratory failure in flail chest is multifaceted. The simplistic notion of pendelluft (ie, movement of air back and forth between the injured and uninjured chest) is not valid. Experimental data and clinical observations suggest that hypoventilation and flail-induced changes in lung and respiratory muscle function likely contribute to respiratory failure. Flail chest is accompanied by substantial pain, which can impair cough, promote regional atelectasis, cause

intercostal muscle spasm, and alter respiratory muscle activation and recruitment patterns. It may also increase the elastic load imposed on the respiratory muscles through local (adjacent to flail segment) or generalized atelectasis (owing to splinting and pain). Associated lung contusion also would increase the elastic load and work of breathing. In addition to these adverse effects, the flail segment may independently impair muscle performance. The paradoxic inward motion of the flail segment during inspiration increases the degree of inspiratory muscle shortening for a given tidal volume. Consequently, during inspiration, the inspiratory muscles shorten more and operate at shorter lengths.[61] Activation at a shorter muscle length will decrease inspiratory muscle efficiency and increase the oxygen cost of breathing.[61] The combination of the added work of breathing, respiratory muscle inefficiency, and hypoxemia owing to atelectasis and pulmonary contusion all combine to predispose to respiratory muscle fatigue and respiratory failure (**Fig. 8**).

ANKYLOSING SPONDYLITIS

Ankylosing spondylitis is a chronic inflammatory disease characterized by inflammation of the spine, and sacroiliac and peripheral joints, as well as involvement of extraarticular organs, including the lungs and the heart.[72] The chronic inflammation of the spinal structures, and costovertebral, apophyseal, and sacroiliac joints causes fibrosis and ossification of these joints and bony ankylosis of the costovertebral and sternoclavicular joints (**Fig. 9**).[73,74]

Respiratory Mechanics

Limited rib cage expansion is the pathophysiologic hallmark of ankylosing spondylitis and is due to stiffening and fusion of the costovertebral and

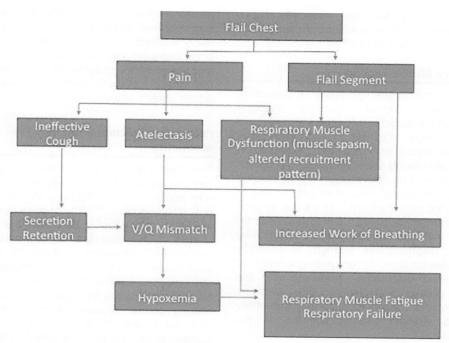

Fig. 8. Pathophysiology of respiratory failure in flail chest. V/Q, ventilation/perfusion.

sternoclavicular articulations, to rigidity of the spine, and possibly to intercostal muscle atrophy with advanced disease.[74,75] Rib cage motion is similar to that in healthy individuals in terms of direction, but the magnitude of motion is severely limited.[75] Rib cage stiffness leads to a decrease in chest wall and total respiratory compliance, but lung compliance remains normal, except in cases of coexisting lung fibrosis.[76,77] Because the rib cage is stiff and the abdomen is compliant, chest wall inflation is primarily accomplished through diaphragmatic displacement of the abdomen (ie, the lung expands along "the path of least resistance"). This pathway accounts for most of the tidal volume change during quiet breathing, speech, or exercise.[74,78,79] This

strategy may minimize the work and energy needed to inflate the lung. Transdiaphragmatic pressure increases by 2.4-fold in levels of ventilation where healthy individuals increase transdiaphragmatic pressure by 1.4-fold.[74]

Despite moderately severe reductions in rib cage mobility, the VC or TLC is only mildly diminished (75%-80% of predicted).[80,81] The mild restrictive impairment is usually proportional to disease activity and duration, and to the degree of spinal and rib cage rigidity.[81–84] The restrictive defect may increase in advanced disease when kyphosis supervenes.[85] Up to 50% of patients with advanced disease and/or osteoporosis may have some degree of kyphosis.[86] Spinal fractures, which may occur with minimal trauma, may further

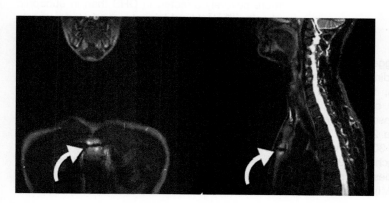

Fig. 9. Chest MRI in a patient with ankylosing spondylitis. Note inflammatory lesions of the chest wall in the manubriosternal joint on coronal (*left*) and sagittal (*right*) images. (*Adapted from* Weber U, Pfirrmann CW, Kissling RO, et al. Whole body MR imaging in ankylosing spondylitis: a descriptive pilot study in patients with suspected early and active confirmed ankylosing spondylitis. BMC Musculoskelet Disord 2007;8:20; with permission.)

impair respiratory function, especially those involving the cervical spine, which can cause tetraplegia and respiratory failure.[87,88]

Respiratory Muscle Function

Respiratory muscle strength (maximal inspiratory pressure and maximal expiratory pressure) may be mildly reduced in individuals with severely limited rib cage expansion.[80,81,89] Respiratory muscle endurance may also be decreased in advanced ankylosing spondylitis. The mild reduction in respiratory muscle strength and endurance may reflect intercostal muscle atrophy related to decreased rib cage mobility,[74] or be due to poor patient performance during the measurement maneuvers.[90] Although the intercostal muscles may be weak, diaphragmatic strength is generally intact in these patients.[74] In ankylosing spondylitis, the increased diaphragm shortening and the relatively greater transdiaphragmatic pressure required to inflate a stiff rib cage may potentially provide a strength training stimulus to the diaphragm.

Gas Exchange and Exercise Capacity

In the absence of parenchymal lung disease, arterial Po_2 and diffusion capacity are either in the normal range or slightly reduced.[81] The mild abnormalities of gas exchange are most likely related to a mild reduction in lung volumes. Exercise capacity may be mildly reduced, especially in patients with marked rib cage restriction.[91,92] The mechanism of reduced exercise capacity is poorly understood. The lack of correlation between the magnitude of rib cage expansion and maximal oxygen consumption or work rate may suggest that exercise capacity is limited by peripheral muscle deconditioning rather than ventilatory constrains.[91] Another explanation for decreased exercise capacity may be through a decrease in cardiac output related to rib cage stiffness, possibly owing to decreased preload from reduced negative swings in intrathoracic pressures.[93,94]

OBESITY

Obesity rates have reached staggering proportions throughout the world, including the United States.[95,96] By recent estimates, two-thirds of adults in the United States are overweight or obese and 1 in 3 children are obese.[97] Body fat, which usually constitutes 15% to 20% of body mass in healthy men and 25% to 30% in healthy women, may increase by as much as 500% in women and 800% in men.[98,99] Obesity is present when the body mass index (BMI) is equal or

greater than 30 kg/m^2 and severe when the BMI is greater than 40 kg/m^2.[100] The associated respiratory morbidity results mainly from alterations in chest wall mechanics and the control of breathing, and the presence of systemic and airway inflammatory and metabolic deregulation, such as that linking obesity to asthma.

Pulmonary Function and Chest Wall Mechanics

The most common abnormalities of pulmonary function are decreases in expiratory reserve volume and FRC.[101–103] TLC and VC are normal or only mildly reduced.[101,104] For each unit increase in BMI from 20 kg/m^2 to 30 kg/m^2, the expiratory reserve volume decreases by approximately 5% and the FRC decreases by about 3%; thereafter, each decreases 1%.[101] FRC is reduced owing to the increased volume of abdominal and thoracic fat compressing the rib cage and abdomen, thus making pleural pressure less subatmospheric and decreasing chest wall compliance.[105–107] Consequently, the balance between the inward recoil of the lung and the outward recoil of the chest wall occurs at a lower lung volume (ie, a lower FRC).[105,106] Other tests of pulmonary function such as the forced expiratory volume in 1 second (FEV$_1$)/FVC ratio, maximal voluntary ventilation, peak inspiratory flow rate, and the ratio of dead space to tidal volume are normal.[108,109] The single breath diffusion capacity is usually normal, even in morbid obesity.[101–103,109]

In obesity hypoventilation syndrome (OHS), the FRC and expiratory reserve volume are more severely reduced than they are in individuals with eucapnic obesity and comparable BMI.[110–112] In OHS and in morbid obesity (BMI >40 kg/m^2), the TLC, VC, and RV may be significantly decreased (<80% of predicted).[104,111] The sizable reductions in TLC and VC in these individuals are probably related to weakness of the respiratory muscles.[113,114] In general, pulmonary function is more severely affected in OHS than in eucapnic obesity.[104,111] In addition to respiratory muscle weakness, differences in the distribution of body fat also are associated with differences in pulmonary function impairment. Central fat distribution (from waist to hips) seems to impair pulmonary function more than lower fat distribution (below hips).[115–117] The correlation of respiratory impairment with upper body fat seems to be more evident in men than in women.[115]

Respiratory system compliance is invariably decreased in obesity, and further decreases as BMI increases or when changing from the upright to supine position.[105–107,118] Surprisingly, the reduction in respiratory system compliance is largely attributed to a decrease in lung compliance rather than reductions in chest wall compliance.[105,107,119] In obesity, the increased volume of intrathoracic and abdominal fat causes a marked increase in the pleural pressures and thus reduces the end-expiratory lung volume (FRC).[105,118] When the FRC is reduced, lung compliance decreases owing to airway closure and development of atelectasis. When measured in anesthetized, paralyzed obese individuals, chest wall compliance was found to be normal.[105,107,118] In this setting, the chest wall pressure–volume curve has the same slope as in nonobese individuals, but is shifted rightward (**Fig. 10**). This rightward shift is consistent with mass loading and not stiffening of the chest wall.[105,119] This mass loading creates a "threshold" load that the inspiratory muscles must overcome before inspiration ensues. The excess chest wall adipose tissue increases end-expiratory intrathoracic and intraabdominal pressures. These high intrathoracic and abdominal pressures need to overcome before any diaphragmatic displacement and occurrence of airflow. Once the threshold load is overcome, the chest wall inflates with a compliance characteristic similar to the normal chest wall.[105,119]

Airway and total respiratory system resistance increase with increasing BMI, with values for airway and respiratory system resistance being double those seen in nonobese individuals.[106,120–122] The increase in airway resistance has been attributed to breathing at low lung volumes.[121,123] Because airway resistance remains elevated after correcting for low lung volume, additional factors other than low lung volumes must be contributing to increased airway resistance.[120,124] The normal FEV_1/FVC ratio suggests that the greatest resistance to airflow may be at the level of the small airways and lung tissue itself, rather than the large airways.[120,124] Transition from an upright to a supine position may further increase respiratory resistance in severe obesity.[120,121]

Expiratory flow limitation during tidal breathing has been described in obese individuals, especially in the supine position.[118,125,126] Flow limitation may be primarily related to lowering FRC to a region on the flow–volume curve where tidal breathing encroaches on the maximal flow–volume envelope.[109] Intrinsic PEEP may develop as a result of expiratory flow limitation, especially in states with reduced expiratory time or increased tidal volume.[125,127]

Control of Breathing and Gas Exchange

In eucapnic obese individuals, the central ventilatory drive is intact. The added elastic and threshold loads increase respiratory drive by approximately 2 to 3 times that of nonobese individuals as measured by the mouth occlusion pressure at 100 msec, ventilatory and electromyographic responses to hypoxia and hypercapnia.[127–129] Unlike the nonobese, obese individuals increase further the respiratory drive when changing from sitting to supine position.[127] The amplified respiratory

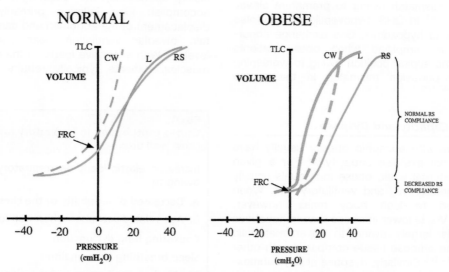

Fig. 10. Theoretic volume–pressure curves in healthy and obese individuals. In the obese, the functional residual capacity (FRC) is reset to a lower lung volume where the lung is less compliant, and tidal breathing occurs at the lower stiffer region of the respiratory system volume–pressure curve. CW, chest wall; L, lung; RS, respiratory system; TLC, total lung capacity.

drive is strongly associated with BMI and is critical in maintaining normocapnia in obesity.[127]

In patients with OHS, the central ventilatory drive is reduced and the mouth occlusion pressure at 100 msec, ventilatory, and electromyographic responses to hypoxia and hypercapnia are blunted when compared with nonobese subjects; the response to hypoxia is blunted to a greater extent than that to hypercapnia.[130–132] The attenuated ventilatory drive in OHS may be related to genetic predisposition or other factors, such as chronic hypoxemia, hypercapnia, or sleep apnea. However, the finding of an intact ventilatory drive in first-degree relatives of patients with OHS argues against a genetic predilection.[133,134] Leptin, a protein produced by adipose tissue that acts in the hypothalamus to decrease appetite and increase the metabolic rate, has been implicated as a possible mediator of the ventilatory response. Serum levels of leptin are generally higher in OHS than in eucapnic obesity, suggesting a central resistance to leptin.[135,136] It is believed that the development of leptin resistance or relative leptin deficiency may contribute to diminished ventilatory responsiveness and hypercapnia in OHS.[137]

In individuals with eucapnic obesity, arterial Po_2 is usually normal or slightly reduced. Severely obese or those with OHS patients have hypoxemia and a widened alveolar–arterial oxygen tension gradient.[109,138–140] Hypercapnia during wakefulness rarely occurs in obese individuals with BMI of less than 30 kg/m². The underlying mechanism responsible for hypoxemia is a ventilation–perfusion mismatch owing to premature airway closure.[140,141] In OHS, hypoventilation may also contribute to hypoxemia. Gas exchange abnormalities are amplified when obese patients assume the supine position owing to worsening ventilation–perfusion mismatch in the supine position.[142,143]

Exercise Capacity and Dyspnea

Individuals with eucapnic obesity usually have near normal exercise capacity.[144] For a given rate of external work, obese individuals usually have a greater $\dot{V}o_2$ and ventilatory rate. When normalized to lean body mass, however, the peak $\dot{V}o_2$ is lower in obese than in nonobese individuals largely owing to lower metabolic rate of the adipose tissue compared with other tissues.[144,145] Similarly, dyspnea at any submaximal work rate seems to be greater in obese individuals, owing to a relatively greater ventilation and metabolic cost.[146,147] However, dyspnea scores at any given ventilatory rate or $\dot{V}o_2$ are not higher in obesity, suggesting that respiratory mechanical factors do not contribute significantly to respiratory discomfort.[144] During exercise, obese individuals adjust respiratory mechanics by increasing end-expiratory volume, which serves to optimize operating lung volumes and attenuate expiratory flow limitation.[144]

PATHOGENIC ASPECTS OF RESPIRATORY FAILURE IN CHEST WALL DISEASES

Elastic loads imposed on the respiratory muscles are the primary cause of ventilatory failure in chest wall diseases (**Box 1**). Hypoventilation may develop acutely if the magnitude of load is excessive and there is loss of integrity of rib cage, as in flail chest, or it may develop after a variable period of time if the load is chronic and progressive, as in KS, thoracoplasty, or obesity. In disorders with chronic elastic loading of the respiratory muscles, the development of respiratory failure depends on a balance between the magnitude of the elastic load and the functional status of respiratory muscles. Minimal decreases in chest wall compliance, as in pectus excavatum or in KS with Cobb angles of less than 120°, do not excessively overload the respiratory muscles and do not cause respiratory failure unless there is concomitant respiratory muscle weakness.[12] Likewise, when decreased distensibility of the chest wall is limited to only one of its compartments, for example, the rib cage in ankylosing spondylitis, the diaphragm adapts to accomplish lung inflation primarily through displacement of the abdomen and can thus sustain alveolar ventilation near normocapnic levels.[78] With excessive loads on the respiratory muscles, patients typically require a greater

---

Box 1
Causes contributing to respiratory failure in chest wall diseases

Increased elastic loads on respiratory muscles owing to

a. Decreased distensibility of the chest wall

b. Age-related decrease in chest wall compliance

Coexisting lung dysfunction

Sleep breathing abnormalities

Mechanical disadvantage of the diaphragm

Age-related impairment of respiratory muscle function

inspiratory pressure to inflate the stiff chest wall with each breath (P_{breath}). In some instances, P_{breath} becomes a significant fraction of maximal inspiratory pressure (>50% of the maximal inspiratory pressure).[9] In this setting, the breathing pattern is altered by decreasing tidal volume and increasing respiratory frequency to decrease P_{breath} and avoid fatigue of the respiratory muscles.[34] Consequently, the proportion of wasted (dead space) ventilation increases, alveolar ventilation decreases, and ultimately hypoventilation and hypercapnia ensue.[34]

Age-related changes to the respiratory system also contribute to the development of respiratory failure in patients with chest wall disorders (**Fig. 11**). Chest wall compliance, lung elastic recoil, and respiratory muscle performance all decrease with aging. The chest wall compliance of elderly individuals in the seated position is approximately 31% lower than that of healthy individuals of a younger group.[19] Lung dysfunction with ventilation–perfusion disturbance and worsening of hypoxemia may occur in restrictive chest wall diseases owing to development of regional microatelectasis,[7] or less frequently owing to bronchial compression by the deformed spine in severe KS.[148]

Sleep breathing abnormalities significantly contribute to development of respiratory failure, with the first signs of respiratory failure invariably manifesting during sleep in these patients.[149] During wakefulness, patients with chest wall disorders typically depend on intercostal and accessory muscle activation to maintain alveolar ventilation.[16] During REM sleep, intercostal and accessory muscle activation is inhibited and, in conjunction with a weakened diaphragm, may lead to hypoventilation.[24,26] Decreased intercostal muscle tone may further reduce FRC and in certain patients may cause chest wall instability. Through disruption of ventilation–perfusion relationships, the reduced FRC and chest wall instability may further contribute to worsening of hypoxemia and hypercapnia.[12] The supine sleep position also lowers tidal volume and worsens gas exchange owing to cephalad movement of abdominal contents and displacement of the diaphragm into the thoracic cavity.[150]

Diaphragm mechanical advantage may be compromised in patients with severe chest wall distortion in the sense that diaphragmatic muscle tension is not converted into effective pressure and muscle shortening into inspiratory flow.[9,151,152] This factor is probably related to the way the diaphragm is coupled to a distorted thoracic cavity, to regional differences in chest wall compliance, or to rib cage muscle dysfunction. Such examples include KS[151] and possibly thoracoplasty and chronic flail chest.[69,70] As a result, the diaphragm has decreased strength and endurance, and is vulnerable to fatigue. Age-related decrease in respiratory muscle mass may further compromise respiratory muscle performance.[153] Over time, the increased work of breathing may lead to respiratory muscle fatigue, an altered breathing pattern with shallow and frequent breathing, and ultimately alveolar hypoventilation, and the development of pulmonary hypertension, cor pulmonale, and death (see **Fig. 11**).

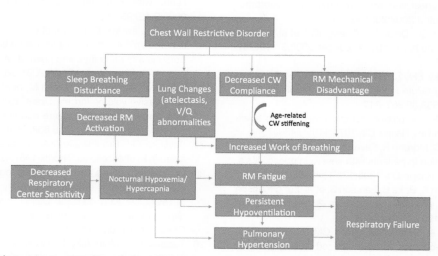

Fig. 11. Pathogenic causes of respiratory failure in restrictive chest wall disorders characterized by chronic loading of respiratory muscles such as kyphoscoliosis or thoracoplasty. CW, chest wall; RM, respiratory muscle; V/Q, ventilation/perfusion.

SUMMARY

Diseases affecting the nonmuscular structures of the chest wall produce restrictive pathophysiology and decrease compliance of the chest wall. Respiratory system compliance may be decreased significantly in KS and little affected in pectus excavatum or ankylosing spondylitis. Obesity decreases total respiratory system compliance primarily through a decrease in lung compliance. Respiratory failure may develop acutely as in flail chest or after a variable period of time depending on the magnitude of the imposed elastic loads on the respiratory muscles. Sleep breathing abnormalities, age-related decreases in chest wall compliance, and associated lung dysfunction usually contribute to the development of respiratory failure.

REFERENCES

1. Tzelepis GE, McCool FD. The respiratory system and chest wall diseases. In: Broaddus VC, Mason RC, Ernst JD, et al, editors. Murray's and Nadel's textbook of respiratory medicine, vol. 2, 6th edition. Philadelphia: Elsevier; 2016. p. 1707–22.
2. Hresko MT. Clinical practice. Idiopathic scoliosis in adolescents. N Engl J Med 2013;368(9): 834–41.
3. Johnston CE, Richards BS, Sucato DJ, et al. Correlation of preoperative deformity magnitude and pulmonary function tests in adolescent idiopathic scoliosis. Spine 2011;36(14):1096–102.
4. Kafer ER. Respiratory and cardiovascular functions in scoliosis. Bull Eur Physiopathol Respir 1977; 13(2):299–321.
5. Shneerson JM, Simonds AK. Noninvasive ventilation for chest wall and neuromuscular disorders. Eur Respir J 2002;20(2):480–7.
6. Weinstein SL, Dolan LA, Cheng JCY, et al. Adolescent idiopathic scoliosis. Lancet 2008;371(9623): 1527–37.
7. Bergofsky EH, Turino GM, Fishman AP. Cardiorespiratory failure in kyphoscoliosis. Medicine (Baltimore) 1959;38:263–317.
8. Kafer ER. Respiratory function in paralytic scoliosis. Am Rev Respir Dis 1974;110(4):450–7.
9. Lisboa C, Moreno R, Fava M, et al. Inspiratory muscle function in patients with severe kyphoscoliosis. Am Rev Respir Dis 1985;132(1):48–52.
10. Pehrsson K, Bake B, Larsson S, et al. Lung function in adult idiopathic scoliosis: a 20 year follow up. Thorax 1991;46(7):474–8.
11. Baydur A, Swank SM, Stiles CM, et al. Respiratory mechanics in anesthetized young patients with kyphoscoliosis. Immediate and delayed effects of corrective spinal surgery. Chest 1990; 97(5):1157–64.
12. Bergofsky EH. Respiratory failure in disorders of the thoracic cage. Am Rev Respir Dis 1979; 119(4):643–69.
13. Sinha R, Bergofsky EH. Prolonged alteration of lung mechanics in kyphoscoliosis by positive pressure hyperinflation. Am Rev Respir Dis 1972; 106(1):47–57.
14. Ting EY, Lyons HA. The relation of pressure and volume of the total respiratory system and its components in kyphoscoliosis. Am Rev Respir Dis 1964;89:379–86.
15. McCool FD, Tzelepis GE, Leith DE, et al. Oxygen cost of breathing during fatiguing inspiratory resistive loads. J Appl Physiol (1985) 1989; 66(5):2045–55.
16. Estenne M, Derom E, De Troyer A. Neck and abdominal muscle activity in patients with severe thoracic scoliosis. Am J Respir Crit Care Med 1998;158(2):452–7.
17. Secker-Walker RH, Ho JE, Gill IS. Observations on regional ventilation and perfusion in kyphoscoliosis. Respiration 1979;38(4):194–203.
18. Conti G, Rocco M, Antonelli M, et al. Respiratory system mechanics in the early phase of acute respiratory failure due to severe kyphoscoliosis. Intensive Care Med 1997;23(5):539–44.
19. Estenne M, Yernault JC, De Troyer A. Rib cage and diaphragm-abdomen compliance in humans: effects of age and posture. J Appl Physiol (1985) 1985;59(6):1842–8.
20. Kafer ER. Idiopathic scoliosis. Mechanical properties of the respiratory system and the ventilatory response to carbon dioxide. J Clin Invest 1975; 55(6):1153–63.
21. Inal-Ince D, Savci S, Arikan H, et al. Effects of scoliosis on respiratory muscle strength in patients with neuromuscular disorders. Spine J 2009;9(12):981–6.
22. Lin MC, Liaw MY, Chen WJ, et al. Pulmonary function and spinal characteristics: their relationships in persons with idiopathic and postpoliomyelitic scoliosis. Arch Phys Med Rehabil 2001;82(3):335–41.
23. Piesiak P, Brzecka A, Kosacka M, et al. Efficacy of noninvasive volume targeted ventilation in patients with chronic respiratory failure due to kyphoscoliosis. Adv Exp Med Biol 2015;838:53–8.
24. Sawicka EH, Branthwaite MA. Respiration during sleep in kyphoscoliosis. Thorax 1987;42(10):801–8.
25. Clinical indications for noninvasive positive pressure ventilation in chronic respiratory failure due to restrictive lung disease, COPD, and nocturnal hypoventilation–a consensus conference report. Chest 1999;116(2):521–34.
26. Tusiewicz K, Moldofsky H, Bryan AC, et al. Mechanics of the rib cage and diaphragm during sleep. J Appl Physiol Respir Environ Exerc Physiol 1977;43(4):600–2.

27. Mezon BL, West P, Israels J, et al. Sleep breathing abnormalities in kyphoscoliosis. Am Rev Respir Dis 1980;122(4):617–21.

28. Guilleminault C, Kurland G, Winkle R, et al. Severe kyphoscoliosis, breathing, and sleep: the "Quasi-modo" syndrome during sleep. Chest 1981;79(6): 626–30.

29. Kearon C, Viviani GR, Killian KJ. Factors influencing work capacity in adolescent idiopathic thoracic scoliosis. Am Rev Respir Dis 1993; 148(2):295–303.

30. Kesten S, Garfinkel SK, Wright T, et al. Impaired exercise capacity in adults with moderate scoliosis. Chest 1991;99(3):663–6.

31. Shen J, Lin Y, Luo J, et al. Cardiopulmonary exercise testing in patients with idiopathic scoliosis. J Bone Joint Surg Am 2016;98(19):1614–22.

32. Martínez-Llorens J, Ramírez M, Colomina MJ, et al. Muscle dysfunction and exercise limitation in adolescent idiopathic scoliosis. Eur Respir J 2010;36(2):393–400.

33. Ramonatxo M, Milic-Emili J, Prefaut C. Breathing pattern and load compensatory responses in young scoliotic patients. Eur Respir J 1988;1(5): 421–7.

34. Roussos C, Koutsoukou A. Respiratory failure. Eur Respir J Suppl 2003;47:3s–14s.

35. Zakynthinos S, Roussos C. Hypercapnic respiratory failure. Respir Med 1993;87(6):409–11.

36. Abid I, Ewais MM, Marranca J, et al. Pectus excavatum: a review of diagnosis and current treatment options. J Am Osteopath Assoc 2017; 117(2):106–13.

37. Haller JA, Kramer SS, Lietman SA. Use of CT scans in selection of patients for pectus excavatum surgery: a preliminary report. J Pediatr Surg 1987; 22(10):904–6.

38. Daunt SW, Cohen JH, Miller SF. Age-related normal ranges for the Haller index in children. Pediatr Radiol 2004;34(4):326–30.

39. Kelly RE, Mellins RB, Shamberger RC, et al. Multicenter study of pectus excavatum, final report: complications, static/exercise pulmonary function, and anatomic outcomes. J Am Coll Surg 2013; 217(6):1080–9.

40. Lawson ML, Mellins RB, Paulson JF, et al. Increasing severity of pectus excavatum is associated with reduced pulmonary function. J Pediatr 2011;159(2):256–61.e2.

41. Jeong JY, Ahn JH, Kim SY, et al. Pulmonary function before and after the Nuss procedure in adolescents with pectus excavatum: correlation with morphological subtypes. J Cardiothorac Surg 2015;10:37.

42. Leith DE, Mead J. Mechanisms determining residual volume of the lungs in normal subjects. J Appl Physiol 1967;23(2):221–7.

43. Binazzi B, Innocenti Bruni G, Coli C, et al. Chest wall kinematics in young subjects with Pectus excavatum. Respir Physiol Neurobiol 2012;180(2–3): 211–7.

44. Mead J, Sly P, Le Souef P, et al. Rib cage mobility in pectus excavatum. Am Rev Respir Dis 1985; 132(6):1223–8.

45. Peterson RJ, Young WG, Godwin JD, et al. Noninvasive assessment of exercise cardiac function before and after pectus excavatum repair. J Thorac Cardiovasc Surg 1985;90(2):251–60.

46. Rowland T, Moriarty K, Banever G. Effect of pectus excavatum deformity on cardiorespiratory fitness in adolescent boys. Arch Pediatr Adolesc Med 2005; 159(11):1069–73.

47. Malek MH, Fonkalsrud EW, Cooper CB. Ventilatory and cardiovascular responses to exercise in patients with pectus excavatum. Chest 2003;124(3): 870–82.

48. Tang M, Nielsen HHM, Lesbo M, et al. Improved cardiopulmonary exercise function after modified Nuss operation for pectus excavatum. Eur J Cardiothorac Surg 2012;41(5):1063–7.

49. Tardy MM, Tardy-Médous MM, Filaire M, et al. Exercise cardiac output limitation in pectus excavatum. J Am Coll Cardiol 2015;66(8):976–7.

50. Narayan RL, Vaishnava P, Castellano JM, et al. Quantitative assessment of right ventricular function in pectus excavatum. J Thorac Cardiovasc Surg 2012;143(5):e41–42.

51. Spiegelhalter E. 68 years-a record breaking thoracoplasty? BMJ 2016;355:i6513.

52. Hazel K, Weyant MJ. Chest wall resection and reconstruction: management of complications. Thorac Surg Clin 2015;25(4):517–21.

53. Icard P, Le Rochais JP, Rabut B, et al. Andrews thoracoplasty as a treatment of post-pneumonectomy empyema: experience in 23 cases. Ann Thorac Surg 1999;68(4):1159–63.

54. Bredin CP. Pulmonary function in long-term survivors of thoracoplasty. Chest 1989;95(1):18–20.

55. Bastos R, Calhoon JH, Baisden CE. Flail chest and pulmonary contusion. Semin Thorac Cardiovasc Surg 2008;20(1):39–45.

56. Wanek S, Mayberry JC. Blunt thoracic trauma: flail chest, pulmonary contusion, and blast injury. Crit Care Clin 2004;20(1):71–81.

57. Paydar S, Mousavi SM, Niakan H, et al. Appropriate management of flail chest needs proper injury classification. J Am Coll Surg 2012;215(5): 743–4.

58. Ahmed Z, Mohyuddin Z. Management of flail chest injury: internal fixation versus endotracheal intubation and ventilation. J Thorac Cardiovasc Surg 1995;110(6):1676–80.

59. LoCicero J, Mattox KL. Epidemiology of chest trauma. Surg Clin North Am 1989;69(1):15–9.

60. Majercik S, Pieracci FM. Chest wall trauma. Thorac Surg Clin 2017;27(2):113–21.

61. Tzelepis GE, McCool FD, Hoppin FG. Chest wall distortion in patients with flail chest. Am Rev Respir Dis 1989;140(1):31–7.

62. Cappello M, De Troyer A. Actions of the inspiratory intercostal muscles in flail chest. Am J Respir Crit Care Med 1997;155(3):1085–9.

63. Cappello M, Legrand A, De Troyer A. Determinants of rib motion in flail chest. Am J Respir Crit Care Med 1999;159(3):886–91.

64. Cappello M, Yuehua C, De Troyer A. Respiratory muscle response to flail chest. Am J Respir Crit Care Med 1996;153(6 Pt 1):1897–901.

65. Borrelly J, Aazami MH. New insights into the pathophysiology of flail segment: the implications of anterior serratus muscle in parietal failure. Eur J Cardiothorac Surg 2005;28(5):742–9.

66. Lardinois D, Krueger T, Dusmet M, et al. Pulmonary function testing after operative stabilisation of the chest wall for flail chest. Eur J Cardiothorac Surg 2001;20(3):496–501.

67. Landercasper J, Cogbill TH, Strutt PJ. Delayed diagnosis of flail chest. Crit Care Med 1990;18(6): 611–3.

68. Kishikawa M, Yoshioka T, Shimazu T, et al. Pulmonary contusion causes long-term respiratory dysfunction with decreased functional residual capacity. J Trauma 1991;31(9):1203–8 [discussion: 1208–10].

69. Beal SL, Oreskovich MR. Long-term disability associated with flail chest injury. Am J Surg 1985; 150(3):324–6.

70. Landercasper J, Cogbill TH, Lindesmith LA. Long-term disability after flail chest injury. J Trauma 1984; 24(5):410–4.

71. Slater MS, Mayberry JC, Trunkey DD. Operative stabilization of a flail chest six years after injury. Ann Thorac Surg 2001;72(2):600–1.

72. Taurog JD, Chhabra A, Colbert RA. Ankylosing spondylitis and axial spondyloarthritis. N Engl J Med 2016;374(26):2563–74.

73. Braun J, Sieper J. Ankylosing spondylitis. Lancet 2007;369(9570):1379–90.

74. Romagnoli I, Gigliotti F, Galarducci A, et al. Chest wall kinematics and respiratory muscle action in ankylosing spondylitis patients. Eur Respir J 2004;24(3):453–60.

75. Jordanoglou J. Rib movement in health, kyphoscoliosis, and ankylosing spondylitis. Thorax 1969; 24(4):407–14.

76. Aggarwal AN, Gupta D, Wanchu A, et al. Use of static lung mechanics to identify early pulmonary involvement in patients with ankylosing spondylitis. J Postgrad Med 2001;47(2):89–94.

77. van Noord JA, Cauberghs M, Van de Woestijne KP, et al. Total respiratory resistance and reactance in ankylosing spondylitis and kyphoscoliosis. Eur Respir J 1991;4(8):945–51.

78. Kalliakosta G, Mandros C, Tzelepis GE. Chest wall motion during speech production in patients with advanced ankylosing spondylitis. J Speech Lang Hear Res 2007;50(1):109–18.

79. Tzelepis GE, Kalliakosta G, Tzioufas AG, et al. Thoracoabdominal motion in ankylosing spondylitis: association with standardised clinical measures and response to therapy. Ann Rheum Dis 2009;68(6):966–71.

80. Er G, Angln E. Determining the relationship of kinesiophobia with respiratory functions and functional capacity in ankylosing spondylitis. Medicine (Baltimore) 2017;96(29):e7486.

81. Vanderschueren D, Decramer M, Van den Daele P, et al. Pulmonary function and maximal transrespiratory pressures in ankylosing spondylitis. Ann Rheum Dis 1989;48(8):632–5.

82. Berdal G, Halvorsen S, van der Heijde D, et al. Restrictive pulmonary function is more prevalent in patients with ankylosing spondylitis than in matched population controls and is associated with impaired spinal mobility: a comparative study. Arthritis Res Ther 2012;14(1):R19.

83. Brambila-Tapia AJL, Rocha-Muñoz AD, Gonzalez-Lopez L, et al. Pulmonary function in ankylosing spondylitis: association with clinical variables. Rheumatol Int 2013;33(9):2351–8.

84. Fisher LR, Cawley MI, Holgate ST. Relation between chest expansion, pulmonary function, and exercise tolerance in patients with ankylosing spondylitis. Ann Rheum Dis 1990;49(11):921–5.

85. Fu J, Zhang G, Zhang Y, et al. Pulmonary function improvement in patients with ankylosing spondylitis kyphosis after pedicle subtraction osteotomy. Spine 2014;39(18):E1116–22.

86. Vosse D, van der Heijde D, Landewé R, et al. Determinants of hyperkyphosis in patients with ankylosing spondylitis. Ann Rheum Dis 2006;65(6): 770–4.

87. Maas F, Spoorenberg A, van der Slik BPG, et al. Clinical risk factors for the presence and development of vertebral fractures in patients with ankylosing spondylitis. Arthritis Care Res 2017;69(5): 694–702.

88. Thumbikat P, Hariharan RP, Ravichandran G, et al. Spinal cord injury in patients with ankylosing spondylitis: a 10-year review. Spine 2007;32(26): 2989–95.

89. Sahin G, Calikoğlu M, Ozge C, et al. Respiratory muscle strength but not BASFI score relates to diminished chest expansion in ankylosing spondylitis. Clin Rheumatol 2004;23(3):199–202.

90. Steier J, Kaul S, Seymour J, et al. The value of multiple tests of respiratory muscle strength. Thorax 2007;62(11):975–80.

91. Carter R, Riantawan P, Banham SW, et al. An investigation of factors limiting aerobic capacity in patients with ankylosing spondylitis. Respir Med 1999;93(10):700–8.

92. Jennings F, Oliveira HA, de Souza MC, et al. Effects of aerobic training in patients with ankylosing spondylitis. J Rheumatol 2015;42(12):2347–53.

93. Coast JR, Cline CC. The effect of chest wall restriction on exercise capacity. Respirology 2004;9(2):197–203.

94. Miller JD, Beck KC, Joyner MJ, et al. Cardiorespiratory effects of inelastic chest wall restriction. J Appl Physiol (1985) 2002;92(6):2419–28.

95. GBD 2015 Obesity Collaborators, Afshin A, Forouzanfar MH, Reitsma MB, et al. Health effects of overweight and obesity in 195 countries over 25 years. N Engl J Med 2017;377(1):13–27.

96. Ng M, Fleming T, Robinson M, et al. Global, regional, and national prevalence of overweight and obesity in children and adults during 1980–2013: a systematic analysis for the Global Burden of Disease Study 2013. Lancet 2014;384(9945):766–81.

97. Ogden CL, Carroll MD, Lawman HG, et al. Trends in obesity prevalence among children and adolescents in the United States, 1988-1994 through 2013-2014. JAMA 2016;315(21):2292–9.

98. Romero-Corral A, Somers VK, Sierra-Johnson J, et al. Normal weight obesity: a risk factor for cardiometabolic dysregulation and cardiovascular mortality. Eur Heart J 2010;31(6):737–46.

99. Strain GW, Zumoff B. The relationship of weight-height indices of obesity to body fat content. J Am Coll Nutr 1992;11(6):715–8.

100. James WPT. The epidemiology of obesity: the size of the problem. J Intern Med 2008;263(4):336–52.

101. Jones RL, Nzekwu MMU. The effects of body mass index on lung volumes. Chest 2006;130(3):827–33.

102. Mehari A, Afreen S, Ngwa J, et al. Obesity and pulmonary function in African Americans. PLoS One 2015;10(10):e0140610.

103. Zhou LN, Wang Q, Gu CJ, et al. Sex differences in the effects of obesity on lung volume. Am J Med Sci 2017;353(3):224–9.

104. Biring MS, Lewis MI, Liu JT, et al. Pulmonary physiologic changes of morbid obesity. Am J Med Sci 1999;318(5):293–7.

105. Behazin N, Jones SB, Cohen RI, et al. Respiratory restriction and elevated pleural and esophageal pressures in morbid obesity. J Appl Physiol (1985) 2010;108(1):212–8.

106. Pelosi P, Croci M, Ravagnan I, et al. Respiratory system mechanics in sedated, paralyzed, morbidly obese patients. J Appl Physiol (1985) 1997;82(3):811–8.

107. Pelosi P, Croci M, Ravagnan I, et al. The effects of body mass on lung volumes, respiratory mechanics, and gas exchange during general anesthesia. Anesth Analg 1998;87(3):654–60.

108. Bedell GN, Wilson WR, Seebohm PM. Pulmonary function in obese persons. J Clin Invest 1958;37(7):1049–60.

109. Salome CM, King GG, Berend N. Physiology of obesity and effects on lung function. J Appl Physiol (1985) 2010;108(1):206–11.

110. Koenig SM. Pulmonary complications of obesity. Am J Med Sci 2001;321(4):249–79.

111. Piper AJ, Grunstein RR. Obesity hypoventilation syndrome: mechanisms and management. Am J Respir Crit Care Med 2011;183(3):292–8.

112. Ray CS, Sue DY, Bray G, et al. Effects of obesity on respiratory function. Am Rev Respir Dis 1983;128(3):501–6.

113. Manuel AR, Hart N, Stradling JR. Correlates of obesity-related chronic ventilatory failure. BMJ Open Respir Res 2016;3(1):e000110.

114. Sahebjami H, Gartside PS. Pulmonary function in obese subjects with a normal FEV1/FVC ratio. Chest 1996;110(6):1425–9.

115. Ceylan E, Cömlekçi A, Akkoçlu A, et al. The effects of body fat distribution on pulmonary function tests in the overweight and obese. South Med J 2009;102(1):30–5.

116. Collins LC, Hoberty PD, Walker JF, et al. The effect of body fat distribution on pulmonary function tests. Chest 1995;107(5):1298–302.

117. Sutherland TJT, Goulding A, Grant AM, et al. The effect of adiposity measured by dual-energy X-ray absorptiometry on lung function. Eur Respir J 2008;32(1):85–91.

118. Steier J, Lunt A, Hart N, et al. Observational study of the effect of obesity on lung volumes. Thorax 2014;69(8):752–9.

119. Banzett RB, Loring SH. Heavy breathing. J Appl Physiol (1985) 2007;102(6):2090–1.

120. Watson RA, Pride NB. Postural changes in lung volumes and respiratory resistance in subjects with obesity. J Appl Physiol (1985) 2005;98(2):512–7.

121. Yap JC, Watson RA, Gilbey S, et al. Effects of posture on respiratory mechanics in obesity. J Appl Physiol (1985) 1995;79(4):1199–205.

122. Zerah F, Harf A, Perlemuter L, et al. Effects of obesity on respiratory resistance. Chest 1993;103(5):1470–6.

123. Nicolacakis K, Skowronski ME, Coreno AJ, et al. Observations on the physiological interactions between obesity and asthma. J Appl Physiol (1985) 2008;105(5):1533–41.

124. King GG, Brown NJ, Diba C, et al. The effects of body weight on airway calibre. Eur Respir J 2005;25(5):896–901.

125. Ferretti A, Giampiccolo P, Cavalli A, et al. Expiratory flow limitation and orthopnea in massively obese subjects. Chest 2001;119(5):1401–8.

126. Pankow W, Podszus T, Gutheil T, et al. Expiratory flow limitation and intrinsic positive end-expiratory pressure in obesity. J Appl Physiol (1985) 1998; 85(4):1236–43.

127. Steier J, Jolley CJ, Seymour J, et al. Neural respiratory drive in obesity. Thorax 2009;64(8):719–25.

128. Burki NK, Baker RW. Ventilatory regulation in eucapnic morbid obesity. Am Rev Respir Dis 1984; 129(4):538–43.

129. Sampson MG, Grassino AE. Load compensation in obese patients during quiet tidal breathing. J Appl Physiol Respir Environ Exerc Physiol 1983;55(4): 1269–76.

130. Leech J, Onal E, Aronson R, et al. Voluntary hyperventilation in obesity hypoventilation. Chest 1991; 100(5):1334–8.

131. Sampson MG, Grassino K. Neuromechanical properties in obese patients during carbon dioxide rebreathing. Am J Med 1983;75(1):81–90.

132. Zwillich CW, Sutton FD, Pierson DJ, et al. Decreased hypoxic ventilatory drive in the obesity-hypoventilation syndrome. Am J Med 1975;59(3):343–8.

133. Javaheri S, Colangelo G, Corser B, et al. Familial respiratory chemosensitivity does not predict hypercapnia of patients with sleep apnea-hypopnea syndrome. Am Rev Respir Dis 1992;145(4 Pt 1): 837–40.

134. Jokic R, Zintel T, Sridhar G, et al. Ventilatory responses to hypercapnia and hypoxia in relatives of patients with the obesity hypoventilation syndrome. Thorax 2000;55(11):940–5.

135. Phipps PR, Starritt E, Caterson I, et al. Association of serum leptin with hypoventilation in human obesity. Thorax 2002;57(1):75–6.

136. Shimura R, Tatsumi K, Nakamura A, et al. Fat accumulation, leptin, and hypercapnia in obstructive sleep apnea-hypopnea syndrome. Chest 2005; 127(2):543–9.

137. Campo A, Frühbeck G, Zulueta JJ, et al. Hyperleptinaemia, respiratory drive and hypercapnic response in obese patients. Eur Respir J 2007; 30(2):223–31.

138. Javaheri S, Simbartl LA. Respiratory determinants of diurnal hypercapnia in obesity hypoventilation syndrome. What does weight have to do with it? Ann Am Thorac Soc 2014;11(6):945–50.

139. Mokhlesi B. Obesity hypoventilation syndrome: a state-of-the-art review. Respir Care 2010;55(10): 1347–62.

140. Rivas E, Arismendi E, Agustí A, et al. Ventilation/ Perfusion distribution abnormalities in morbidly obese subjects before and after bariatric surgery. Chest 2015;147(4):1127–34.

141. Zavorsky GS, Hoffman SL. Pulmonary gas exchange in the morbidly obese. Obes Rev 2008; 9(4):326–39.

142. Hakala K, Mustajoki P, Aittomäki J, et al. Improved gas exchange during exercise after weight loss in morbid obesity. Clin Physiol 1996; 16(3):229–38.

143. Tucker DH, Sieker HO. The effect of change in body position on lung volumes and intrapulmonary gas mixing in patients with obesity, heart failure, and emphysema. Am Rev Respir Dis 1960;82: 787–91.

144. Ofir D, Laveneziana P, Webb KA, et al. Ventilatory and perceptual responses to cycle exercise in obese women. J Appl Physiol (1985) 2007;102(6): 2217–26.

145. Salvadori A, Fanari P, Mazza P, et al. Work capacity and cardiopulmonary adaptation of the obese subject during exercise testing. Chest 1992;101(3): 674–9.

146. Babb TG, Ranasinghe KG, Comeau LA, et al. Dyspnea on exertion in obese women: association with an increased oxygen cost of breathing. Am J Respir Crit Care Med 2008;178(2):116–23.

147. Bernhardt V, Babb TG. Exertional dyspnoea in obesity. Eur Respir Rev 2016;25(142):487–95.

148. Qiabi M, Chagnon K, Beaupré A, et al. Scoliosis and bronchial obstruction. Can Respir J 2015; 22(4):206–8.

149. Perrin C, D'Ambrosio C, White A, et al. Sleep in restrictive and neuromuscular respiratory disorders. Semin Respir Crit Care Med 2005;26(1): 117–30.

150. Hudgel DW, Martin RJ, Johnson B, et al. Mechanics of the respiratory system and breathing pattern during sleep in normal humans. J Appl Physiol Respir Environ Exerc Physiol 1984;56(1): 133–7.

151. Cooper DM, Rojas JV, Mellins RB, et al. Respiratory mechanics in adolescents with idiopathic scoliosis. Am Rev Respir Dis 1984;130(1):16–22.

152. Giordano A, Fuso L, Galli M, et al. Evaluation of pulmonary ventilation and diaphragmatic movement in idiopathic scoliosis using radioaerosol ventilation scintigraphy. Nucl Med Commun 1997;18(2):105–11.

153. Polkey MI, Harris ML, Hughes PD, et al. The contractile properties of the elderly human diaphragm. Am J Respir Crit Care Med 1997; 155(5):1560–4.

Pathophysiology of Neuromuscular Respiratory Diseases

Joshua O. Benditt, MD

KEYWORDS

- Neuromuscular disease • Pathophysiology of neuromuscular disease • Respiratory failure
- Pulmonary function assessment • Amyotrophic lateral sclerosis • Muscular dystrophies
- Spinal cord injury

KEY POINTS

- The respiratory pump is designed to bring oxygen into the body to fuel energy generation and remove carbon dioxide as a waste product of cellular metabolism.
- The system is made up of the cortex of the brain that controls voluntary breathing; the brainstem, which is involved with automatic breathing; and the spinal cord and motor neurons that transmit nerve impulses.
- The effects of neuromuscular diseases on the respiratory system range from isolated and mild to protean and severe.
- An understanding of the pathophysiology of specific diseases as well as adopting a general approach to patients with one of these disorders can be helpful and in many cases lead to improvement in quality and quantity of life.

NORMAL PHYSIOLOGY

The respiratory pump is designed to bring oxygen into the body to fuel energy generation and remove carbon dioxide as a waste product of cellular metabolism.[1–3] The system is made up of the cortex of the brain that controls voluntary breathing; the brainstem, which is involved with automatic breathing; the spinal cord and motor neurons that transmit nerve impulses; the respiratory muscles that are the effectors of the system; and a complex system of feedback receptors and nerves that regulate ventilation (**Fig. 1**). The system is remarkably flexible and can precisely maintain CO_2 and acid-base balance. This article discusses each of the components of this complex network.

CENTRAL NERVOUS SYSTEM
Voluntary Breathing Controllers

Voluntary breathing is initiated by signals from the cerebral cortex. Centers located within the parietal cortex send signals that initiate inspiration and expiration.[4] These cortical areas project to the motor neurons in the spinal cord via the corticospinal tracts.

Automatic Breathing Controllers

Automatic breathing is controlled by a complex system that includes respiratory centers in the pons and medulla, nerve tracts in the lower brainstem, pathways in the spinal cord, and the feedback mechanisms that are both chemical and mechanical in nature. There are believed 3 centers that generate the rhythm and drive to breathe: 1 located in the pons and 2 in the medulla. More detailed reviews of this topic are available.[5]

Spinal Cord

The spinal cord and motor nerves conduct nerve impulses from the cortex and brainstem to the anterior horn cells of the motor neurons supplying

Department of Medicine, University of Washington School of Medicine, 1959 NE Pacific Street, Seattle, WA 98119, USA
E-mail address: benditt@uw.edu

Clin Chest Med 39 (2018) 297–308
https://doi.org/10.1016/j.ccm.2018.01.011
0272-5231/18/© 2018 Elsevier Inc. All rights reserved.

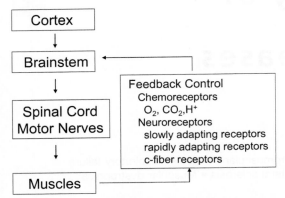

Fig. 1. Schematic of respiratory system, including controllers, effectors, and receptor feedback inputs.

Table 1		
Respiratory muscles and their innervation		
Muscle Group	**Spinal Cord Level**	**Nerve (s)**
Inspiratory muscles		
Diaphragm	C3–C5	Phrenic
Parasternal intercostals	T1–T7	Intercostal
Lateral external intercostals	T1–T12	Intercostal
Scalenes	C4–C8	
Sternoclydomastoids		
Expiratory muscles		
Lateral internal intercostals	T1–T12	Intercostal
Rectus abdominis	T7–L1	Lumbar
External and internal obliques	T7–L1	Lumbar
Transversus abdominis	T7–L1	Lumbar
Upper airway muscles		
Muscles of mastication		CN V, VII
Laryngeal and pharyngeal		
Abductors		CN IX–XII
Adductors		CN IX–XII

the respiratory muscles. The fibers in both these tracts travel through the spinal cord to synapse with the lower motor neurons.

PERIPHERAL NERVOUS SYSTEM
Lower Motor Neurons

The lower motor neuron has its cell body in the spinal cord (anterior horn cell) but exits the spinal cord to become the spinal nerve roots and the nerves that supply the respiratory muscles. When the nerves arrive at the muscle, they divide into branches known as twigs that, on reaching the muscle fiber, further divide into bulbous projections called boutons that apply themselves to the muscle membrane at a specialized anatomic junction called the motor end plate. These boutons contain acetylcholine, which is the chemical transmitter that serves to excite the muscle to contract. With nerve firing, there is release of acetylcholine at the motor end plate into the cleft between the nerve and the muscle. The acetylcholine binds to receptors on the muscle side of the motor end plate, which results in a suprathreshold excitatory end plate potential and depolarization of the muscle membrane.[6] A muscle action potential then results in contraction of the muscle fiber.

Respiratory Muscles

The respiratory muscles are the mechanical effectors of the breathing system. They are often divided into 3 major groups: (1) the inspiratory muscles, (2) the expiratory muscles, and (3) the accessory muscles of respiration. The muscles that maintain patency of the upper airway during the respiratory cycle are sometimes also considered muscles of respiration because of their close interaction with the other respiratory muscles. **Table 1** shows the innervation of the inspiratory muscles.

The diaphragm is the major muscle of inspiration and accounts for approximately 70% of the inhaled tidal volume in the normal individual.[7] Contraction of the diaphragm results in a downward piston motion of the muscle as well as outward and upward movement of the ribs through the zone of apposition (**Fig. 2**).

The intercostal muscles are thin sheets of muscular fibers that run between the ribs in the costal spaces.[8] There are 2 sheets of muscle fibers, the external and internal intercostals. The external intercostals function to expand the rib cage during inspiration. The internal intercostals are deeper and function to decrease rib cage size during expiration. The orientation of the muscle fibers with respect to the ribs results in the increase or decrease in the size of the rib cage, as the muscles contract (**Fig. 3**).

The abdominal muscles (rectus abdominis, internal oblique, external oblique, and transversus abdominis) serve several functions in respiration that mainly assist expiration but also can function in inspiration. The abdominal muscles also may play a minor role in inspiration if their contraction reduces lung volume below function residual capacity; abdominal muscles can store elastic recoil energy in the chest wall that then assists

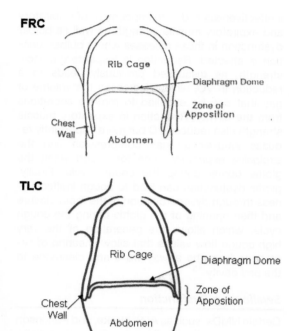

Fig. 2. Diagram of chest wall and the mechanical effects and position of the diaphragm at function residual capacity (FRC) and total lung capacity (TLC).

expansion of the chest wall during the next inspiration.[9] This inspiratory assist may be seen during exercise where expiration becomes active.

The accessory muscles of respiration (sternocleidomastoid, scalenes, trapezii, latissimus dorsi, platysma, and pectoralis major and minor muscles) can expand the rib cage and assist

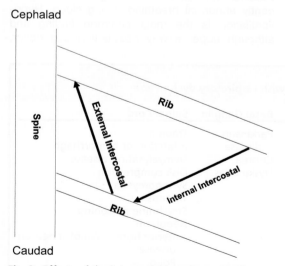

Fig. 3. Effects of the intercostal muscle contraction on ribcage motion. Vectors indicate the direction of rib movement with contraction.

inspiration during situations of increased ventilatory demand, such as during exercise or when other inspiratory muscles are impaired, as in tetraplegia or chronic obstructive pulmonary disease.

The muscles of the upper airway are also considered muscles of respiration because they maintain patency of the upper airway and allow air to flow into and out of the lungs without interruption.[10] These muscles are innervated by cranial nerves V, VII, and IX–XII. The central control centers for these muscles are the same as those described previously for the more commonly considered ventilatory muscles.

CONTROLLER FEEDBACK

The respiratory control mechanisms depend on both neural and chemical receptors found in peripheral and central sites.[5] The automatic respiratory centers in the brainstem respond to feedback from these receptors and adjust neural output to the ventilatory and upper airway muscles that expand the chest wall and maintain upper airway patency.

Neural receptors are present in the upper airway, respiratory muscles, lungs, and pulmonary vessels. Once stimulated, these receptors project signals to the central respiratory controller via the vagus nerve. The respiratory centers then adjust their output to the respiratory muscles to alter ventilation and modulate reflexes, such as cough and sneeze.

Chemical receptors or chemoreceptors are located both peripherally as well as in the central nervous system. The peripheral chemoreceptors, which include the carotid and aortic bodies, are the primary site for sensing low levels of Pao_2 and also respond to a lesser extent to changes in $Paco_2$ and pH. Although the control of ventilation during exercise is not completely understood, the predominant stimulus for increased ventilation is believed to arise from the peripheral receptors. The central chemoreceptors are crucial in the adjustments of ventilation to acid-base disturbances and $Paco_2$.[5] The central chemoreceptors are responsible for most of the response to carbon dioxide. They respond to increases in $Paco_2$ by their detection of the fall in pH of the cerebrospinal fluid associated with an increase in cerebrospinal fluid $Paco_2$, which closely follows an increase in serum $Paco_2$.

RESPIRATORY PATHOPHYSIOLOGY OF NEUROMUSCULAR DISEASE

Although each neuromuscular disease (NMD) has a specific natural history and pathophysiologic effects on the respiratory system, there are some generalized patterns that are often seen. These include negative effects on respiratory muscle strength resulting in a reduction in vital capacity (VC) and cough strength as well as effects on bulbar musculature and swallowing, sleep quality, and control of breathing. This discussion focuses on more chronic NMDs. **Tables 2** and **3** illustrate some of the more common NMDs and their primary site of pathologic effect.

Effects on Respiratory Muscle Strength

The effects on respiratory muscle strength vary with the type of NMD and whether and where the disease effects nerves, muscles, and controllers of breathing. In general, almost all NMDs result in a decrease in VC due to effects on inspiratory and expiratory muscles. The effect on VC is variable and may be mild (eg, hemidiaphragm paralysis) or severe (eg, advanced amyotrophic lateral sclerosis [ALS]). The onset of respiratory muscle weakness and reduction in VC as a function of time can also be variable and may be hyperacute (eg, cervical and thoracic spinal cord injury [SCI]), acute (Guillain-Barré syndrome or myasthenia gravis) or more gradual (muscular dystrophies or ALS) **(Fig. 4)**. In addition to weakness of the breathing muscles, there are often associated changes in chest wall and lung mechanics. In a study of 25 patients with a variety of NMDs, De Troyer and colleagues[11] found that VC was significantly less than would be predicted by decreased muscle strength alone and that there was a decrease in lung compliance of 40% on average. In addition, for reasons that are not entirely clear, the chest wall seems less compliant in those with NMDs.[12]

Effects on Cough Function

Most NMDs reduce cough effectiveness, an important lung defense mechanism. Cough ineffectiveness is due to impairment of inspiratory and expiratory muscle strength as well as bulbar dysfunction in those diseases where bulbar function is affected. Reduction in inspiratory muscle strength, as discussed previously, leads to a reduction in VC, which decreases the volume of gas that can be expelled to remove secretions from the airway. Reduction in expiratory muscle strength also reduces VC but more importantly reduces intra-airway gas compression and the explosive expiratory force for cough when the glottis opens during the cough cycle. Finally, glottis dysfunction can lead to cough ineffectiveness through dyscoordination of the rapid closure and then opening of the glottis during the cough cycle, which allows the generation of the very high cough flow values that allow shearing of secretions from the airway walls and clearance to the oral cavity.[13]

Swallowing Dysfunction

Certain NMDs, such as ALS, stroke, and Parkinson disease, can affect bulbar muscles substantially. In this case, dysfunction of the lips, tongue and, in particular, the pharyngeal and laryngeal muscles results in an increased risk of aspiration, which often leads to bacteria from the oral cavity entering the lower airways and sometimes large bolus aspiration with choking. This can lead to pneumonia, respiratory failure, and death. In addition, malnutrition can occur because of decreased ability to take in enough calories via the mouth.[14]

Sleep Disturbance

Patients with NMDs are at high risk of significantly abnormal breathing during sleep. Hypoventilation is the most common finding and although upper airway obstruction can occur,

---

Table 2
Diseases of the central nervous system associated with respiratory dysfunction

Cerebral Cortex	Brainstem	Basal Ganglia	Spinal Cord
Stroke	Stroke	Parkinson disease	Trauma
Neoplasm	Neoplasm	Chorea	Infarction or hemorrhage
Cerebral degeneration	Drugs	Dyskinesias	Demyelinating disease
Seizures	Hemorrhage		Disk compression
	Progressive bulbar palsy		Syringomyelia
	Multiple system atrophy		Tetanus
	Poliomyelitis		Strychnine poisoning
	Anoxic encephalopathy		Neoplasm
	Encephalitis		Anterior horn Cell/motor neuron disease
	MS		Polio
	Primary alveolar hypoventilation		Motor neuron Disease
			Epidural abscess

Table 3
Diseases of the peripheral nervous system associated with respiratory dysfunction

Motor Nerves	Neuromuscular Junction	Myopathies
Motor neuron disease	Drugs	DM
ALS	Antibiotics	Muscular dystrophies
SMA	Neuromuscular junction blockers	Polymyositis and dermatomyositis
Guillain-Barré syndrome	Anticholinesterase inhibitors	Thick filament myopathy
Critical illness neuropathy	Corticosteroids	Glycogen storage diseases
Vasculitides	Lidocaine	Pompe disease
Toxins (eg, lithium,	Quinidine	McArdle disease
arsenic, gold)	Lithium	Tarui disease
Metabolic	Antirheumatics	Severe hypokalemia
Diabetes	Toxins	Hypophosphatemia
Porphyria	Botulism	Mitochondrial myopathy
Uremia	Snake venoms	Nemaline body myopathy
Lymphoma	Scorpion bites	Acid maltase deficiency
Diphtheria	Shellfish	
	Crab poisoning	
	Myasthenia gravis	
	LEMS	

hypoventilation-related hypercarbia is the more common finding.[15] Sleep-disordered breathing is most commonly seen during rapid eye movement (REM) sleep, where hypotonia of skeletal muscles other than the diaphragm is occurs. Pre-existing weakness of the diaphragm leaves this muscle unable to maintain normal ventilation resulting in hypoventilation and hypercarbia during sleep. In addition to hypercarbia, significant hypoxemia and hemoglobin desaturation occur, related to the hypoventilation, described previously, and to the rapid shallow breathing pattern that is seen during REM sleep, which leads to an increased in respiratory system dead space, wasted ventilation, and worsened hypercarbia and hypoxemia.

Control of Breathing

Individuals with NMDs show a rapid shallow breathing pattern compared with normal subjects. This pattern persists when patients are exposed to hypoxic or hypercapenic gas mixtures, and the breathing pattern seems due to muscle weakness

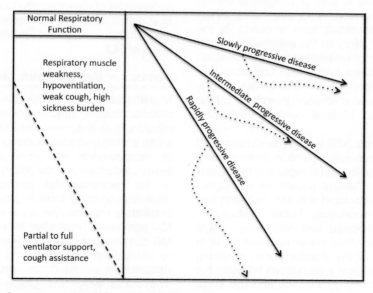

Fig. 4. Schematic of common natural histories of NMDs.

rather than central respiratory drive.[16] The measurement of mouth occlusion pressure during the first 100 milliseconds of inspiration, which is a measure of central ventilatory drive, is actually higher in those with NMDs compared with normal subjects.[16,17]

PATHOPHYSIOLOGY OF SPECIFIC DISEASES

Some of the more common diseases that may be seen in clinical practice are reviewed.

Central Nervous System Diseases

Several disorders can affect the pathways that connect the voluntary respiratory centers of the cortex to the spinal motor neurons. A midpontine stroke can cause what is known as the locked-in syndrome that results in total muscle paralysis (aside from eye movement) and loss of voluntary breathing control.[17] Extrapyramidal disorders, such as Parkinson disease, can also affect voluntary breathing. In these disorders, patients may be unable to voluntarily affect the breathing pattern, and they may also show a Cheyne-Stokes respiratory pattern. Respiratory muscle weakness, restrictive physiology, and upper airway obstruction have been reported in Parkinson disease and other extrapyramidal disorders.[18] Hemispheric lesions can also affect breathing. In hemiplegia after stroke, chest wall and diaphragm movements on the contralateral side of the cortical injury can be decreased resulting in restrictive physiology.[19]

The classic disruption of automatic but not voluntary breathing is that of congenital central alveolar hypoventilation, or Ondine curse, which is now known to result from a defect in the PHOX2B gene.[20] Injury to the automatic respiratory centers in the brainstem leads to central sleep apnea when a patient falls asleep and loses triggering of respiration. This can also be seen in unilateral and bilateral medullary infarction, bulbar poliomyelitis, and bilateral cervical tractotomy (for chronic pain).

Multiple sclerosis (MS) is a primary disorder of the central nervous system and is characterized by recurrent demyelination in regions of the central nervous system. Several causes of respiratory impairment are associated with MS, including respiratory muscle weakness, bulbar dysfunction, obstructive sleep apnea, and respiratory control dysfunction. Respiratory impairment can occur in the early course of the disease during or during acute attacks. There is a correlation between the degree of pulmonary dysfunction and the stage of neurologic disability although no correlation

has been found between pulmonary dysfunction and the duration of the disease.[21]

The potential for central or obstructive sleep-disordered breathing and nocturnal ventilatory dysfunction in MS should prompt a continued assessment of sleep-disordered breathing symptoms and consideration of polysomnography because MS patients have been found to have a higher incidence of sleep-disordered breathing than the general population.[22]

Diseases of the Spinal Cord

Diseases of the spinal cord often dramatically affect breathing because of their direct impact on control of motor nerves that control respiratory muscles. Although traumatic injury is the major cause of spinal cord pathology, other causes include tumor, vascular accident, transverse myelitis, and syringomyelia. Cervical SCI often results in a requirement for long-term ventilation. Thoracic SCI and lumbar SCI rarely cause respiratory failure but may still affect cough function because of the importance of the abdominal muscles in effective cough function.

For patients with SCI who require chronic ventilator support, tracheostomy is an option although several effective nontracheostomy approaches are available, including mouthpiece and mask ventilation and potentially phrenic nerve pacing.[23]

Sleep apnea is more common in SCI than in the general population and it seems that the higher the level of injury, the more likely it is that an individual develops sleep apnea.[24] The cause of this increased risk is not clear but possible causes include more time sleeping in the supine position, hypertrophy of neck muscles increasing the risk of obstruction, the use of sedating antispasticity medications, or an as-yet undefined central neural effect of SCI.

Diseases of the Neuromuscular Junction

Myasthenia gravis (MG), the most common chronic disease affecting neuromuscular transmission, is an autoimmune disease characterized by an antibody-mediated immune attack directed at acetylcholine receptors and/or receptor-associated proteins in the postsynaptic membrane of the neuromuscular junction. It results in weakness of many muscle groups, including the respiratory muscles. An acute crisis can result in ICU admission, respiratory failure, and death.[25,26] MG can also occur as a paraneoplastic syndrome in association with thymoma. Removal of the thymoma may result in amelioration of the myasthenia symptoms. Outpatient management of with corticosteroids, cholinergic agents, and immunosuppressants are aimed at relieving symptoms and preventing acute crises.

The Lambert-Eaton myasthenic syndrome (LEMS) is associated with small cell lung cancer that can affect the respiratory muscles in a fashion similar to MG. LEMS differs from MG in that it affects the presynaptic neuromuscular junction rather than the postsynaptic membrane as in MG. Although respiratory involvement is often a late finding, frank respiratory failure can be a manifestation of LEMS and this disorder should be considered in individuals with unexplained neuromuscular weakness.

Diseases of the Motor Nerves

ALS is a disease that can affect upper and lower motor neurons. The disease has a peak incidence in the seventh and eighth decades of life and affects men more than women.[27] ALS often affects all of the respiratory muscles, including those for airway protection and cough. Pneumonia and respiratory failure are the leading cause of death in this disease. Sleep-disordered breathing is common in ALS, is associated with respiratory muscle weakness and diaphragm weakness in particular, and increases in frequency as the disease progresses. Strong consideration of noninvasive positive-pressure ventilation (NPPV) is suggested for all patients with FVC less than 50% predicted, maximal inspiratory pressure (MIP) greater than -60 cm H_2O, sniff nasal inspiratory pressure (SNIP) less than 40 cm H_2O, or sleep evaluation showing desaturation at nighttime or a positive sleep study.[28] As ALS progresses with bulbar involvement, NPPV may cease to be effective and a decision needs to be made concerning the appropriateness of tracheostomy and long-term invasive ventilation. Tracheostomy can prolong life substantially but does not affect progression of the underlying disease, and fewer than 10% of patients in the United States choose this option.[29]

Spinal muscular atrophy (SMA) is a genetic disease of that resembles ALS in its effects on the motor neurons but has an onset in infancy. It occurs in several forms SMA types 1 to 4 range from most to least severe muscle impairment. In SMA type 1, intercostal muscles are more significantly affected and the diaphragm is relatively spared, resulting in paradoxic movement of the chest wall during inspiration with inward movement of the ribcage and outward movement of the abdominal wall. Left untreated, there is a progressive respiratory failure beginning with anatomic changes that lead to repeated respiratory infections, progressive respiratory failure initially at night but later during the day, and

ultimately complete respiratory failure. NPPV or tracheostomy ventilation for children with SMA type 1 has been successfully used.[30]

Nocturnal support of sleep-disordered breathing may be necessary for those with SMA type 2. Invasive ventilation is not required chronically for SMA types 2, 3, and 4. A "Consensus Statement for Standard of Care in Spinal Muscular Atrophy" has been developed to aid in standardizing clinical care and also to make uniform study protocols.[31]

Acute polio still exists in the developing world, but in the developed world, the major health issue arising from polio is the postpolio syndrome (PPS), in which new weakness develops in survivors of the polio epidemics of the mid-twentieth century.[32] The cause of PPS is unknown although theories of pathogenesis include: (1) progressive degeneration of reinnervated motor units, (2) persistence of poliovirus in neural tissue, and (3) induction of autoimmunity with subsequent destruction of neural structures. The average time to onset from the time of the initial infection is 35 years but ranges from 8 years to 71 years.

PPS effects on the respiratory system include: restrictive disease caused by weakness of respiratory muscles and chest wall deformities, obstructive and central sleep apnea, and hypercarbic respiratory failure. Known risk factors for restrictive disease include ventilation at the acute polio onset, acute polio infection over 10 years of age, and time from acute polio episode to development of weakness less than 35 years.[33] Sleep-disordered breathing is common and in 1 series was noted to occur in 65% of patients.[34]

Diaphragm paralysis or weakness can be caused by both motor nerve and muscle problems (see **Tables 2** and **3**) and may be either unilateral or bilateral. In unilateral diaphragm paralysis, patients may be asymptomatic at rest but have dyspnea with exertion.[35] Orthopnea may be present but is not as common or severe as in bilateral paralysis. The diagnosis is often suggested by an elevated hemidiaphragm on chest radiograph and confirmed with fluoroscopic sniff test.[36] Ultrasonographic imaging of the diaphragm in the zone of apposition provides an alternate means of diagnosing chronic unilateral diaphragm paralysis by demonstrating a thin diaphragm that fails to thicken with inspiration.[37]

Bilateral diaphragm paralysis is most often seen in the setting of a disease producing severe generalized muscle weakness. The most common causes are diffuse muscle diseases or motor neuron disease, such as ALS. In bilateral diaphragm paralysis orthopnea, dyspnea with exertion and dyspnea on immersion into water due to water pressure on the abdominal wall and upward displacement of the diaphragm are notable symptoms.[38] Sleep-disordered breathing with hypoventilation and hypoxemia is common.[39] Pulmonary function is impaired with a reduction in VC associated and a significant drop in the supine position of up to 50% and reduction MIP.[35,40] Disability can be pronounced. Physical examination may reveal paradoxic breathing in a resting or sleeping supine patient. Bilateral diaphragmatic paralysis can be difficult to diagnose radiographically because there is no normal hemidiaphragm to use for comparison with an abnormal one. As a result, chest radiography and fluoroscopic sniff testing can yield false-negative results. Two-dimensional ultrasound to assess the movement of the diaphragm dome shares the same limitations as fluoroscopy.[41] The gold standard diagnostic test is measuring transdiaphragmatic pressure using thin balloon-tipped polyethylene catheters placed in the esophagus and stomach to demonstrate the lack of ability to generate a transdiaphragmatic pressure. Bilateral diaphragm paralysis is not often reversible unless the underlying disease is treatable.

Diseases Affecting the Respiratory Muscles

There are many causes of chronic muscle disease resulting in respiratory muscle dysfunction, including genetic muscular dystrophies, myopathies, and myotonias as well as inflammatory myopathies and those associated with systemic diseases.

Duchenne muscular dystrophy (DMD)and Becker muscular dystrophy are both progressive myopathies caused by mutations of the dystrophin gene on chromosome Xp21. Dystrophin is a protein on the cytoplasmic face of the plasma membrane of muscle fibers, functioning as 1 component of a large, tightly associated glycoprotein complex. It provides mechanical reinforcement to the sarcolemma and stabilizes the glycoprotein complex.

In DMD, dystrophin is absent whereas in Becker muscular dystrophy, a milder variant, dystrophin is reduced in quantity or quality. Both disorders are inherited as X-linked traits and are characterized by progressive muscle wasting and weakness of all skeletal and ultimately cardiac muscle in male patients.

Respiratory effects of muscle weakness result in restrictive pulmonary deficit and inspiratory and expiratory muscle weakness predisposes these individuals to developing respiratory complications such as atelectasis and pneumonia. As the respiratory muscles further weaken and the restriction becomes severe, patients often need nocturnal ventilatory assistance due to hypoventilation and obstructive sleep apneas.[42] Daytime NPPV may be provided to individuals with DMD as the disease progresses. If individuals with DMD or Becker muscular dystrophy require surgery, they may be at higher risk of respiratory complications and a preventive team approach has been suggested.[43]

Myotonic dystrophy (DM) is an autosomal dominant disorder that is genetically heterogeneous with variable phenotypic expression. It is caused by mutations in the dystrophia myotonic protein kinase gene.[44] The disease results from processing defects involving the mRNAs of several genes affecting skeletal muscle chloride channel function, the insulin receptor, and cardiac troponin T.[45] There are 2 major classifications, including DM1, formerly known as Steinert disease, and DM2, a more mild disease form. DM differs from other muscular dystrophies with multisystem effects, including cardiac conduction abnormalities, cataracts, infertility, and insulin resistance. DM1 presents at birth through adulthood in its milder form. Only adult onset has been seen in DM2. A characteristic phenotypic feature of skeletal muscle weakness is facial muscle weakness Limb weakness is associated with the weakness of thigh, hip flexor, and extensor muscles. Cardiac abnormalities include both conduction disturbances and structural defects.[46] Respiratory muscle weakness is common in DM1, resulting in variable restrictive pulmonary impairment and alveolar hypoventilation. Oropharyngeal muscle weakness can result in dysphagia and the liability of chronic aspiration but is more commonly associated with sleep-disordered breathing. Sleep-disordered breathing with a prominent central apnea component and nocturnal hypoxemia has been shown to be common in DM. Daytime hypercapnea has also been observed.[47] Sudden death in DM is associated with ventricular arrhythmias and nocturnal hypoxemia secondary to sleep-disordered breathing is a significant risk factor for cardiac arrhythmia. DM patients with severe oropharyngeal muscle weakness may develop chronic upper airway airflow restriction or aspiration.

Other muscular dystrophies, such as limb-girdle muscular dystrophy, facioscapulohumeral dystrophy, and DM, can affect the respiratory muscles but do not generally cause respiratory impairment until later in the course of the disease.

Inflammatory myopathies, such as dermatomyositis, polymyositis, and inclusion body myositis, are systemic inflammatory diseases of unknown etiology, which cause profound skeletal muscle weakness. Symptoms related to respiratory muscle weakness usually are not the presenting complaints; however, respiratory muscle weakness can occur in 5% to 10% of the patients with dermatomyositis and polymyositis[48] and may be found in as many as 75% of individuals if respiratory muscle function is carefully evaluated.[49] Interstitial lung disease may occur in up to 70% of patients with dermatomyositis or polymyositis.[50] Individuals diagnosed with dermatomyositis or polymyositis should be evaluated for the presence of restrictive pulmonary disease, which may be due to respiratory muscle weakness as well as interstitial lung 2disease. If respiratory muscle weakness is pronounced (maximal inspiratory pressure <30% of predicted), ventilatory failure may ensue.[48]

Several genetic metabolic myopathies can affect the respiratory muscles, including glycogen storage diseases and lipid metabolism disorders. Acid maltase deficiency (type II glycogenosis, or Pompe disease) is a disease that involves respiratory muscles and may come to the attention of the respiratory practitioner. It is due to the deficiency of acid α-glucosidase, an enzyme responsible for the degradation of glycogen polymers to glucose. Deficiency of this enzyme leads to accumulation of glycogen within cardiac and skeletal muscle lysosomes resulting in myopathy. Although typically involving infants, this disease can manifest in adulthood. Other metabolic myopathies can be caused by defects of lipid metabolism or disorders involving the mitochondria directly.[51]

CLINICAL ASSESSMENT OF PATHOPHYSIOLOGIC EFFECTS OF NEUROMUSCULAR DISEASE

A clinically helpful manner to assess dysfunction of the neuromuscular respiratory system is to divide it into 3 main areas of function[52] (Fig. 5):

1. Ventilatory function determined predominantly by the inspiratory muscles
2. Cough function, which is determined by inspiratory, expiratory, and glottic function
3. Swallowing and airway protection determined by glottic muscles

Each 1 of these 3 functional parts of the system may show evidence of impairment and contribute to neuromuscular respiratory failure although dysfunction in each of the system is not always present at the same time. Evidence for dysfunction in each of the 3 areas should be sought at each clinic visit by eliciting historical data, performing a thorough physical examination, and laboratory testing. Recent respiratory society statements have underscored the need for regular and thorough evaluation in this manner.[53]

Assessing Ventilatory Muscle Function

The best measures of respiratory muscle strength and function in NMD remain and area of discussion and investigation. MIP and maximal expiratory pressure have been traditional measures for respiratory muscle strength. FVC has also been used as a measure of global respiratory muscle strength in that both inspiratory and expiratory muscles are involved. Supine VC seems more sensitive than upright VC in revealing diaphragm weakness. SNIP seems to be a reproducible and accurate measure of inspiratory muscle strength. It has been shown an accurate predictor of the presence nocturnal desaturations and respiratory failure in patients with ALS.[54] Because no 1 test accurately predicts clinical sequelae of NMD, it has been suggested that ongoing testing with multiple modalities is important to identify those at risk for sleep-disordered breathing and hypoventilation.[55]

Hypoventilation in NMD often first presents at night during sleep, in particular the REM stage, as discussed previously. Symptoms consistent with sleep-disordered breathing include more frequent nocturnal awakenings, nocturia, vivid nightmares, night sweats, daytime hypersomnolence, morning headaches, nausea, depression, decreased concentration, and diminished daytime performance. Polysomnography can be used to evaluate sleep in patients with NMD but an overnight stay in a sleep laboratory may be especially difficult for such individuals if they require a personal care attendant, position changes, or help with toileting. Thus, assuring a high pretest probability prior to ordering a sleep study is important. Baseline values of daytime $Paco_2$ greater than or equal to 45 or base excess

Neuromuscular Respiratory Disease

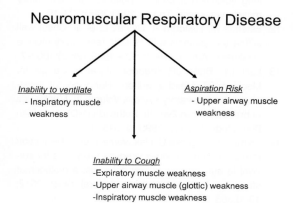

Inability to ventilate
- Inspiratory muscle weakness

Aspiration Risk
- Upper airway muscle weakness

Inability to Cough
-Expiratory muscle weakness
-Upper airway muscle (glottic) weakness
-Inspiratory muscle weakness

Fig. 5. The 2 major effects of NMD on the respiratory system.

of greater than or equal to 4 mEq may correlate with sleep hypoventilation.[55]

An unattended sleep study in the home or overnight oximetry and partial pressure of exhaled carbon dioxide levels monitoring may substitute for a full laboratory polysomnogram; however, the sensitivity and specificity of these portable tests are unclear in this population.[56] For patients who have elevated $Paco_2$ despite adequate nocturnal therapy, dyspnea during the daytime or hypoxemia due to recurrent respiratory infections associated with atelectasis, diurnal ventilatory support may be needed as well.

Assessing Cough Function

Cough insufficiency may be suspected if a patient describes an inability to bring secretions to the mouth for expectoration or if there is a history of frequent respiratory infections. Cough function is best assessed by measuring peak cough flow rate (PCF). This can be easily measured with an asthma peak flow meter or office spirometer connected to a facemask or mouthpiece (see **Fig. 4**). Normal values range from 360 L/min to 960 L/min[13]; a value below 160 L/min may place individuals at high risk for cough insufficiency and ventilator dependence. During a respiratory infection, PCF may drop substantially and a PCF of less than 270 L/min during a healthy period can drop below 160 L/min during infection, so should trigger cough augmentation procedures.[57]

Assessing Swallowing Function

Swallowing dysfunction is a frequent finding in patients with NMDs. Impaired swallowing and ingesting adequate nutrition can be challenging for patients. Choking is common and may even be triggered by aspiration of saliva. Malnutrition or rapid weight loss should signal the clinician to assess the swallowing mechanism. Historical points, such as choking episodes, particularly with thin liquids such as water, should be sought. Questions concerning ability to adequately clear airway secretions with colds or bronchitis should be asked as well as inquiring about frequency of pneumonia. Swallowing may be tested by barium swallow or direct visualization of swallowing endoscopically.[58] Consultation with speech and swallowing experts can be helpful.

SUMMARY

The effects of NMDs on the respiratory system can range from isolated and mild to protean and severe. An understanding of the pathophysiology of specific diseases as well as adopting a general approach to the patient with 1 of these disorders can be helpful and in many cases can lead to improvement in quality and quantity of life.

REFERENCES

1. Bergofsky EH. Respiratory failure in disorders of the thoracic cage. Am Rev Respir Dis 1979;119:643–69.
2. Perrin C, Unterborn JN, Ambrosio CD, et al. Pulmonary complications of chronic neuromuscular diseases and their management. Muscle Nerve 2004; 29(1):5–27.
3. Benditt JO, Boitano LJ. Pulmonary issues in patients with chronic neuromuscular disease. Am J Respir Crit Care Med 2013;187(10):1046–55.
4. Evans KC, Shea SA, Saykin AJ. Functional MRI localisation of central nervous system regions associated with volitional inspiration in humans. J Physiol 1999;520(Pt 2):383–92.
5. Guyenet PG, Bayliss DA. Neural control of breathing and CO2 Homeostasis. Neuron 2015;87(5):946–61.
6. Fagerlund MJ, Eriksson LI. Current concepts in neuromuscular transmission. Br J Anaesth 2009; 103(1):108–14.
7. De Troyer A, Kelly S, Zin WA. Mechanical action of the intercostal muscles on the ribs. Science 1983; 220:87–8.
8. Legrand A, Schneider E, Gevenois PA, et al. Respiratory effects of the scalene and sternomastoid muscles in humans. J Appl Physiol (1985) 2003;94(4): 1467–72.
9. Mesquita Montes A, Maia J, Crasto C, et al. Abdominal muscle activity during breathing in different postures in COPD "Stage 0" and healthy subjects. Respir Physiol Neurobiol 2017;238:14–22.
10. Tachikawa S, Nakayama K, Nakamura S, et al. Coordinated respiratory motor activity in nerves innervating the upper airway muscles in rats. PLoS One 2016;11(11):e0166436.
11. De Troyer A, Borenstein S, Cordier R. Analysis of lung volume restriction in patients with respiratory muscle weakness. Thorax 1980;35(8):603–10.
12. Estenne M, Heilporn A, Delhez L, et al. Chest wall stiffness in patients with chronic respiratory muscle weakness. Am Rev Respir Dis 1983;128(6):1002–7.
13. Leith DE, Butler JP, Sneddon SL, et al. Cough. In: Macklem PT, Mead J, editors. Handbook of physiology: the respiratory system. Volume III. Mechanics of breathing, Part 2vol. III. Bethesda (MD): American Physiologic Society; 1990. p. 315–36.
14. Shimizu T, Nagaoka U, Nakayama Y, et al. Reduction rate of body mass index predicts prognosis for survival in amyotrophic lateral sclerosis: a multicenter study in Japan. Amyotroph Lateral Scler 2012; 13(4):363–6.
15. Fermin AM, Afzal U, Culebras A. Sleep in neuromuscular diseases. Sleep Med Clin 2016;11(1):53–64.

16. Baydur A. Respiratory muscle strength and control of ventilation in patients with neuromuscular disease. Chest 1991;99(2):330–8.

17. Plum F, Posner JB. The diagnosis of stupor and coma. 1st edition. Philadelphia: FA Davis; 1966.

18. Baille G, De Jesus AM, Perez T, et al. Ventilatory dysfunction in Parkinson's disease. J Parkinsons Dis 2016;6(3):463–71.

19. Fluck DC. Chest movements in hemiplegia. Clin Sci 1966;31(3):383–8.

20. Patwari PP, Carroll MS, Rand CM, et al. Congenital central hypoventilation syndrome and the PHOX2B gene: a model of respiratory and autonomic dysregulation. Respir Physiol Neurobiol 2010;173(3): 322–35.

21. Buyse B, Demedts M, Meekers J, et al. Respiratory dysfunction in multiple sclerosis: a prospective analysis of 60 patients. Eur Respir J 1997;10(1):139–45.

22. Tantucci C, Massucci M, Piperno R, et al. Control of breathing and respiratory muscle strength in patients with multiple sclerosis. Chest 1994;105(4): 1163–70.

23. Bach JR. Noninvasive respiratory management of high level spinal cord injury. J Spinal Cord Med 2012;35(2):72–80.

24. Berlowitz DJ, Brown DJ, Campbell DA, et al. A longitudinal evaluation of sleep and breathing in the first year after cervical spinal cord injury. Arch Phys Med Rehabil 2005;86(6):1193–9.

25. Gajdos P, Chevret S, Toyka K. Intravenous immunoglobulin for myasthenia gravis. Cochrane Database Syst Rev 2008;(1):CD002277.

26. Lee SJ, Hur J, Lee TW, et al. Myasthenia gravis presenting initially as acute respiratory failure. Respir Care 2015;60(1):e14–6.

27. Worms PM. The epidemiology of motor neuron diseases: a review of recent studies. J Neurol Sci 2001;191(1–2):3–9.

28. Wolfe LF, Joyce NC, McDonald CM, et al. Management of pulmonary complications in neuromuscular disease. Phys Med Rehabil Clin N Am 2012;23(4): 829–53.

29. Rabkin J, Ogino M, Goetz R, et al. Tracheostomy with invasive ventilation for ALS patients: neurologists' roles in the US and Japan. Amyotroph Lateral Scler Frontotemporal Degener 2013;14(2):116–23.

30. Oskoui M, Levy G, Garland CJ, et al. The changing natural history of spinal muscular atrophy type 1. Neurology 2007;69(20):1931–6.

31. Wang CH, Finkel RS, Bertini ES, et al. Consensus statement for standard of care in spinal muscular atrophy. J Child Neurol 2007;22(8):1027–49.

32. Trojan DA, Cashman NR. Post-poliomyelitis syndrome. Muscle Nerve 2005;31(1):6–19.

33. Dean E, Ross J, Road JD, et al. Pulmonary function in individuals with a history of poliomyelitis. Chest 1991;100(1):118–23.

34. Dahan V, Kimoff RJ, Petrof BJ, et al. Sleep-disordered breathing in fatigued postpoliomyelitis clinic patients. Arch Phys Med Rehabil 2006;87(10): 1352–6.

35. McCool FD, Tzelepis GE. Dysfunction of the diaphragm. N Engl J Med 2012;366(10):932–42.

36. Gierada DS, Slone RM, Fleishman MJ. Imaging evaluation of the diaphragm. Chest Surg Clin N Am 1998;8(2):237–80.

37. Gottesman E, McCool FD. Ultrasound evaluation of the paralyzed diaphragm. Am J Respir Crit Care Med 1997;155(5):1570–4.

38. McCool F, Mead J. Dyspnea on immersion: mechanisms in patients with bilateral diaphragm paralysis. Am Rev Respir Dis 1989;139:275–6.

39. Khan A, Morgenthaler TI, Ramar K. Sleep disordered breathing in isolated unilateral and bilateral diaphragmatic dysfunction. J Clin Sleep Med 2014; 10(5):509–15.

40. Mier-Jedrzelowicz A, Brophy C, Moxham J, et al. Assessment of diaphragm weakness. Am Rev Resp Dis 1988;137:877–83.

41. Miller SG, Brook MM, Tacy TA. Reliability of two-dimensional echocardiography in the assessment of clinically significant abnormal hemidiaphragm motion in pediatric cardiothoracic patients: comparison with fluoroscopy. Pediatr Crit Care Med 2006; 7(5):441–4.

42. Bourke SC, Gibson GJ. Sleep and breathing in neuromuscular disease. Eur Respir J 2002;19(6): 1194–201.

43. Birnkrant DJ, Panitch HB, Benditt JO, et al. American College of Chest Physicians consensus statement on the respiratory and related management of patients with Duchenne muscular dystrophy undergoing anesthesia or sedation. Chest 2007; 132(6):1977–86.

44. Brook JD, McCurrach ME, Harley HG, et al. Molecular basis of myotonic dystrophy: expansion of a trinucleotide (CTG) repeat at the 3' end of a transcript encoding a protein kinase family member. Cell 1992;69(2):385.

45. Savkur RS, Philips AV, Cooper TA. Aberrant regulation of insulin receptor alternative splicing is associated with insulin resistance in myotonic dystrophy. Nat Genet 2001;29(1):40–7.

46. Groh WJ. Arrhythmias in the muscular dystrophies. Heart Rhythm 2012;9(11):1890–5.

47. Thil C, Agrinier N, Chenuel B, et al. Longitudinal course of lung function in myotonic dystrophy type 1. Muscle Nerve 2017;56(4):816–8.

48. Braun NMT, Aurora NS, Rochester DF. Respiratory muscle and pulmonary function in poliomyositis and other proximal myopathies. Thorax 1983;38: 316–23.

49. Teixeira A, Cherin P, Demoule A, et al. Diaphragmatic dysfunction in patients with idiopathic

inflammatory myopathies. Neuromuscul Disord 2005;15(1):32–9.

50. Fathi M, Lundberg IE, Tornling G. Pulmonary complications of polymyositis and dermatomyositis. Semin Respir Crit Care Med 2007;28(4):451–8.

51. Adler M, Shieh PB. Metabolic myopathies. Semin Neurol 2015;35(4):385–97.

52. Benditt JO. The neuromuscular respiratory system: physiology, pathophysiology, and a respiratory care approach to patients. Respir Care 2006;51(8): 829–37 [discussion: 837–9].

53. McKim DA, Road J, Avendano M, et al. Home mechanical ventilation: a Canadian Thoracic Society clinical practice guideline. Can Respir J 2011; 18(4):197–215.

54. Morgan RK, McNally S, Alexander M, et al. Use of Sniff nasal-inspiratory force to predict survival in amyotrophic lateral sclerosis. Am J Respir Crit Care Med 2005;171(3):269–74.

55. Hukins CA, Hillman DR. Daytime predictors of sleep hypoventilation in Duchenne muscular dystrophy. Am J Respir Crit Care Med 2000;161(1):166–70.

56. Kirk VG, Flemons WW, Adams C, et al. Sleep-disordered breathing in Duchenne muscular dystrophy: a preliminary study of the role of portable monitoring. Pediatr Pulmonol 2000;29(2):135–40.

57. Bach JR, Saporito LR. Criteria for extubation and tracheostomy tube removal for patients with ventilatory failure. A different approach to weaning. Chest 1996;110(6):1566–71.

58. Tilton AH, Miller MD, Khoshoo V. Nutrition and swallowing in pediatric neuromuscular patients. Semin Pediatr Neurol 1998;5(2):106–15.

Sleep-Disordered Breathing in Neuromuscular and Chest Wall Diseases

Janet Hilbert, MD

KEYWORDS

- Sleep-disordered breathing • Sleep hypoventilation • Neuromuscular diseases • Thoracic wall

KEY POINTS

- Sleep-disordered breathing occurs frequently in neuromuscular and chest wall disorders as a result of the effects of normal sleep on ventilation and additional challenges imposed by specific disorders.
- Sleep-disordered breathing patterns include sleep hypoventilation, obstructive sleep apnea, central sleep apnea, and overlapping syndromes.
- Sleep hypoventilation precedes diurnal respiratory failure and clinical presentation is often nonspecific.
- Diagnostic polysomnography can identify patterns and severity of sleep-disordered breathing.
- Therapeutic polysomnography is recommended for titration of optimal noninvasive ventilation settings and minimizing patient-noninvasive ventilator asynchrony.

INTRODUCTION

Sleep-disordered breathing is common in neuromuscular and chest wall diseases, collectively known as restrictive thoracic disorders. These disorders include a diverse group of conditions that share common risk factors for sleep-disordered breathing, including respiratory muscle weakness and/or thoracic restriction. Sleep-disordered breathing results from both the effects of normal sleep on ventilation and the superimposed challenges imposed by the underlying disorder. Patterns of sleep-disordered breathing vary with the specific diagnosis and stage of disease. Sleep hypoventilation precedes diurnal hypoventilation and is difficult to recognize clinically because symptoms are nonspecific. Treatment with noninvasive positive-pressure ventilation (NPPV) is associated with improved outcomes. Polysomnography has a role in both the diagnosis

of sleep-disordered breathing and in the titration of effective NPPV while potentially avoiding patient-ventilator asynchrony. This review focuses primarily on the intersection of sleep and breathing in neuromuscular and chest wall disorders.

EPIDEMIOLOGY OF SLEEP-DISORDERED BREATHING IN NEUROMUSCULAR AND CHEST WALL DISORDERS

Restrictive thoracic disorders comprise a diverse group of conditions[1,2] (**Box 1**) that vary based on anatomic distribution of neuromuscular involvement, underlying cause, clinical presentation, and rate of progression but are commonly associated with alveolar hypoventilation and, ultimately, hypercapnic respiratory failure. These disorders are also distinguished by the presence/absence of risk factors for obstructive or central

Disclosures: No commercial or financial conflicts of interest.
Department of Internal Medicine, Section of Pulmonary, Critical Care, and Sleep Medicine, Yale University, Yale University School of Medicine, 300 Cedar Street, PO Box 208057, New Haven, CT 06520-8057, USA
E-mail address: janet.hilbert@yale.edu

Clin Chest Med 39 (2018) 309–324
https://doi.org/10.1016/j.ccm.2018.01.009
0272-5231/18/© 2018 Elsevier Inc. All rights reserved.

monitoring techniques and definitions used to detect and define sleep-disordered breathing.

In a study of 60 adult and pediatric patients with diverse neuromuscular disorders, most of whom had symptoms of daytime dysfunction, the prevalence of a respiratory disturbance index greater than or equal to 5, greater than or equal to 10, and greater than or equal to 15 was 83%, 63%, and 42%, respectively. More than 90% of the respiratory disturbances were hypopneas; 23% of patients had a decrease in mean oxygen saturation as measured by pulse oximetry (Sp_{O_2}) during sleep, suggesting hypoventilation. These patients were studied at home with a device monitoring airflow, chest effort, heart rate, body position, Sp_{O_2}, and tracheal sounds, but no sleep or carbon dioxide assessment was performed.[4] In a retrospective case series of patients with diverse neuromuscular disorders, home-based transcutaneous capnometry identified nocturnal hypoventilation (defined as transcutaneous carbon dioxide [$P_{tc}CO_2$] ≥ 50 for $\geq 5\%$ monitoring time) in 7 of 16 patients (44%) with normal daytime end-tidal carbon dioxide ($P_{ET}CO_2$) and in 3 of 4 patients (75%) with elevated daytime $P_{ET}CO_2$.[5] In another retrospective study of 232 adult patients with neuromuscular disease who underwent nocturnal capno-oximetry, prevalence rates for hypoventilation varied from 10% to 60%, depending on the criteria used to define hypoventilation.[6] Overall, prevalence of sleep-disordered breathing is high in most of these disorders, and chronic respiratory failure occurs with disease progression.[7,8]

PATHOPHYSIOLOGY OF SLEEP-DISORDERED BREATHING IN NEUROMUSCULAR AND CHEST WALL DISORDERS
Effects of Sleep on Breathing in Normal Individuals

Sleep is a normal, regularly occurring, reversible state characterized behaviorally by "perceptual disengagement from and unresponsiveness to the environment."[9] Sleep is divided into rapid eye movement (REM) and non-REM (NREM) sleep, which are as different physiologically from each other as either is from wake. In simple terms, REM can be thought of as an active mind in a quiet body whereas NREM is a quiet mind in an active body. NREM sleep is further subdivided into stages N1, N2, and N3 and REM is subdivided into phasic REM and tonic REM.[10] During sleep, there are ultradian cycles of NREM and REM sleep that repeat every 90 minutes or so, with REM periods lengthening as sleep progresses. There are characteristic changes in sleep from infancy though the geriatric years, but normal adults

sleep-disordered breathing (such as craniofacial abnormalities or upper airway muscle involvement associated with obstructive sleep apnea, cardiomyopathy associated with Cheyne-Stokes respiration, or spinal cord disease associated with central sleep apnea).[3] The prevalence of sleep-disordered breathing depends on the specific disease and stage of that disease as well as the spend approximately 20% to 25% of sleep time in REM.

Sleep affects both control of breathing and pulmonary function. With the onset of sleep (which occurs through NREM in adults), there is loss of the wakefulness drive to breathe as well as reduction in mechanical and behavioral inputs to ventilation.[11] Breathing falls under purely metabolic control.[12] Ventilatory responsiveness to both hypoxia and hypercapnia are diminished, particularly in REM sleep.[13–16] Additionally, in normal REM sleep, there is active inhibition of skeletal muscle, including accessory muscles of respiration, with sparing of the diaphragm. Functional residual capacity falls, in part due to supine posture and cephalad movement of the diaphragm, with decreased compensation by intercostal muscles during REM sleep.[17,18] Finally, upper airway resistance increases during sleep, more so in REM sleep than NREM sleep.[19,20] The end result is that during sleep in normal healthy individuals, although metabolic rate falls, minute ventilation falls further, resulting in a normal increase in mean carbon dioxide tension in sleep of approximately 4 mm Hg and normal increase in peak carbon dioxide tension of 9 mm Hg.[21,22] Breathing is stable in NREM sleep with regular rate and tidal volume but becomes irregular in REM with pauses and decreased ventilation during phasic REM.[23,24] These changes in respiration with sleep (**Box 2**) may be insignificant in healthy individuals but predispose to sleep-disordered breathing in susceptible individuals.

Additional Challenges in Sleep in Restrictive Thoracic Disorders

The cardinal feature of restrictive thoracic disorders is weakness or mechanical disadvantage of the diaphragm, the major muscle of respiration. Hypoventilation due to diaphragm dysfunction is initially most pronounced in REM sleep, when there is lack of compensation by accessory muscles of respiration.[18] In general, there is a predicable temporal pattern to the development of hypoventilation, first occurring in REM sleep, then occurring in both REM and NREM sleep (but worse in REM), and finally occurring while awake.[7] The rate of progression from mild REM-related hypoventilation to diurnal respiratory failure depends on the underlying disease (eg, fairly slow in Duchenne muscular dystrophy and more rapid in amyotrophic lateral sclerosis [ALS]). Weakness of accessory muscles further compounds generalized hypoventilation as well as results in poor cough, atelectasis, and further hypoxemia. Dysfunction of upper air muscles contributes to

---

> **Box 2**
> **Factors contributing to sleep-disordered breathing in neuromuscular and chest wall disease**
>
> *Effects of sleep on breathing in normal individuals*
> - Loss of wakefulness drive to breathe
> - Reduction in nonmetabolic inputs to ventilation
> - Decreased chemoresponsiveness to hypoxia and hypercapnia
> - REM-related skeletal muscle atonia
> - Reduced lung volumes
> - Increased upper airway resistance
>
> *Superimposed loads in individuals with restrictive thoracic disorders*
> - Diaphragm weakness
> - Weakness of accessory muscles of respiration
> - Upper airway muscle weakness
> - Obesity
> - Macroglossia
> - Craniofacial abnormalities
> - Associated cardiomyopathy
> - Atelectasis
> - Chest wall abnormality
> - Further decreased chemoresponsiveness

---

obstructive sleep-disordered breathing. Additional factors, such as the development of obesity due to inactivity or the development of scoliosis or chest wall abnormalities, contribute to hypoventilation.[25] Both obesity and upper airway anatomic abnormalities if present (eg, macroglossia and craniofacial abnormalities) contribute to obstructive sleep apnea. Cardiomyopathy, which can occur with the muscular dystrophies, may be associated with central sleep apnea in the form of Cheyne-Stokes respiration.[26] Reduced ventilatory responses to hypoxia and hypercapnia may be a primary feature of the underlying disease.[27] Rising bicarbonate to compensate for hypoventilation may lead to further decreased chemoresponsiveness, thus compounding hypoventilation.[28]

PATTERNS OF SLEEP-DISORDERED BREATHING IN NEUROMUSCULAR AND CHEST WALL DISORDERS
Definitions

Diurnal hypoventilation is generally accepted to be an awake partial pressure of carbon dioxide in arterial blood (Pa_{CO_2}) greater than or equal to 45 mm Hg. The definition of sleep hypoventilation has varied over time, however, among studies, and with different age groups, thus affecting prevalence statistics.[6] The American Academy of Sleep Medicine (AASM) has published scoring rules for sleep hypoventilation in adults and children (**Box 3**).[10] In patients with neuromuscular disease without daytime hypercapnia at baseline, both the AASM definition for sleep-related hypoventilation and a simpler definition (peak $P_{tc}CO_2 \geq$ 49 mm Hg) predicted subsequent need for assisted ventilation (as determined either by meeting the 1999 National Association for the Medical Direction of Respiratory Care [NAMDRC] National Consensus Conference criteria for NPPV [**Box 6**] or emergent need following acute ventilatory failure) over a median follow-up of 2.5 years, with the simpler definition having a higher sensitivity (62.9% versus 25.7%) and lower specificity (35.3% versus 80%).[29]

The scoring criteria for discrete sleep-disordered breathing events have also varied over time, with most recent AASM scoring rules for apneas (obstructive, central, and mixed), hypopneas, and respiratory effort-related arousals) outlined in the AASM scoring manual.[10] Pseudocentral apneas are not listed in the AASM scoring manual but these are respiratory pauses, often occurring in phasic REM, that appear central by usual scoring criteria (because of apparent lack of effort, often more pronounced on thoracic than abdominal belt) but are due to respiratory muscle weakness, not decreased central drive.[30] Pseudocentral pauses in REM sleep are commonly seen with neuromuscular disorders and have been called the canary in the coal mine warning sign of future hypoventilation.[31] Difficulty classifying respiratory disturbances as central versus obstructive in neuromuscular disease is well documented and clearly affects prevalence statistics.[30] Other clues (in addition to usual scoring criteria) to distinguish central versus obstructive apneas often need to be used, including (1) the presence of snoring (indicating obstruction); (2) the pattern of breaths between apneas (decrescendo in obstructive apnea and crescendo-decrescendo in central apnea, in particular Cheyne-Stokes respiration); (3) the timing of arousals (with first breath after termination of apnea with obstructive apnea but at maximal ventilation in Cheyne-Stokes respiration); (4) the distribution of apneas (obstructive and pseudocentral apneas worse in REM and central apneas worse in NREM), and (5) intercostal electromyographic activity (if monitored).

Summary metrics for discrete sleep-disordered breathing events include (1) the apnea-hypopnea index (AHI) (apneas plus hypopneas per hour of sleep) for polysomnography, (2) the respiratory event index (apneas plus hypopneas per hour of scorable monitoring time) for home sleep apnea testing, and (3) the respiratory disturbance index (apneas plus hypopneas plus respiratory effort–related arousals per hour of sleep) for polysomnography. The presence of discrete sleep-disordered breathing events with or without symptoms defines clinical syndromes. AASM consensus definitions for clinical syndromes of sleep-disordered breathing have been updated in the third edition of the *International Classification of Sleep Disorders*.[32]

Patterns of Sleep-Disordered Breathing in Neuromuscular and Restrictive Thoracic Disorders

The classic sleep-disordered breathing pattern in restrictive thoracic disorders is hypoventilation, initially most pronounced in REM sleep, but over time, hypoventilation tends to occur throughout sleep, and then finally in wake.[7,12] There are disorders, however, that also present with obstructive or central sleep disordered breathing (**Table 1**). Some examples of disorders that may lead to findings on diagnostic polysomnography other than or in addition to hypoventilation are noted below.

Isolated diaphragmatic paralysis

Diaphragmatic dysfunction may occur as part of underlying progressive neuromuscular disease or

---

Box 3
Current American Academy of Sleep Medicine scoring criteria for sleep-related hypoventilation in adults and children

Adult criteria

- $\geq$10 min of sleep with Pa_{CO_2} (or surrogate) >55 mm Hg OR

- $\geq$10 mm Hg increase in Pa_{CO_2} (or surrogate) during sleep (in comparison to an awake supine value) to a value exceeding 50 mm Hg for $\geq$10 min

Pediatric criteria

- Greater than 25% of the total sleep time as measured by either the arterial P_{CO_2} or surrogate is spent with a Pa_{CO_2} greater than 50 mm Hg

Data from Berry RB, Budhiraja R, Gottlieb, DJ, et al. Rules for scoring respiratory events in sleep: update of the 2007 AASM manual for the scoring of sleep and associated events. Deliberations of the sleep apnea definitions task force of the american academy of sleep medicine. J Clin Sleep Med 2012;8(5):597–619.

Table 1
Patterns of sleep-disordered breathing in neuromuscular and chest wall diseases

	Hypoventilation	Obstructive Apnea	Central Apnea
Isolated diaphragm paralysis	Yes, particularly if bilateral paralysis If unilateral, more pronounced supine and on unaffected side	No	No
Duchenne muscular dystrophy	Yes (late)	Yes (early)	Yes (if cardiomyopathy)
ALS	Yes	Variably reported	Pseudocentral
Spinal cord disease	Variable, depending on level	Yes	Yes

may occur in isolation (eg, due to trauma, infection, or unknown cause as in neuralgic amyotrophy).[33] Bilateral diaphragmatic paralysis may have a significant impact on ventilation (particularly in REM sleep) and result in diurnal respiratory failure whereas unilateral diaphragmatic paralysis may present incidentally.[34] In a case series of 5 patients with unilateral diaphragm paralysis, hypopneas associated with sustained oxygen desaturation were seen in REM sleep, and these were most pronounced when patients were sleeping supine or on the unaffected side.[35] In a more recent retrospective study of 66 patients with isolated unilateral and bilateral diaphragmatic paralysis, elevated AHI in REM was noted but no differences in AHI or nocturnal oxygenation were found between groups.[36] The lack of differences was attributed to patients being referred in for suspected sleep-disordered breathing rather than evaluation of diaphragmatic paralysis. Most patients with diaphragmatic paralysis required bilevel positive airway pressure as opposed to continuous positive airway pressure (CPAP), more so in the bilateral diaphragmatic paralysis group.

Duchenne muscular dystrophy
In Duchenne muscular dystrophy, prevalence rates of sleep apnea vary from 18% to 81% whereas prevalence rates of sustained oxygen desaturation less than 90% in sleep vary from 14% to 62%.[37–40] Sleep-disordered breathing follows a bimodal pattern with obstructive apnea occurring early and hypoventilation occurring later. A bimodal pattern has also been described for acid maltase deficiency.[41] Additionally, muscular dystrophies, myotonic dystrophies, and glycogen storage diseases may be associated with cardiomyopathy, which may increase the risk for central sleep apnea.[42]

Amyotrophic lateral sclerosis
In an early study of sleep-disordered breathing in ALS, sleep hypoventilation consisting of nonobstructive hypopneas in REM sleep was the most common finding (8/18 patients) with no obstructive apneas seen despite bulbar weakness.[43] In a more recent study of 65 patients with ALS who underwent polysomnography, $P_{tc}CO_2$ greater than 50 mm Hg occurred in 60% of patients and sleep hypoventilation as defined by $P_{tc}CO_2$ increase of greater than 10 mm Hg above baseline occurred in 39%[44]; 54% of this cohort had sleep apnea based on AHI of at least 5/h, with most of these respiratory disturbances classified as obstructive. Due to inherent difficulties in classifying respiratory disturbances in neuromuscular disease, pseudocentral apneas may be the most common abnormality in ALS.[42]

Charcot-Marie-Tooth disease
Obstructive sleep apnea was initially reported in a family with Charcot-Marie-Tooth disease (presumably related to pharyngeal neuropathy), and a more recent case-control study found a prevalence of an AHI of at least 5/h in 38% in patients with Charcot-Marie-Tooth disease, significantly higher than controls.[45,46]

Spinal cord disease
Up to 79% of patients with spinal cord injury have sleep-disordered breathing, with more frequent central sleep apnea in cervical spine injury and more frequent obstructive sleep apnea in thoracic spine injury.[3,47] Sleep-onset hypoventilation occurs more frequently in cervical spine injury and may contribute to the development of sleep-disordered breathing.[48]

CLINICAL PRESENTATION OF SLEEP-DISORDERED BREATHING IN NEUROMUSCULAR AND CHEST WALL DISORDERS

The clinical presentation of sleep-disordered breathing in restrictive thoracic disorders is most often nonspecific although individuals with obstructive or central sleep apnea may present with witnessed apnea in addition to disrupted sleep and daytime sleepiness. Symptoms of nocturnal hypoventilation (**Box 4**) may be attributed to the underlying disease and often develop insidiously. Sleep is disrupted by physical discomfort, inability to change position, difficulty handling secretions, or other reasons. Patients may have gasping awakenings from sleep or may have orthopnea even while awake, a symptom that can occur acutely and be particularly severe in acute disorders affecting diaphragm function, such as neuralgic amyotrophy.[49] In addition to postural effects, dyspnea may be increased by immersion in water.[50] Fatigue is often reported. Morning headache may reflect hypercapnia. Sleepiness may occur related to sleep-disordered breathing or may be a primary phenomenon (eg, myotonic dystrophy is associated with central hypersomnia).[51,52] The Epworth Sleepiness Scale score is a validated measure for sleepiness but has not been studied in neuromuscular disease.[53] Other sleep-disordered breathing questionnaires that are useful for obstructive sleep apnea, such as the Berlin Questionnaire and STOP-Bang Questionnaire, have also not been validated for hypoventilation.[54–56] The Sleep-Disordered Breathing in Neuromuscular Disease Questionnaire is a simple 5-question questionnaire with possible scores ranging from 0 to 10 (**Box 5**).[57] In the initial study, a score of 5 or more points had a sensitivity of 86%, specificity of 88%, positive predictive value of 69%, and negative predictive value of 95% to identify neuromuscular disease combined with sleep-disordered breathing.

Signs of respiratory insufficiency include tachypnea, rapid shallow breathing, use of accessory muscles, and paradoxic breathing (particularly when supine).[33,58] Signs of cor pulmonale resulting from hypoventilation may occur late in the disease. Physical examination findings suggesting obstructive sleep apnea may include macroglossia, low or narrow palate, short thick neck with neck circumference > 40 cm (16 in) in women and > 43 cm (17 in) in men, and obesity.[59,60] Signs of left heart failure due to coexistent cardiomyopathy may indicate increased risk for Cheyne-Stokes respiration. Scoliosis may be associated with increased risk for nocturnal hypoventilation.[25]

Other studies that are often readily available may be helpful (see **Box 4**). Baseline awake SpO_2 is often normal in restrictive thoracic disorders but, if low, could indicate increased risk for hypoventilation. In chronic obstructive pulmonary disease, nocturnal oxygen desaturation is much more common in individuals with lower SpO_2 ($\leq$93%) than in those with higher SpO_2 ($\geq$95%), but degree of nocturnal oxygen desaturation is poorly predicted by awake SpO_2.[61,62] Some investigators suggest that in patients with neuromuscular and chest wall disorders, awake SpO_2 of less than 95% should trigger further investigation.[63] Serum bicarbonate (at a threshold value of 27 mEq/L), although nonspecific, has a sensitivity of 92% and specificity of 50% in obesity-hypoventilation syndrome, a syndrome in part defined by daytime hypercapnia.[64] Arterial blood gas is the gold standard to establish the diagnosis of diurnal hypoventilation but is not adequate to screen for sleep-related hypoventilation because sleep-related hypoventilation precedes daytime hypercapnia.[7,8,65] Even a morning arterial blood gas is not adequate to rule out sleep-related hypoventilation.[66] In 1 study, however, daytime $PaCO_2$ greater than 40 mm Hg was predictive of nocturnal hypoventilation in children and adolescents with neuromuscular disorders.[67] In another study, $PaCO_2$ ($\geq$45 mm Hg) and base excess ($\geq$4 mmol/L) were predictive of nocturnal oxygen desaturation.[68] Polycythemia, a late finding, may indicate significant hypoxemia.[67] Electrocardiography and echocardiography may suggest right or left heart disease.

Box 4
Clinical presentation of hypoventilation in neuromuscular and chest wall disorders

Symptoms

- Orthopnea
- Dyspnea bending forward or when immersed in water
- Morning headache
- Poor sleep quality
- Fatigue

Signs

- Tachypnea
- Rapid shallow breathing
- Use of accessory muscles of respiration
- Paradoxic breathing (particularly when supine)
- Cor pulmonale (late)

Laboratory studies

- Reduced awake SpO_2
- Elevated serum bicarbonate
- Polycythemia (late)

Pulmonary function

- Low vital capacity (particularly supine)
- Low negative inspiratory force or sniff nasal inspiratory force

Pulmonary function testing (reviewed in Eric J. Gartman's article, "Pulmonary function Testing in Neuromuscular and Chest Wall Disorders," in this issue) typically demonstrates a restrictive pattern. Decreased muscle strength is often the first indicator of disease and needs to fall significantly before an appreciable fall in vital capacity (which, in turn, precedes the fall in total lung capacity).[69] Upright vital capacity is often easily measured and helpful. A supine fall in vital capacity by greater than or equal to 25% is more sensitive and specific for diaphragmatic weakness in neuromuscular disorders.[70] Tests of respiratory muscle strength may be difficult for patients with bulbar weakness to perform and sniff nasal inspiratory pressure may have better prognostic value in these patients.[71–73] In general, as lung function declines with progressive disorders, there is increased risk of progression of sleep-disordered breathing from REM hypopneas to REM hypoventilation, to continuous sleep-related hypoventilation, to diurnal hypoventilation. Vital capacity and maximal inspiratory muscle pressure have been shown to predict sleep-disordered breathing onset, continuous hypoventilation, and diurnal respiratory failure in primary myopathies at thresholds of less than 60% and less than 4.5 kPa, less than 40% and less than 4.0 kPa, and less than 25% and less than 3.5 kPa, respectively.[7,67] In children with progressive neuromuscular disease, vital capacity less than 70%, and forced expiratory volume in 1 second less than 65% were shown to predict nocturnal hypoventilation.[25] Other studies have failed to show a correlation between daytime pulmonary function and sleep-disordered breathing or nocturnal oxygen desaturation.[30] The 1999 NAMDRC National Consensus Conference (convened and organized by the NAMDRC with representation from multiple other respiratory, sleep, and medical organizations [Box 6]) developed guidelines for the initiation of NPPV in progressive neuromuscular disease (Box 6) which ultimately informed Centers for Medicare and Medicaid coverage decisions, (Box 7). These guidelines include maximal inspiratory pressure less than 60 cm H_2O and forced vital capacity less than 50% among the physiologic criteria to initiate NPPV.[74] Other guidelines suggest similar, but slightly different criteria (see Box 6).[74]

DIAGNOSIS OF SLEEP-DISORDERED BREATHING IN NEUROMUSCULAR AND CHEST WALL DISORDERS

Diagnostic studies to evaluate sleep-disordered breathing include nocturnal SpO_2 monitoring, nocturnal capnometry ($P_{ET}CO_2$ or $P_{tc}CO_2$), respiratory polygraphy, and polysomnography. Each has advantages and limitations (Table 2).

Continuous nocturnal pulse oximetry monitoring is often readily available and can detect nocturnal oxygen desaturation. Although the mechanism underlying desaturation cannot be determined by oximetry, nocturnal desaturation in chronic respiratory disease is usually due to sleep hypoventilation.[75] The 1999 NAMDRC National Consensus Conference guidelines include oxygen saturation less than or equal to 88% for 5 continuous minutes as one of the physiologic criteria to initiate NPPV in restrictive thoracic disorders.[74] British Thoracic Society guidelines for respiratory management of children with neuromuscular weakness suggest that technically adequate SpO_2 greater than or equal to 93% is considered sufficient to exclude clinically significant hypoventilation in asymptomatic children with neuromuscular disease but abnormal results should be followed-up with more detailed studies.[76] Clear-cut thresholds of nocturnal oxygen desaturation indicating hypoventilation have not been established. Additionally, the absence of nocturnal desaturation does not necessarily exclude hypoventilation, particularly in patients who have well-preserved awake baseline oxygen saturation and are still on the upper flat portion of the sigmoidal oxyhemoglobin dissociation curve, those who have reduced or absent REM sleep, or those who are on supplemental oxygen.[66] Finally, although nocturnal oximetry with an adequate averaging rate of 3 seconds can detect transient desaturations suggesting sleep apnea, oximetry is neither sensitive nor specific for sleep apnea, cannot distinguish central versus

---

Box 5
Questions included in the Sleep-Disordered Breathing in Neuromuscular Disease Questionnaire

Do you feel breathless if you lie down (eg, on your bed)?

Do you feel breathless if you bend forward (eg, to tie your shoelaces)?

Do you feel breathless if you swim in water or lay in a bath?

Have you changed your position in bed?

Have you noticed a change in your sleep (waking more, getting up, poor quality sleep)?

From Steier J, Jolley CJ, Seymour J, et al. Screening for sleep-disordered breathing in neuromuscular disease using a questionnaire for symptoms associated with diaphragm paralysis. Eur Respir J 2011;37(2):401; with permission.

Box 6
Guidelines for initiation of noninvasive positive-pressure ventilation in neuromuscular and chest wall disorders

NAMDRC National consensus conference,[a] 1999,[74] restrictive thoracic disorders
- Symptoms of hypoventilation (fatigue, dyspnea, and morning headache) AND
- One of
  - $Paco_2 \geq 45$ mm Hg
  - Nocturnal oximetry with $Spo_2 \leq 88\%$ for 5 consecutive minutes
  - For NMD only: MIP less than 60 cm H_2O or FVC less than 50%

American Thoracic Society, 2004,[82] DMD
- Sleep-related upper airway obstruction OR
- Chronic respiratory insufficiency

American Academy of Neurology, 2009,[95] ALS
- One of
  - Orthopnea
  - SNP less than 40 cm H_2O or MIP less than 60 cm H_2O
  - Abnormal nocturnal oximetry
  - FVC less than 50%

International Standard of Care Committee for Congenital Muscular Dystrophy, 2010,[108] MD
- Symptomatic daytime hypercapnia
- Symptomatic nocturnal hypoventilation
- Nonsymptomatic nocturnal hypercapnia and hypopneas
- Failure to thrive
- Recurrent chest infections (>3/y)
- Fatigue
- Respiratory muscle weakness as documented by pulmonary function tests

German Society for Pneumology, 2010,[114] neuromuscular diseases
- Clinical signs of chronic respiratory failure and at least one of
  - Chronic daytime hypercapnia $Paco_2 \geq 45$ mm Hg
  - Nocturnal hypercapnia with rise in $P_{tc}co_2$ of ≥ 10 mm Hg during the night
  - Rapid significant reduction in vital capacity

Canadian Thoracic Society, 2011,[96] ALS
- Any one of
  - Orthopnea
  - Daytime hypercapnia
  - Symptomatic sleep-disordered breathing
  - FVC less than 50%
  - SNP less than 40 cm H_2O or MIP less than 40 cm H_2O

Canadian Thoracic Society, 2011,[96] kyphoscoliosis
- Chronic hypercapnic respiratory failure

Canadian Thoracic Society, 2011,[96] DMD
- Diurnal hypercapnia ($Paco_2$ >45 mm Hg) OR
- Nocturnal hypercapnia and symptoms consistent with hypoventilation

Canadian Thoracic Society, 2011,[96] MD
- Daytime hypercapnia OR
- Symptomatic nocturnal hypoventilation

Canadian Thoracic Society, 2011,[96] postpolio syndrome
- Chronic hypoventilation

British Thoracic Society, 2012,[76] children with neuromuscular weakness
- Symptomatic nocturnal hypoventilation OR
- Daytime hypercapnia

European Federation of Neurological Societies, 2012,[97] ALS
- Symptoms/signs related to respiratory muscle weakness. At least one of
  - Dyspnea
  - Tachypnea
  - Orthopnea
  - Disturbed sleep due to nocturnal desaturation/arousals
  - Morning headache
  - Use of accessory muscles at rest
  - Paradoxic respiration
  - Daytime fatigue
  - Excessive daytime sleepiness (ESS >9)
- Abnormal respiratory function tests. At least one of
  - FVC <80%
  - SNP<40 cm H_2O
  - MIP <60 cm H_2O
  - Significant nocturnal desaturation on overnight oximetry
  - Morning blood gas $Paco_2$ >45 mm Hg

Abbreviations: DMD, Duchenne muscular dystrophy; ESS, Epworth Sleepiness Scale; Fio_2, fraction of inspired oxygen; FVC, forced vital capacity; MD, myotonic dystrophy; MIP, maximal inspiratory pressure; NMD, neuromuscular disease; SNP, sniff nasal pressure.

[a] Note: The NAMDRC National Consensus Conference (1999) was convened and organized by the National Association for the Medical Direction of Respiratory Care (NAMDRC) and included representatives from American Academy of Home Care Physicians, American Association for Respiratory Care, American College of Chest Physicians, American College of Physicians, American Sleep Disorders Association, American Thoracic Society, Mayo Clinic, and National Association for Medical Direction of Respiratory Care.

Reproduced with permission of the © ERS 2018: European Respiratory Journal 2011;37(2):400–5; DOI: 10.1183/09031936.00036210.

obstructive apnea, and is not a recommended test for the diagnosis of sleep apnea.

Methods for continuous noninvasive monitoring of carbon dioxide include $P_{ET}co_2$ and $P_{tc}co_2$. $P_{ET}co_2$ measures breath-to-breath changes in exhaled carbon dioxide whereas $P_{tc}co_2$ assesses arterialized capillary CO_2. Comparable results have been found during sleep testing in children.[77] Conflicting validation data have been reported in adults, although recent advances in technology have been associated with increased reliability of $P_{tc}co_2$.[78–80] Although both $P_{ET}co_2$ and $P_{tc}co_2$ have limitations (see **Table 1**), those associated

with $P_{ET}co_2$ are more likely to be seen in a sleep laboratory setting, particularly in adults. Because pediatric obstructive sleep apnea in children may present with sustained hypoventilation, assessment of CO_2 with either $P_{ET}co_2$ or $P_{tc}co_2$ is recommended during routine pediatric polysomnography. The $P_{ET}co_2$ waveform can demonstrate adult OSA, but this is not a current recommended airflow sensor for this indication. The AASM clinical practice guideline for NPPV titration in hypoventilation syndromes suggests that CO_2 monitoring with either $P_{ET}co_2$ or $P_{tc}co_2$ may be useful.[81]

Box 7
Centers for Medicare and Medicaid Services coverage criteria for respiratory assist devices in restrictive thoracic disorders (Local Coverage Determination 33800, effective 10/1/15)

- Progressive neuromuscular disease or severe thoracic cage abnormality AND
- Chronic obstructive pulmonary disease does not contribute significantly AND
- One of
  ○ $Paco_2$ ≥45 mm Hg while awake and on prescribed Fio_2
  ○ Nocturnal oximetry with Spo_2 ≤88% for ≥5 min on prescribed Fio_2 (minimum recording time 2 h)
  ○ For neuromuscular disease only: maximal inspiratory pressure less than 60 cm H_2O
  ○ For neuromuscular disease only: forced vital capacity less than 50%

Abbreviation: Fio_2, fraction of inspired oxygen.

Respiratory polygraphy (cardiorespiratory study) incorporates a variable number of sensors depending on the institution and age of the patient. In pediatric studies, measurement channels typically include airflow, respiratory effort, oxygen saturation, carbon dioxide monitoring, heart rate, and sometimes a position sensor but no sleep monitoring. Limited channel monitoring (home sleep apnea testing) incorporates measures of airflow, respiratory effort, oxygen saturation, heart rate, and often position and snoring but does not include sleep or carbon dioxide monitoring. These studies can detect both oxygen desaturation and discrete respiratory disturbances. Respiratory polygraphy is included in multiple guidelines as an option for periodic monitoring in children with neuromuscular disease.[76,82,83] Limited channel monitoring performs well in establishing the diagnosis of obstructive sleep apnea in adult patients with a high index of suspicion for moderate-severe obstructive sleep apnea but is well known to result in an underestimation of sleep apnea compared with polysomnography.[84] It is not a recommended test in adults with neuromuscular disease or known or suspected hypoventilation.[85]

Diagnostic polysomnography is the gold standard test to detect sleep-disordered breathing and remains the recommended test in children with suspicion for any sleep-disordered breathing and in adults with suspected complicated sleep-disordered breathing.[85–88] Additional sensors can be added, such as capnometry (to assess hypoventilation) and intercostal electromyography (to assess work of breathing).[81] Even in the absence of daytime hypercapnia, nocturnal hypercapnia may predict the subsequent need for NPPV.[29,65] Discrete respiratory disturbances can be better characterized as central, obstructive, or pseudocentral.[31] Sleep architecture and nonrespiratory sleep disorders can be evaluated. Characteristic polysomnographic findings in restrictive thoracic disorders include sleep disruption and fragmented, reduced, or absent REM sleep, which generally improve with NPPV.[44] Some restrictive thoracic disorders, such as myotonic dystrophy, may be associated with periodic limb movements or primary hypersomnia, which requires laboratory testing for diagnosis.[51,52,89] Polysomnography, however, is costly and labor intensive and may be difficult for patients with limited mobility. Although sleep testing is required for the diagnosis of sleep apnea, current practice guidelines and third-party payers do not require formal sleep testing for the initiation of NPPV for hypoventilation in restrictive thoracic disorders (see **Box 6**).

TREATMENT OF SLEEP-DISORDERED BREATHING IN NEUROMUSCULAR AND CHEST WALL DISORDERS

CPAP is the treatment of choice for significant obstructive sleep apnea whereas bilevel modes of positive airway pressure therapy incorporating a backup rate or adaptive servo-ventilation are generally required for central sleep apnea.[90–92] Neither CPAP nor adaptive servo-ventilation is adequate for hypoventilation due to neuromuscular or chest wall disease. NPPV (reviewed in Dean R. Hess' article, "Noninvasive Ventilation for Neuromuscular Disease," in this issue) is the treatment of choice for sleep-disordered breathing in neuromuscular disease as it has been shown to improve important outcomes including mortality, rate of lung function decline, quality of life, daytime gas exchange, and symptoms, as well as chest wall deformity in children.[76,93–97] Additionally, NPPV has also been shown to improve sleep-related hypoventilation and sleep quality, effects that are maintained over time.[44,98] By consensus, the timing of NPPV initiation is determined by symptoms, lung function, and ventilation (see **Box 6**). Increased mortality was seen in an early study of Duchenne muscular dystrophy with early initiation of NPPV, but this may have been related to increased left ventricular hypokinesia in the control group.[99] There has been clear improvement in survival since NPPV became standard practice for this disorder.[100,101] Early initiation of NPPV in ALS is associated with improved survival.[102] The first randomized,

Table 2
Diagnostic studies to evaluate sleep-disordered breathing

	Advantages	Limitations
Nocturnal oximetry	• Readily available • Inexpensive • Can be performed at home • Can detect significant oxygen desaturation • Pattern of desaturation may suggest hypoventilation or sleep apnea	• Not sensitive or specific for either hypoventilation or sleep apnea • Cannot determine mechanism for desaturation • Accuracy falls at low Sp_{O_2} levels • Cannot rule out sleep-disordered breathing
End-tidal carbon dioxide monitoring	• Often available • Can detect hypoventilation	• May be inaccurate with mouth breathing, pulmonary disorders characterized by significant ventilation-perfusion mismatch, high respiratory rates, moisture in tubing, or use of supplemental oxygen • May be poorly tolerated in younger children • Less expensive than $P_{tc}CO_2$ • Cannot rule out sleep-disordered breathing
Transcutaneous carbon dioxide monitoring	• Can detect hypoventilation • May be more accurate than $P_{ET}CO_2$ in many common situations	• May be inaccurate with hypoperfusion, skin disease, edema, or hypovolemia • More expensive than $P_{ET}CO_2$ • Cannot rule out sleep-disordered breathing
Nocturnal respiratory polygraphy	• Can detect uncomplicated sleep apnea and may discriminate between obstructive and central events • Can detect significant oxygen desaturation • Can detect hypoventilation (if $P_{tc}CO_2$ or $P_{ET}CO_2$ monitored) • Less expensive than polysmnography	• Underestimates sleep apnea compared with polysomnography • Cannot rule out sleep-disordered breathing
Nocturnal diagnostic polysomnography (with $P_{tc}CO_2$ or $P_{ET}CO_2$ monitoring)	• Can detect hypoventilation • Can detect sleep apnea and better discriminate between different types of respiratory disturbances (obstructive, central, and pseudocentral) • Can detect other sleep disorders • Can rule out sleep-disordered breathing assuming REM sleep adequately sampled	• Expensive • Labor intensive • May be difficult for patients

placebo-controlled trial (using sham NPPV vs active NPPV) of very early NPPV initiation in ALS with preserved pulmonary function (ie, before usual criteria met, patients excluded if forced vital capacity <50% predicted) showed a slower rate of change in forced vital capacity.[103] There are no randomized controlled trials of outcomes when NPPV is initiated early based solely on sleep-related hypoventilation. In patients with restrictive thoracic disorders with nocturnal hypercapnia and daytime normocapnia who otherwise fulfill usual criteria to initiate NIV, however, the presence of nocturnal hypoventilation seems to predict the subsequent need for NPPV.[29,65]

NPPV is often initiated at empiric settings without sleep study guidance but there is a potential role for therapeutic polysomnography. Many patients treated with NPPV, although improved, have residual hypercapnia.[5] In a retrospective study of 179 patients with ALS, those who were inadequately ventilated or who had residual upper airway respiratory disturbances had worse survival.[104] Additionally, patient-ventilator asynchrony is common with NPPV, which, in turn, may affect overall effectiveness and adherence.[105,106] Respiratory disturbances seen during NPPV may result from the patient, the ventilator, or patient-ventilator interaction; an identification and scoring system for these events has been proposed.[107]

In-laboratory titration of NPPV settings (with CO_2 monitoring) can theoretically result in more effective control of discrete sleep-disordered breathing events as well as sleep-related hypoventilation and allows for the systematic detection (and correction if possible) of asynchrony. The 2010 AASM best clinical practices guideline for NPPV in stable chronic alveolar hypoventilation syndromes recommends therapeutic polysomnography both for titration of optimal noninvasive ventilation settings and for minimizing patient-ventilator asynchrony.[81] Suggested titration guidelines and targets are provided but technologists and clinicians are advised to use clinical judgment in applying the recommendations. Data are lacking to show that long-term outcomes are improved in restrictive thoracic disorders when therapeutic polysomnography is used. Most current practice guidelines (other than AASM and pediatric guidelines) and third-party payers do not recommend or mandate therapeutic polysomnography for the titration of NPPV. A prospective observational study in ALS, however, showed that intensive NPPV titration (including baseline polysomnography, acclimation to NPPV during naps, 3 therapeutic polysomnographies, support, and trouble-shooting over a 5-day hospitalization) resulted in significant improvement in ventilation, sleep quality, and quality of life at 1 month, with excellent adherence. The additional effect of intensive education and support on outcomes has not been specifically studied.

The 2010 AASM best clinical practices guideline for NPPV in stable chronic alveolar hypoventilation syndromes recommends close follow-up after initiation of NPPV to establish effective utilization patterns (ideally using objective data), to remediate problems, including NPPV side effects and interface issues, and to ensure that the equipment is maintained.[81] Additionally, it is recommended that respiratory function be assessed with measures of oxygenation and ventilation on a regular basis or if signs of clinical deterioration are present.[81]

Follow-up of patients treated with NPPV is generally clinical with assessment of symptoms, pulmonary function, and daytime and nocturnal ventilation. Follow-up sleep studies are recommended in pediatric guidelines. Although polysomnography is often preferred, polygraphy, nocturnal capnometry, or nocturnal oximetry may be substituted depending on availability.[76,82,108] Systematic review of data downloaded from NPPV devices may also be helpful to assess efficacy (eg, exhaled tidal volume, respiratory rate, frequency/tidal volume ratio, and minute ventilation), adherence, leak, and potential asynchrony.[109–111] Validity of device software-derived leak and tidal volume measurements were shown to vary with the specific device in a bench study.[112] AHI seems accurately detected by device software, assuming low leak and low asynchrony index.[113] An algorithm for patient follow-up incorporating noninvasive assessments, device software data, and therapeutic polysomnography has been proposed.[111]

SUMMARY

Sleep-disordered breathing is common in neuromuscular and chest wall diseases and results from both the effects of normal sleep on ventilation and the superimposed challenges imposed by the underlying disorder. Patterns of sleep-disordered breathing vary with the specific diagnosis and stage of disease. Treatment with NPPV is associated with improved outcomes. Polysomnography has a role in both the diagnosis of sleep-disordered breathing and in the titration of NPPV. Long-term follow-up, including review of data downloaded from NPPV devices, is recommended.

REFERENCES

1. Benditt JO, Boitano LJ. Pulmonary issues in patients with chronic neuromuscular disease. Am J Respir Crit Care Med 2013;187(10):1046–55.
2. Wolfe LF, Patwari PP, Mutlu G. Sleep hypoventilation in neuromuscular and chest wall disorders. Sleep Med Clin 2014;9(3):409–23.
3. Sankari A, Bascom A, Oomman S, et al. Sleep disordered breathing in chronic spinal cord injury. J Clin Sleep Med 2014;10(1):65–72.
4. Labanowski M, Schmidt-Nowara W, Guilleminault C. Sleep and neuromuscular disease: frequency of sleep-disordered breathing in a neuromuscular

disease clinic population. Neurology 1996;47(5): 1173–80.

5. Bauman KA, Kurili A, Schmidt SL, et al. Home-based overnight transcutaneous capnography/pulse oximetry for diagnosing nocturnal hypoventilation associated with neuromuscular disorders. Arch Phys Med Rehabil 2013;94(1):46–52.

6. Ogna A, Quera Salva MA, Prigent H, et al. Nocturnal hypoventilation in neuromuscular disease: prevalence according to different definitions issued from the literature. Sleep Breath 2016; 20(2):575–81.

7. Ragette R, Mellies U, Schwake C, et al. Patterns and predictors of sleep disordered breathing in primary myopathies. Thorax 2002;57(8):724–8.

8. Hillman D, Singh B, McArdle N, et al. Relationships between ventilatory impairment, sleep hypoventilation and type 2 respiratory failure. Respirology 2014;19(8):1106–16.

9. Carskadon MA, Dement WC. Normal human sleep: an overview. In: Kryger M, Roth T, Dement WC, editors. Principles and practice of sleep medicine. 6th edition. Philadelphia: Elsevier; 2017. p. 15–24.

10. Budhiraja R, Gottlieb DJ, et al. Rules for scoring respiratory events in sleep: update of the 2007 AASM manual for the scoring of sleep and associated events. Deliberations of the sleep apnea definitions task force of the american academy of sleep medicine. J Clin Sleep Med 2012;8(5): 597–619.

11. Fink BR. Influence of cerebral activity in wakefulness on regulation of breathing. J Appl Physiol 1961;16:15–20.

12. Sowho M, Amatoury J, Kirkness JP, et al. Sleep and respiratory physiology in adults. Clin Chest Med 2014;35(3):469–81.

13. Berthon-Jones M, Sullivan CE. Ventilatory and arousal responses to hypoxia in sleeping humans. Am Rev Respir Dis 1982;125(6):632–9.

14. White DP, Douglas NJ, Pickett CK, et al. Hypoxic ventilatory response during sleep in normal premenopausal women. Am Rev Respir Dis 1982; 126(3):530–3.

15. Douglas NJ, White DP, Weil JV, et al. Hypoxic ventilatory response decreases during sleep in normal men. Am Rev Respir Dis 1982;125(3):286–9.

16. Douglas NJ, White DP, Weil JV, et al. Hypercapnic ventilatory response in sleeping adults. Am Rev Respir Dis 1982;126(5):758–62.

17. Tusiewicz K, Moldofsky H, Bryan AC, et al. Mechanics of the rib cage and diaphragm during sleep. J Appl Physiol Respir Environ Exerc Physiol 1977;43(4):600–2.

18. Tabachnik E, Muller NL, Bryan AC, et al. Changes in ventilation and chest wall mechanics during sleep in normal adolescents. J Appl Physiol Respir Environ Exerc Physiol 1981;51(3):557–64.

19. Hudgel DW, Martin RJ, Johnson B, et al. Mechanics of the respiratory system and breathing pattern during sleep in normal humans. J Appl Physiol Respir Environ Exerc Physiol 1984;56(1):133–7.

20. Tangel DJ, Mezzanotte WS, White DP. Influence of sleep on tensor palatini EMG and upper airway resistance in normal men. J Appl Physiol (1985) 1991;70(6):2574–81.

21. White DP, Weil JV, Zwillich CW. Metabolic rate and breathing during sleep. J Appl Physiol (1985) 1985;59(2):384–91.

22. Robin ED, Whaley RD, Crump CH, et al. Alveolar gas tensions, pulmonary ventilation and blood pH during physiologic sleep in normal subjects. J Clin Invest 1958;37(7):981–9.

23. Gould GA, Gugger M, Molloy J, et al. Breathing pattern and eye movement density during REM sleep in humans. Am Rev Respir Dis 1988;138(4):874–7.

24. Douglas NJ, White DP, Pickett CK, et al. Respiration during sleep in normal man. Thorax 1982; 37(11):840–4.

25. Katz SL, Gaboury I, Keilty K, et al. Nocturnal hypoventilation: predictors and outcomes in childhood progressive neuromuscular disease. Arch Dis Child 2010;95(12):998–1003.

26. Lemay J, Series F, Senechal M, et al. Unusual respiratory manifestations in two young adults with Duchenne muscular dystrophy. Can Respir J 2012;19(1):37–40.

27. Carroll JE, Zwillich CW, Weil JV. Ventilatory response in myotonic dystrophy. Neurology 1977; 27(12):1125–8.

28. Simonds AK. Chronic hypoventilation and its management. Eur Respir Rev 2013;22(129):325–32.

29. Orlikowski D, Prigent H, Quera Salva MA, et al. Prognostic value of nocturnal hypoventilation in neuromuscular patients. Neuromuscul Disord 2017;27(4):326–30.

30. Smith PE, Calverley PM, Edwards RH. Hypoxemia during sleep in Duchenne muscular dystrophy. Am Rev Respir Dis 1988;137(4):884–8.

31. Aboussouan LS. Sleep-disordered breathing in neuromuscular disease. Am J Respir Crit Care Med 2015;191(9):979–89.

32. American Academy of Sleep Medicine. International classification of sleep disorders. 3rd edition. Darien (IL): American Academy of Sleep Medicine; 2014.

33. McCool FD, Tzelepis GE. Dysfunction of the diaphragm. N Engl J Med 2012;366(10):932–42.

34. Stradling JR, Kozar LF, Dark J, et al. Effect of acute diaphragm paralysis on ventilation in awake and sleeping dogs. Am Rev Respir Dis 1987;136(3): 633–7.

35. Baltzan MA, Scott AS, Wolkove N. Unilateral hemidiaphragm weakness is associated with positional hypoxemia in REM sleep. J Clin Sleep Med 2012; 8(1):51–8.

36. Khan A, Morgenthaler TI, Ramar K. Sleep disordered breathing in isolated unilateral and bilateral diaphragmatic dysfunction. J Clin Sleep Med 2014;10(5):509–15.

37. Khan Y, Heckmatt JZ. Obstructive apnoeas in Duchenne muscular dystrophy. Thorax 1994; 49(2):157–61.

38. Kirk VG, Flemons WW, Adams C, et al. Sleep-disordered breathing in Duchenne muscular dystrophy: a preliminary study of the role of portable monitoring. Pediatr Pulmonol 2000;29(2):135–40.

39. Suresh S, Wales P, Dakin C, et al. Sleep-related breathing disorder in Duchenne muscular dystrophy: disease spectrum in the paediatric population. J Paediatr Child Health 2005;41(9–10):500–3.

40. Nozoe KT, Moreira GA, Tolino JR, et al. The sleep characteristics in symptomatic patients with Duchenne muscular dystrophy. Sleep Breath 2015;19(3):1051–6.

41. Kansagra S, Austin S, DeArmey S, et al. Polysomnographic findings in infantile Pompe disease. Am J Med Genet A 2013;161A(12):3196–200.

42. Aboussouan LS, Mireles-Cabodevila E. Sleep-disordered breathing in neuromuscular disease: diagnostic and therapeutic challenges. Chest 2017;152(4):880–92.

43. Ferguson KA, Strong MJ, Ahmad D, et al. Sleep-disordered breathing in amyotrophic lateral sclerosis. Chest 1996;110(3):664–9.

44. Boentert M, Brenscheidt I, Glatz C, et al. Effects of non-invasive ventilation on objective sleep and nocturnal respiration in patients with amyotrophic lateral sclerosis. J Neurol 2015;262(9):2073–82.

45. Dematteis M, Pepin JL, Jeanmart M, et al. Charcot-Marie-Tooth disease and sleep apnoea syndrome: a family study. Lancet 2001;357(9252): 267–72.

46. Boentert M, Knop K, Schuhmacher C, et al. Sleep disorders in Charcot-Marie-Tooth disease type 1. J Neurol Neurosurg Psychiatry 2014;85(3):319–25.

47. Sankari A, Martin JL, Bascom AT, et al. Identification and treatment of sleep-disordered breathing in chronic spinal cord injury. Spinal Cord 2015; 53(2):145–9.

48. Bascom AT, Sankari A, Goshgarian HG, et al. Sleep onset hypoventilation in chronic spinal cord injury. Physiol Rep 2015;3(8) [pii:e12490].

49. Kumar A, Mireles-Cabodevila E, Mehta AC, et al. Sudden onset of dyspnea preceded by shoulder and arm pain. Ann Am Thorac Soc 2016;13(12): 2261–5.

50. Schoenhofer B, Koehler D, Polkey MI. Influence of immersion in water on muscle function and breathing pattern in patients with severe diaphragm weakness. Chest 2004;125(6):2069–74.

51. Gilmartin JJ, Cooper BG, Griffiths CJ, et al. Breathing during sleep in patients with myotonic

52. Udd B, Krahe R. The myotonic dystrophies: molecular, clinical, and therapeutic challenges. Lancet Neurol 2012;11(10):891–905.

53. Johns MW. A new method for measuring daytime sleepiness: the Epworth sleepiness scale. Sleep 1991;14(6):540–5.

54. Netzer NC, Stoohs RA, Netzer CM, et al. Using the Berlin Questionnaire to identify patients at risk for the sleep apnea syndrome. Ann Intern Med 1999; 131(7):485–91.

55. Chung F, Yegneswaran B, Liao P, et al. STOP questionnaire: a tool to screen patients for obstructive sleep apnea. Anesthesiology 2008;108(5):812–21.

56. Prasad KT, Sehgal IS, Agarwal R, et al. Assessing the likelihood of obstructive sleep apnea: a comparison of nine screening questionnaires. Sleep Breath 2017;21(4):909–17.

57. Steier J, Jolley CJ, Seymour J, et al. Screening for sleep-disordered breathing in neuromuscular disease using a questionnaire for symptoms associated with diaphragm paralysis. Eur Respir J 2011;37(2):400–5.

58. Gibson GJ. Diaphragmatic paresis: pathophysiology, clinical features, and investigation. Thorax 1989;44(11):960–70.

59. Davies RJ, Stradling JR. The relationship between neck circumference, radiographic pharyngeal anatomy, and the obstructive sleep apnoea syndrome. Eur Respir J 1990;3(5):509–14.

60. Katz I, Stradling J, Slutsky AS, et al. Do patients with obstructive sleep-apnea have thick necks. Am Rev Respir Dis 1990;141(5):1228–31.

61. Little SA, Elkholy MM, Chalmers GW, et al. Predictors of nocturnal oxygen desaturation in patients with COPD. Respir Med 1999;93(3):202–7.

62. Mohsenin V, Guffanti EE, Hilbert J, et al. Daytime oxygen saturation does not predict nocturnal oxygen desaturation in patients with chronic obstructive pulmonary disease. Arch Phys Med Rehabil 1994;75(3):285–9.

63. Piper AJ, Gonzales-Bermejo J, Janssens J. Sleep hypoventilation: diagnostic considerations and technological limitations. Sleep Med Clin 2014;9: 301–13.

64. Mokhlesi B, Tulaimat A, Faibussowitsch I, et al. Obesity hypoventilation syndrome: prevalence and predictors in patients with obstructive sleep apnea. Sleep Breath 2007;11(2):117–24.

65. Ward S, Chatwin M, Heather S, et al. Randomised controlled trial of non-invasive ventilation (NIV) for nocturnal hypoventilation in neuromuscular and chest wall disease patients with daytime normocapnia. Thorax 2005;60(12):1019–24.

66. Paiva R, Krivec U, Aubertin G, et al. Carbon dioxide monitoring during long-term noninvasive

respiratory support in children. Intensive Care Med 2009;35(6):1068–74.

67. Mellies U, Ragette R, Schwake C, et al. Daytime predictors of sleep disordered breathing in children and adolescents with neuromuscular disorders. Neuromuscul Disord 2003;13(2):123–8.

68. Hukins CA, Hillman DR. Daytime predictors of sleep hypoventilation in Duchenne muscular dystrophy. Am J Respir Crit Care Med 2000; 161(1):166–70.

69. Braun NM, Arora NS, Rochester DF. Respiratory muscle and pulmonary function in polymyositis and other proximal myopathies. Thorax 1983; 38(8):616–23.

70. Fromageot C, Lofaso F, Annane D, et al. Supine fall in lung volumes in the assessment of diaphragmatic weakness in neuromuscular disorders. Arch Phys Med Rehabil 2001;82(1):123–8.

71. Heritier F, Rahm F, Pasche P, et al. Sniff nasal inspiratory pressure. A noninvasive assessment of inspiratory muscle strength. Am J Respir Crit Care Med 1994;150(6 Pt 1):1678–83.

72. Morgan RK, McNally S, Alexander M, et al. Use of Sniff nasal-inspiratory force to predict survival in amyotrophic lateral sclerosis. Am J Respir Crit Care Med 2005;171(3):269–74.

73. Lyall RA, Donaldson N, Polkey MI, et al. Respiratory muscle strength and ventilatory failure in amyotrophic lateral sclerosis. Brain 2001;124(Pt 10):2000–13.

74. Clinical indications for noninvasive positive pressure ventilation in chronic respiratory failure due to restrictive lung disease, COPD, and nocturnal hypoventilation—a consensus conference report. Chest 1999;116(2):521–34.

75. Becker HF, Piper AJ, Flynn WE, et al. Breathing during sleep in patients with nocturnal desaturation. Am J Respir Crit Care Med 1999;159(1): 112–8.

76. Hull J, Aniapravan R, Chan E, et al. British Thoracic Society guideline for respiratory management of children with neuromuscular weakness. Thorax 2012;67(Suppl 1):i1–40.

77. Kirk VG, Batuyong ED, Bohn SG. Transcutaneous carbon dioxide monitoring and capnography during pediatric polysomnography. Sleep 2006; 29(12):1601–8.

78. Sanders MH, Kern NB, Costantino JP, et al. Accuracy of end-tidal and transcutaneous PCO2 monitoring during sleep. Chest 1994;106(2):472–83.

79. Storre JH, Steurer B, Kabitz HJ, et al. Transcutaneous PCO2 monitoring during initiation of noninvasive ventilation. Chest 2007;132(6):1810–6.

80. Storre JH, Magnet FS, Dreher M, et al. Transcutaneous monitoring as a replacement for arterial PCO(2) monitoring during nocturnal non-invasive ventilation. Respir Med 2011;105(1):143–50.

81. Berry RB, Chediak A, Brown LK, et al. Best clinical practices for the sleep center adjustment of noninvasive positive pressure ventilation (NPPV) in stable chronic alveolar hypoventilation syndromes. J Clin Sleep Med 2010;6(5):491–509.

82. Finder JD, Birnkrant D, Carl J, et al. Respiratory care of the patient with Duchenne muscular dystrophy: ATS consensus statement. Am J Respir Crit Care Med 2004;170(4):456–65.

83. Wang CH, Finkel RS, Bertini ES, et al. Consensus statement for standard of care in spinal muscular atrophy. J Child Neurol 2007;22(8): 1027–49.

84. Bianchi MT, Goparaju B. Potential underestimation of sleep apnea severity by at-home kits: rescoring in-laboratory polysomnography without sleep staging. J Clin Sleep Med 2017;13(4):551–5.

85. Kapur VK, Auckley DH, Chowdhuri S, et al. Clinical practice guideline for diagnostic testing for adult obstructive sleep apnea: an American academy of sleep medicine clinical practice guideline. J Clin Sleep Med 2017;13(3):479–504.

86. Wise MS, Nichols CD, Grigg-Damberger MM, et al. Executive summary of respiratory indications for polysomnography in children: an evidence-based review. Sleep 2011;34(3):389–398AW.

87. Aurora RN, Zak RS, Karippot A, et al. Practice parameters for the respiratory indications for polysomnography in children. Sleep 2011;34(3): 379–88.

88. Kushida CA, Littner MR, Morgenthaler T, et al. Practice parameters for the indications for polysomnography and related procedures: an update for 2005. Sleep 2005;28(4):499–521.

89. Quera Salva MA, Blumen M, Jacquette A, et al. Sleep disorders in childhood-onset myotonic dystrophy type 1. Neuromuscul Disord 2006; 16(9–10):564–70.

90. Epstein LJ, Kristo D, Strollo PJ Jr, et al. Clinical guideline for the evaluation, management and long-term care of obstructive sleep apnea in adults. J Clin Sleep Med 2009;5(3):263–76.

91. Aurora RN, Chowdhuri S, Ramar K, et al. The treatment of central sleep apnea syndromes in adults: practice parameters with an evidence-based literature review and meta-analyses. Sleep 2012;35(1): 17–40.

92. Aurora RN, Bista SR, Casey KR, et al. Updated adaptive servo-ventilation recommendations for the 2012 AASM guideline: "the treatment of central sleep apnea syndromes in adults: practice parameters with an evidence-based literature review and meta-analyses". J Clin Sleep Med 2016; 12(5):757–61.

93. Bourke SC, Tomlinson M, Williams TL, et al. Effects of non-invasive ventilation on survival and quality of life in patients with amyotrophic lateral sclerosis: a

randomised controlled trial. Lancet Neurol 2006; 5(2):140–7.

94. Berlowitz DJ, Howard ME, Fiore JF Jr, et al. Identifying who will benefit from non-invasive ventilation in amyotrophic lateral sclerosis/motor neurone disease in a clinical cohort. J Neurol Neurosurg Psychiatry 2016;87(3):280–6.

95. Miller RG, Jackson CE, Kasarskis EJ, et al. Practice parameter update: the care of the patient with amyotrophic lateral sclerosis: drug, nutritional, and respiratory therapies (an evidence-based review): report of the Quality Standards Subcommittee of the American Academy of Neurology. Neurology 2009;73(15):1218–26.

96. McKim DA, Road J, Avendano M, et al. Home mechanical ventilation: a Canadian Thoracic Society clinical practice guideline. Can Respir J 2011; 18(4):197–215.

97. EFNS Task Force on Diagnosis and Management of Amyotrophic Lateral Sclerosis, Andersen PM, Abrahams S, Borasio GD, et al. EFNS guidelines on the clinical management of amyotrophic lateral sclerosis (MALS)–revised report of an EFNS task force. Eur J Neurol 2012;19(3):360–75.

98. Vrijsen B, Buyse B, Belge C, et al. Noninvasive ventilation improves sleep in amyotrophic lateral sclerosis: a prospective polysomnographic study. J Clin Sleep Med 2015;11(5):559–66.

99. Raphael JC, Chevret S, Chastang C, et al. Randomised trial of preventive nasal ventilation in Duchenne muscular dystrophy. French Multicentre Cooperative Group on Home Mechanical Ventilation Assistance in Duchenne de Boulogne Muscular Dystrophy. Lancet 1994;343(8913): 1600–4.

100. Simonds AK, Muntoni F, Heather S, et al. Impact of nasal ventilation on survival in hypercapnic Duchenne muscular dystrophy. Thorax 1998; 53(11):949–52.

101. Eagle M, Baudouin SV, Chandler C, et al. Survival in Duchenne muscular dystrophy: improvements in life expectancy since 1967 and the impact of home nocturnal ventilation. Neuromuscul Disord 2002;12(10):926–9.

102. Lechtzin N, Scott Y, Busse AM, et al. Early use of non-invasive ventilation prolongs survival in subjects with ALS. Amyotroph Lateral Scler 2007; 8(3):185–8.

103. Jacobs TL, Brown DL, Baek J, et al. Trial of early noninvasive ventilation for ALS: a pilot placebo-controlled study. Neurology 2016;87(18):1878–83.

104. Georges M, Attali V, Golmard JL, et al. Reduced survival in patients with ALS with upper airway obstructive events on non-invasive ventilation. J Neurol Neurosurg Psychiatry 2016;87(10): 1045–50.

105. Atkeson AD, RoyChoudhury A, Harrington-Moroney G, et al. Patient-ventilator asynchrony with nocturnal noninvasive ventilation in ALS. Neurology 2011;77(6):549–55.

106. Carlucci A, Pisani L, Ceriana P, et al. Patient-ventilator asynchronies: may the respiratory mechanics play a role? Crit Care 2013;17(2):R54.

107. Gonzalez-Bermejo J, Perrin C, Janssens JP, et al. Proposal for a systematic analysis of polygraphy or polysomnography for identifying and scoring abnormal events occurring during non-invasive ventilation. Thorax 2012;67(6):546–52.

108. Wang CH, Bonnemann CG, Rutkowski A, et al. Consensus statement on standard of care for congenital muscular dystrophies. J Child Neurol 2010;25(12):1559–81.

109. Nicholson TT, Smith SB, Siddique T, et al. Respiratory pattern and tidal volumes differ for pressure support and volume-assured pressure support in amyotrophic lateral sclerosis. Ann Am Thorac Soc 2017;14(7):1139–46.

110. Pasquina P, Adler D, Farr P, et al. What does built-in software of home ventilators tell us? An observational study of 150 patients on home ventilation. Respiration 2012;83(4):293–9.

111. Janssens JP, Borel JC, Pepin JL, et al. Nocturnal monitoring of home non-invasive ventilation: the contribution of simple tools such as pulse oximetry, capnography, built-in ventilator software and autonomic markers of sleep fragmentation. Thorax 2011;66(5):438–45.

112. Contal O, Vignaux L, Combescure C, et al. Monitoring of noninvasive ventilation by built-in software of home bilevel ventilators: a bench study. Chest 2012;141(2):469–76.

113. Georges M, Adler D, Contal O, et al. Reliability of apnea-hypopnea index measured by a home bilevel pressure support ventilator versus a polysomnographic assessment. Respir Care 2015;60(7): 1051–6.

114. Windisch W, Walterspacher S, Siemon K, et al. Guidelines for non-invasive and invasive mechanical ventilation for treatment of chronic respiratory failure. Published by the German Society for Pneumology (DGP). Pneumologie 2010;64(10): 640–52.

Pulmonary Function Testing in Neuromuscular and Chest Wall Disorders

Eric J. Gartman, MD*

KEYWORDS

- Pulmonary function testing • Neuromuscular disease • Chest wall disorders

KEY POINTS

- Patients with neuromuscular and chest wall disorders may have no respiratory symptoms and limited signs of skeletal muscle weakness, but can have significant respiratory muscle weakness.
- A single testing modality may fail to elucidate true respiratory compromise, and often a combination of tests is recommended to fully evaluate these patients.
- Common tests performed on this population include measurement of flow rates, lung volumes, maximal pressures, and airway resistance.
- Most tests needed to evaluate these patients are available through a standard pulmonary function laboratory, but occasionally referral to a specialty laboratory may be required.

Neuromuscular diseases (NMDs) and chest wall disorders have a wide range of effects on the respiratory system, and unfortunately these lead to significant disability and/or progressive respiratory failure in many patients. Respiratory disorders can develop as a consequence of the multitude of functional limitations that may arise in these varied conditions, and are implicated as a leading cause of mortality for many patients.[1,2] Alterations in respiratory system physiology can arise from a combination of effects on the brain, spinal cord, peripheral nervous system, neuromuscular junction, skeleton, and musculature. Further, each disease may have a unique pattern of effect on the respiratory system, and may progress differently over time.

Given the consequential respiratory system morbidity in these conditions, it is imperative to have a thorough understanding of the physiologic effects of each disease (discussed in detail in other articles). In turn, one then may have a better understanding of how to investigate and interpret the battery of physiologic tests that have been developed. It is important to recognize that given the diversity of dysfunction that may arise from these disorders, the same test or parameter that is helpful in 1 condition may not prove as useful in another. Further, patients often may not present with typical respiratory symptoms and may need to have significant functional impairment or weakness before standard pulmonary function tests demonstrate clear abnormalities.[3–6]

This article focuses on the various testing modalities that have been studied in the evaluation of these patients (**Table 1**), with the goal of understanding that it is often a pattern of findings, not just the extent of dysfunction, that is the key to assessing and following these patients over time.[7] Although some effects on the respiratory system are more obvious (eg, muscle weakness,

Disclosure Statement: The author has no relationship with a commercial company that has a direct financial interest in subject matter or materials discussed in article or with a company making a competing product.
Department of Medicine, Division of Pulmonary, Critical Care, and Sleep Medicine, Warren Alpert Medical School of Brown University, Providence, RI, USA
* Providence VA Medical Center, 830 Chalkstone Avenue, Providence, RI 02908.
E-mail address: eric_gartman@brown.edu

Clin Chest Med 39 (2018) 325–334
https://doi.org/10.1016/j.ccm.2018.01.005
0272-5231/18/Published by Elsevier Inc.

Table 1
Pulmonary function tests performed in neuromuscular and chest wall disorders

Commonly Available	Availability Usually Limited to More Advanced Laboratories or Research Centers
Spirometry	Sniff nasal pressures
Lung volumes	Invasive catheter
Static mouth pressures (MIP/MEP)	measurement of pressures
Maximal voluntary ventilation (MVV)	Phrenic nerve stimulation (eg, magnetic)
Positional Testing (eg, supine)	Impulse oscillometry
Flow-volume loops	
Bronchoprovocation testing (eg, methacholine)	

decreased flows), others may secondarily arise and may lead to the deleterious outcomes that are observed (eg, poor cough, swallowing and upper airway dysfunction, skeletal and chest wall abnormalities, and sleep-disordered breathing).[8–11] There are no set guidelines to dictate the frequency of testing, and generally this is determined by the rapidity of clinical progression.[12]

SPIROMETRY

The most commonly utilized testing modality, likely because of its ubiquitous availability, is spirometry, with the hallmark parameter being the vital capacity (VC) (and less so the maximal voluntary ventilation [MVV]). The performance of spirometry is standardized and meant to follow outlined quality controls, which enables it to serve as a reliable and repeatable measurement.[13] However, it is important to recognize that patients with neuromuscular diseases may not be able to perform the maneuvers as intended, and adaptation of the standards or accommodation may be necessary.[14,15]

The value of spirometry when used alone to test for impairment has long been debated, because it has been shown that significant muscle weakness may be present even though the vital capacity is normal.[16,17] However, it also has been recognized that patients may have little clinically perceived respiratory dysfunction, but when formally assessed they are clearly impaired. In 2 studies of patients with motor neuron disease (mostly ALS) totaling 254 participants, significant declines in lung function were evident even though they expressed few or no symptoms (sometimes as low as 50% of predicted).[4,5]

Spirometry's most consistent role is in the longitudinal assessment of patients and in determining prognosis. In multiple neuromuscular conditions, it has been shown to be a predictor of disease disability scores, disease-related complications, need for assisted ventilation, and survival time.[4,5,18–20] Further, improvements in spirometric parameters have been used as evidence of treatment response in Parkinson's disease and myasthenia gravis.[21–23]

In patients with cervical spinal cord injury, it has been recognized that bronchial hyperresponsiveness can develop, likely because of loss of sympathetic innervation.[24–27] This can be investigated using a broncho-provocation challenge, most commonly conducted by having the patient inhale increasing doses of methacholine and repeating spirometry following each dose. A positive test is achieved by observing more than a 20% decline in the baseline forced expiratory volume in 1 second (FEV1).

Supine Positioning

One valuable maneuver in the evaluation of certain neuromuscular disorders is comparing the vital capacities between seated and supine positioning. With significant diaphragm weakness or paralysis, the vital capacity will be observed to fall in the supine position, and the extent of the decline will depend on both the severity of weakness and whether one or both diaphragms are affected. In unilateral disease, the vital capacity can decline 15% to 25% (with right-sided issues being more significant because of the weight of liver) and can fall 40% or more in bilateral disease.[28–30]

It should be recognized, however, that certain conditions lead to an increase in vital capacity in the supine position, often leading to confusion clinically. Conditions that leave the diaphragm neurologically intact but the chest wall and abdominal muscles impaired can lead to such a scenario (eg, high spinal cord injuries and large ventral hernias with loss of functional abdominal musculature). The decrease in vital capacity in the upright position results from increased abdominal compliance leading to diaphragmatic dysfunction caused by effects on the length-tension properties of the diaphragm and on the normal chest wall configuration afforded by the abdominal muscles' actions on the rib cage. This has led to the suggestion that reducing the abdominal compliance by binding the abdominal wall can improve upright inspiratory function in such patients.[11,31–38]

Use in the Inpatient Setting

In general, pulmonary function testing is best performed in the outpatient setting in patients not undergoing current exacerbation of their disease or affected by infection. However, serial measurements of spirometry and surrogates of respiratory muscle strength may be of benefit in predicting which patients may require higher levels of respiratory support during an acute worsening of a neuromuscular disease. The majority of data relating to this topic is in patients with Guillain-Barre Syndrome (GBS) and myasthenia gravis (MG), and it has yielded conflicting results. The value of measuring vital capacity (and other bedside tests of respiratory muscle strength) for predicting impending respiratory failure has been shown best in GBS. Parameters that have been shown to be associated with progression to respiratory failure include VC less than 20 cc/kg, VC less than 60% predicted, reduction in VC greater than 30%, maximal inspiratory pressure greater than −30 cmH2O, and maximal expiratory pressure less than 40 cm H_2O.[39,40] In contrast, in patients with MG, some authors have described similar predictive value in these parameters, while others have found them less useful.[41,42]

It is important to recognize that the results of bedside respiratory testing should be incorporated into a composite clinical picture, and not be viewed in isolation. For example, it has been shown that in addition to progressive reductions in vital capacity and maximal mouth pressures, other clinical features have been shown to be predictive of impending respiratory failure in GBS (eg, onset to admission < 7 days, inability to cough, inability to lift elbows or head, liver enzyme elevations, bulbar dysfunction, bilateral facial weakness, and dysautonomia).[39,40]

FLOW-VOLUME LOOPS

The flow-volume loop (FVL) generally is obtained during standard spirometry, and should conform to American Thoracic Society (ATS)/European Respiratory Society (ERS) guidelines.[13] The FVL represents a full inspiratory and expiratory effort in a single maneuver, and is generated by having the patient take a rapid full inhalation to total lung capacity and perform a maximal expiratory maneuver (without hesitation) to residual volume, followed by a rapid maximal inspiration (Fig. 1A). Given the nature of this maneuver, it is obvious that those affected by NMDs may have characteristic abnormalities that can be recognized and useful clinically.

An early report describing the relationship between FVL changes and respiratory muscle weakness was published in the late 1970s. Kreitzer and colleagues[6] showed in ALS patients that those with reduced respiratory muscle strength (decreased maximal pressures, decreased VC, and decreased maximal flows) had a drop-off in expiratory flow as they approached RV (concavity in the curve toward the volume axis). Further research into the utility of the FVL in recognizing respiratory dysfunction emerged in the mid-1980s in Parkinson's disease patients.[43,44] Vincken and colleagues[43] performed pulmonary function testing on 27 patients with Parkinson's disease and found that 24 of them had abnormal FVL contours, characterized by either regular or irregular oscillations in flow that were directly visualized to be resulting from rhythmic or irregular involuntary movements of glottic and supraglottic structures. Further, they described 2 patterns of FVLs – types A and B – with type A representing consecutive flow decelerations and accelerations, and type B showing more of a rounded shape with a shift in peak expiratory flow to lower lung volumes, an abrupt drop in flow approaching residual volume, and a truncated peak inspiratory flow (Fig. 1B, C). In a similar manner, Schiffman reported such a sawtooth pattern in a patient with Parkinson's disease, which likely represented the type A pattern described by Vincken.[44]

In order to investigate this described upper airway obstruction further in Parkinson's disease patients, Bogaard and colleagues[45] studied the effect of stage of disease on the maximal FVL and static mouth pressures. In their 31 subjects, they confirmed a significant number of abnormal FVLs (4 type A, 18 type B, remainder normal), that a combination of upper airway obstruction and impaired respiratory muscle force were responsible for these curves, and that the proportion of normal FVLs decreased with increasing disease severity. The frequency of FVL abnormalities, of both types, was confirmed in another study by Izquierdo-Alonso and colleagues,[46] who found that approximately 50% of Parkinson's disease patients (all severity levels) had evidence of an abnormal FVL (21 type A, 9 type B).

Vincken and colleagues[47] expanded the examination of the FVL in other NMDs to assess for upper airway muscle involvement in 2 further studies. First, in 30 patients with various NMDs (10 with apparent bulbar involvement, 20 without), they assessed the value of the FVL in defining bulbar and upper airway muscle involvement. They found abnormal FVLs (flow oscillations, flow plateaus) significantly more often in patients with clinically apparent bulbar involvement (90% vs 15%), and all the patients who

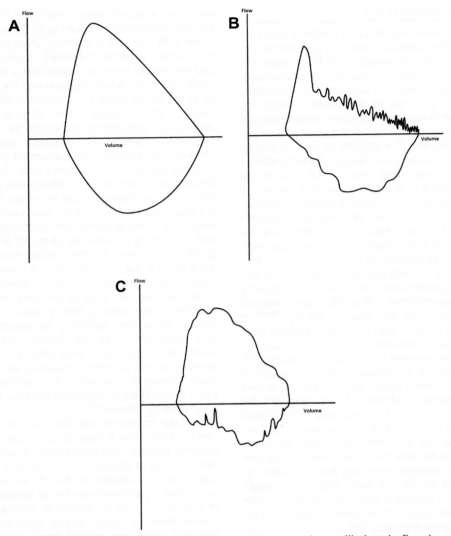

Fig. 1. (A) normal flow-volume loop; (B) flow-volume loop demonstrating oscillations in flow in a Parkinson's disease patient, similar to type A[43]; (C) flow-volume loop demonstrating sudden changes in flow with occasional near-complete cutoffs in flow as seen in multiple NMDs with significant respiratory muscle weakness, similar to type B.[43]

subsequently developed severe respiratory complications had had abnormal FVL contours. Subsequently, this same group investigated 20 patients with various NMDs in 2 groups, those with and without reduced maximal inspiratory and expiratory pressures (ie, respiratory muscle weakness). They found that those with evidence of weakness had significantly more abnormal pulmonary function and that 4 parameters on the FVL correlated with reduced maximal pressures. These parameters were low peak expiratory flow, reduced slope of the ascending limb of the expiratory curve, a dropoff in expiratory flow near residual volume, and low inspiratory flow at 50% of vital capacity. A score was developed (number of parameters) and found to be significantly higher in those with signs of weakness; additionally, it was found that a score of 2 or more had 80% specificity and 90% sensitivity in predicting muscle weakness.[48]

In MG patients, in addition to the well-known diaphragmatic and chest wall muscle weakness issues, it has been demonstrated that the effects on the bulbar and upper airway muscles lead to upper airway obstruction. Putman and Wise showed that over half of their patients who had performed FVLs showed evidence of airway obstruction.[49]

LUNG VOLUMES

No matter the method used for determining lung volumes, the measurement of functional residual capacity (FRC) serves as the basis for calculating the other volumes. FRC represents the lung volume at which the forces of lung elastic recoil and outward chest wall expansion are balanced, and then other values obtained during spirometry are added or subtracted to calculate the full spectrum of lung volumes (**Fig. 2**).[50] As such, both the resting lung volume (FRC) and lung volumes dependent on an intact neuromuscular system can be characteristically affected in patients with NMDs. In general, FRC declines with progressive disease and is mostly due to an increase in chest wall stiffness, although in some conditions a reduction in lung compliance has been described (attributed to either microatelectasis and/or alteration in alveolar elastic properties).[8,11,51–54]

As a result of these physiologic changes, the usual pattern of lung volumes in this population is one of restriction. The resting lung volume (FRC) is generally low, and in NMDs, mostly as a result of respiratory muscle weakness, the calculated volumes are low (eg, TLC will be low because of a low inspiratory capacity). However, it should be noted that residual volume (RV) has been shown to increase in some progressive NMD because of expiratory muscle weakness. In fact, this change in RV has been shown to be an early sign of muscular weakness in several conditions.[1,4,6,55]

TESTS OF RESPIRATORY MUSCLE STRENGTH

Tests of respiratory muscle strength are an extremely important component in the pulmonary function evaluation, given that progressive failure of the respiratory pump will culminate in the negative clinical outcomes that are seen. As noted previously, significant weakness can exist without an evident decline in spirometry, so formal evaluation of strength is required.[16,17] Various tests have been developed to assess respiratory muscle strength, ranging from easily accessed and noninvasive to relatively invasive and limited in availability to special centers or research settings.

Static Maximal Mouth Pressures

Maximal inspiratory and expiratory pressures (MIPs, MEPs) are the most commonly performed tests of respiratory muscle strength. It is important to understand the method by which they are performed, since there exists variability in the literature (and in pulmonary function laboratories). MIPs initiated from lower lung volumes will be higher given the added outward chest wall recoil force and better length-tension relationship of the inspiratory muscles at low lung volumes. MEPs will be higher if performed from higher lung volumes given the addition of significant inward lung and chest wall recoil, as well as better length-tension relationship of expiratory muscles at higher lung volumes. However, despite recommendations that MIP be performed from RV and MEP be performed from TLC, there remains significant variation in starting volumes (mostly from FRC).[3,56] In addition, because of this variation (and the nature of the test itself), there is a wide range of reported normalcy that can lead to uncertainty in its interpretation.[57–59]

Despite these recognized limitations, there can be great value in performing these tests. In patients with stable disease, it has been recognized that significant reductions in MIP and MEP can exist without a correlation to the degree of generalized muscle weakness, arguing for the incorporation of this testing into the neurologic

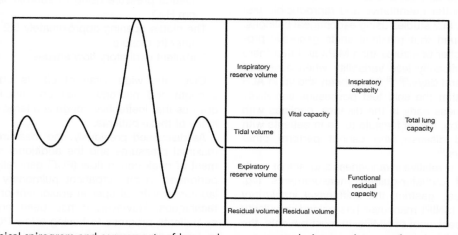

Fig. 2. Typical spirogram and components of lung volumes measure during a pulmonary function test.

examination.[7] Further, a proximal distribution of muscle weakness in myopathic patients portended a greater risk of respiratory muscle weakness, and the demonstration of reduced maximal static efforts was associated with poorer pulmonary function, higher RV, retention of carbon dioxide, and a greater likelihood of respiratory infections and failure.[7,55] In amyotrophic lateral sclerosis (ALS) patients, Schiffman and Belsh similarly affirmed that there can be significant respiratory muscle weakness in the absence of symptoms, documented the rate of decline in MIP/MEP, and suggested that these measures could be used to guide prognosis.[5] The pattern of MIP and MEP can also be useful, especially in conditions affecting the diaphragm, where a significant reduction in MIP and relative preservation of MEP would be expected. The ratio of MIP:MEP has been found to provide an alternative to supine testing in patients unable to tolerate such positioning.[60]

It is worth noting, however, that it has been recognized that maximal mouth pressures may be low in the absence of true respiratory muscle weakness, and if there is clinical need to confirm weakness, additional testing modalities may be needed.[61–64]

Maximal Sniff Pressures

Given issues in the performance of maximal static mouth pressures, especially as patients develop severe weakness (air leak, submaximal efforts), other techniques have been developed to assess respiratory muscle strength. The maximal sniff is performed from FRC and a variety of pressures can be measured depending on the equipment used (eg, transdiaphragmatic [Pdi], esophageal [Pes], or nasal [Pn]).[56] The sniff maneuver comes naturally to all people and thus has been found to be a better quantitative and reproducible test than MIP. In 2 studies using esophageal balloons, it was found that maximal sniffs generally produced higher pressures than MIPs and that there was significantly less variability when assessed over several days.[65,66] It has been shown in ALS patients that the sniff test possesses sensitivity for weakness early in the disease, declines with progression, and is feasible to do in patients with advanced disease who cannot perform other maneuvers.[67]

Given the relative invasiveness and lack of availability of catheter-guided measurements (eg, esophageal, gastric), the sniff nasal inspiratory pressure (SNIP) maneuver has gained popularity in the assessment of NMDs. In most patients, the SNIP is reflective of esophageal pressure and a good marker of inspiratory muscle strength.[64,68] Caution is recommended, however, in patients with obstructive lung diseases (eg, chronic obstructive pulmonary disease [COPD], cystic fibrosis), since the SNIP can underestimate muscle strength significantly.[69,70]

The SNIP is performed by inserting a nostril plug with a pressure-sensing probe, and the subject sniffs maximally from FRC. The contralateral nostril usually remains open during the maneuver, although it has been argued recently that higher pressures are measured with it closed and should be the preferred method.[71] There can be a learning effect for this maneuver, with the highest pressures being obtained on sniffs 11 through 20.[72]

Nonvolitional Maneuvers

In certain patients, maximal volitional maneuvers may be unobtainable or unreliable, and phrenic nerve stimulators are employed. The most common method used currently is magnetic stimulation because of its reproducibility, relative technical ease, and patient tolerance compared with electrical stimulation.[73] Following stimulation, similar to the volitional tests, a variety of pressures can be measured depending on the testing modalities being employed.

ASSESSMENT OF COUGH

The orchestrated maneuver of coughing has several components that act in sequence to produce the end result of airway and secretion clearance. Following the nervous system's reception of a cough trigger, a cough then is produced by:

Inhaling to a volume above FRC
The glottis closing
The expiratory muscles contracting and intrapleural pressure rising to approximately 100 cm H_2O
The glottis opening approximately 0.2 seconds after its closure
Turbulent expiratory flow ensues[74]

Given the wide array of effects on muscle strength and neuromuscular coordination, it is obvious that ineffective cough is a large issue for many of these patients.

As discussed previously, the measurement of maximal pressures and the additional measurement of peak cough flow (PCF) generally can be performed in an outpatient pulmonary function laboratory without special equipment or invasive techniques. However, it has been noted that as patients progress to having a low PCF, there is less agreement between a spirometer and pneumotachometer, and caution is needed as to not overestimate PCF using a spirometer in such patients.[75]

The first factor that is recognized to limit cough flow and effectiveness is reduced maximal inspiratory volumes, due to the combination of decreased inspiratory muscle strength and decreased chest wall (and lung) compliance, as discussed previously. It has been shown that NMD patients with ineffective cough can have an approximately 50% reduction in their FVC compared with subjects with an effective cough, and that augmentation of inspiration (ie, increase inspiration capacity and vital capacity) leads to an improvement in PCF.[76–78]

The generation of expiratory muscle force is a problem that progressively worsens in many patients and has been associated with declining PCF. The easiest and most widely available modality is measurement of MEP. Not surprisingly, a decreased MEP is associated with poor cough and inability to generate effective flows.[79] However, given some of the issues with measurement of MEP in this population and the possibility that gastric pressures may be more reflective of true cough strength, invasive catheter testing has been advocated.[62,80] Polkey and colleagues[81] showed that in ALS patients, expiratory muscle weakness was associated with ineffective cough and that cough flow spikes were absent when cough gastric pressures (Pga) were less than 50 cm H_2O. Aiello and colleagues[82] showed that reduced cough Pga (and other pressure measurements) were related to increased disability scores in MS patients. Further, it has been shown that as patients lose the ability to generate cough, there is an association with increased mortality in motor neuron disease.[83]

FORCED OSCILLATION TECHNIQUE (IMPULSE OSCILLOMETRY)

Impulse oscillometry (IOS) is a testing technique that superimposes small pressure changes on the normal tidal breathing to measure respiratory impedance over a spectrum of frequencies. From this measure, it is possible to assess the relative contributions of respiratory system elastance and inertance, as well as respiratory resistance. Further, by examining the frequency-dependence of these parameters patterns of disease may be inferred. Importantly, this testing is performed at normal operating lung volumes and does not require volitional efforts above regular breathing, so it is well-suited for patients who have difficulty following directions and/or performing spirometry or other maximal maneuvers. For this reason,

IOS may be useful in detecting progressive abnormalities associated with changes in physiology over time in patients otherwise unable to perform reliable ongoing respiratory testing.

IOS' ability to detect such changes has been examined experimentally, showing that strapping of the respiratory system of normal subjects resulted in a change in respiratory impedance reflecting the alteration in chest wall mechanics.[84] Similarly, it has been shown that in patients with more severe restriction caused by chest wall disorders, there are elevations in respiratory resistance (with modest frequency dependence) and more prominent negative total respiratory system reactance (with resonant frequency occurring at much higher frequencies).[85] Wesseling and colleagues[86] used this technique in 27 patients with NMDs to assess its ability to discern airflow obstruction, and found that although resistance values were somewhat higher than normal, the resistance pattern and overall impedance characteristics were similar to normal, concluding that this was a useful modality in these patients. IOS has also been used in spinal cord injury patients to assess for changes in airway physiology resulting from the administration of cholinergic agents. Radulovic and colleagues[87] showed that following the administration of neostigmine there was a significant rise in respiratory resistance, and this effect was nullified by coadministration of glycopyrrolate. Although IOS is an attractive measurement option in patients who cannot perform more standard maneuvers, the technology is not available in most pulmonary function laboratories.

SUMMARY

Respiratory complications are extremely common in patients with neuromuscular and chest wall disorders; formal functional testing is required, since patients may be asymptomatic despite having significant impairment. In general, a battery of tests is preferred – especially when ruling out impairment – because significant respiratory system dysfunction can be present despite normal values on limited testing. Following diagnosis, serial testing can provide important guidance regarding effectiveness of therapy, trajectory of progressive impairment, risk of complications, and concern for impending respiratory failure. Most of the tests described can be obtained through a standard pulmonary function laboratory; if more advanced or invasive techniques are required, referral to a specialized center is warranted.

ACKNOWLEDGMENTS

The author would like to thank Henry Del Rosario, MD, and Steven Shurtleff for their assistance with figure illustration. The contents do not represent the views of the U.S. Department of Veterans Affairs or the United States Government.

REFERENCES

1. Perrin C, Unterborn JN, Ambrosio CD, et al. Pulmonary complications of chronic neuromuscular diseases and their management. Muscle Nerve 2004; 29(1):5–27.

2. Miller RG, Rosenberg JA, Gelinas DF, et al. Practice parameter: the care of the patient with amyotrophic lateral sclerosis (an evidence-based review). Muscle Nerve 1999;22(8):1104–18.

3. American Thoracic Society/European Respiratory Society. ATS/ERS statement on respiratory muscle testing. Am J Respir Crit Care Med 2002;166(4):518–624.

4. Fallat RJ, Jewitt B, Bass M, et al. Spirometry in amyotrophic lateral sclerosis. Arch Neurol 1979; 36(2):74–80.

5. Schiffman PL, Belsh JM. Pulmonary function at diagnosis of amyotrophic lateral sclerosis. Rate of deterioration. Chest 1993;103(2):508–13.

6. Kreitzer SM, Saunders NA, Tyler HR, et al. Respiratory muscle function in amyotrophic lateral sclerosis. Am Rev Respir Dis 1978;117(3):437–47.

7. Vincken W, Elleker MG, Cosio MG. Determinants of respiratory muscle weakness in stable chronic neuromuscular disorders. Am J Med 1987;82(1):53–8.

8. Smith PE, Calverley PM, Edwards RH, et al. Practical problems in the respiratory care of patients with muscular dystrophy. N Engl J Med 1987;316(19): 1197–205.

9. Benditt JO, Boitano LJ. Pulmonary issues in patients with chronic neuromuscular disease. Am J Respir Crit Care Med 2013;187(10):1046–55.

10. Rochester DF, Esau SA. Assessment of ventilatory function in patients with neuromuscular disease. Clin Chest Med 1994;15(4):751–63.

11. Estenne M, De Troyer A. The effects of tetraplegia on chest wall statics. Am Rev Respir Dis 1986;134(1): 121–4.

12. Hill NS. Ventilator management for neuromuscular disease. Semin Respir Crit Care Med 2002;23(3): 293–305.

13. Miller MR, Hankinson J, Brusasco V, et al. Standardisation of spirometry. Eur Respir J 2005;26(2): 319–38.

14. Hardiman O. Management of respiratory symptoms in ALS. J Neurol 2011;258(3):359–65.

15. Kelley A, Garshick E, Gross ER, et al. Spirometry testing standards in spinal cord injury. Chest 2003; 123(3):725–30.

16. Smeltzer SC, Skurnick JH, Troiano R, et al. Respiratory function in multiple sclerosis. Utility of clinical assessment of respiratory muscle function. Chest 1992;101(2):479–84.

17. Black LF, Hyatt RE. Maximal static respiratory pressures in generalized neuromuscular disease. Am Rev Respir Dis 1971;103(5):641–50.

18. Phillips MF, Quinlivan RC, Edwards RH, et al. Changes in spirometry over time as a prognostic marker in patients with Duchenne muscular dystrophy. Am J Respir Crit Care Med 2001;164(12): 2191–4.

19. Wang Y, Shao WB, Gao L, et al. Abnormal pulmonary function and respiratory muscle strength findings in Chinese patients with Parkinson's disease and multiple system atrophy–comparison with normal elderly. PLoS One 2014;9(12):e116123.

20. Polatli M, Akyol A, Cildag O, et al. Pulmonary function tests in Parkinson's disease. Eur J Neurol 2001;8(4):341–5.

21. Nakano KK, Bass H, Tyler HR. Levodopa in Parkinson's disease: effect on pulmonary function. Arch Intern Med 1972;130(3):346–8.

22. Radwan L, Strugalska M, Koziorowski A. Changes in respiratory muscle function after neostigmine injection in patients with myasthenia gravis. Eur Respir J 1988;1(2):119–21.

23. Chiu HC, Yeh JH, Chen WH. Pulmonary function study of myasthenia-gravis patients treated with double-filtration plasmapheresis. J Clin Apher 2003;18(3):125–8.

24. Dicpinigaitis PV, Spungen AM, Bauman WA, et al. Bronchial hyperresponsiveness after cervical spinal cord injury. Chest 1994;105(4):1073–6.

25. Singas E, Lesser M, Spungen AM, et al. Airway hyperresponsiveness to methacholine in subjects with spinal cord injury. Chest 1996;110(4):911–5.

26. Grimm DR, Arias E, Lesser M, et al. Airway hyperresponsiveness to ultrasonically nebulized distilled water in subjects with tetraplegia. J Appl Physiol (1985) 1999;86(4):1165–9.

27. Mateus SR, Beraldo PS, Horan TA. Cholinergic bronchomotor tone and airway caliber in tetraplegic patients. Spinal Cord 2006;44(5):269–74.

28. Mier-Jedrzejowicz A, Brophy C, Moxham J, et al. Assessment of diaphragm weakness. Am Rev Respir Dis 1988;137(4):877–83.

29. Celli BR. Respiratory management of diaphragm paralysis. Semin Respir Crit Care Med 2002;23(3):275–81.

30. Fromageot C, Lofaso F, Annane D, et al. Supine fall in lung volumes in the assessment of diaphragmatic weakness in neuromuscular disorders. Arch Phys Med Rehabil 2001;82(1):123–8.

31. Koo P, Gartman EJ, Sethi JM, et al. Physiology in medicine: physiological basis of diaphragmatic dysfunction with abdominal hernias-implications for therapy. J Appl Physiol (1985) 2015;118(2):142–7.

32. Baydur A, Adkins RH, Milic-Emili J. Lung mechanics in individuals with spinal cord injury: effects of injury level and posture. J Appl Physiol (1985) 2001;90(2): 405–11.

33. Schilero GJ, Spungen AM, Bauman WA, et al. Pulmonary function and spinal cord injury. Respir Physiol Neurobiol 2009;166(3):129–41.

34. Mier A, Brophy C, Estenne M, et al. Action of abdominal muscles on rib cage in humans. J Appl Physiol (1985) 1985;58(5):1438–43.

35. Celli BR, Rassulo J, Berman JS, et al. Respiratory consequences of abdominal hernia in a patient with severe chronic obstructive pulmonary disease. Am Rev Respir Dis 1985;131(1):178–80.

36. Goldman M. Mechanical interaction between diaphragm and rib cage. Boston view. Am Rev Respir Dis 1979;119(2 Pt 2):23–6.

37. Crompton CH, MacLusky IB, Geary DF. Respiratory function in the prune-belly syndrome. Arch Dis Child 1993;68(4):505–6.

38. McCool FD, Pichurko BM, Slutsky AS, et al. Changes in lung volume and rib cage configuration with abdominal binding in quadriplegia. J Appl Physiol (1985) 1986;60(4):1198–202.

39. Lawn ND, Fletcher DD, Henderson RD, et al. Anticipating mechanical ventilation in Guillain-Barre syndrome. Arch Neurol 2001;58(6):893–8.

40. Sharshar T, Chevret S, Bourdain F, et al. Early predictors of mechanical ventilation in Guillain-Barre syndrome. Crit Care Med 2003;31(1): 278–83.

41. Thieben MJ, Blacker DJ, Liu PY, et al. Pulmonary function tests and blood gases in worsening myasthenia gravis. Muscle Nerve 2005;32(5):664–7.

42. Rieder P, Louis M, Jolliet P, et al. The repeated measurement of vital capacity is a poor predictor of the need for mechanical ventilation in myasthenia gravis. Intensive Care Med 1995;21(8):663–8.

43. Vincken WG, Gauthier SG, Dollfuss RE, et al. Involvement of upper-airway muscles in extrapyramidal disorders. A cause of airflow limitation. N Engl J Med 1984;311(7):438–42.

44. Schiffman PL. A "saw-tooth" pattern in Parkinson's disease. Chest 1985;87(1):124–6.

45. Bogaard JM, Hovestadt A, Meerwaldt J, et al. Maximal expiratory and inspiratory flow-volume curves in Parkinson's disease. Am Rev Respir Dis 1989;139(3):610–4.

46. Izquierdo-Alonso JL, Jimenez-Jimenez FJ, Cabrera-Valdivia F, et al. Airway dysfunction in patients with Parkinson's disease. Lung 1994;172(1):47–55.

47. Vincken W, Elleker G, Cosio MG. Detection of upper airway muscle involvement in neuromuscular disorders using the flow-volume loop. Chest 1986;90(1): 52–7.

48. Vincken WG, Elleker MG, Cosio MG. Flow-volume loop changes reflecting respiratory muscle weakness in chronic neuromuscular disorders. Am J Med 1987;83(4):673–80.

49. Putman MT, Wise RA. Myasthenia gravis and upper airway obstruction. Chest 1996;109(2):400–4.

50. Wanger J, Clausen JL, Coates A, et al. Standardisation of the measurement of lung volumes. Eur Respir J 2005;26(3):511–22.

51. Gibson GJ, Pride NB, Davis JN, et al. Pulmonary mechanics in patients with respiratory muscle weakness. Am Rev Respir Dis 1977;115(3):389–95.

52. De Troyer A, Borenstein S, Cordier R. Analysis of lung volume restriction in patients with respiratory muscle weakness. Thorax 1980;35(8):603–10.

53. Estenne M, Heilporn A, Delhez L, et al. Chest wall stiffness in patients with chronic respiratory muscle weakness. Am Rev Respir Dis 1983;128(6):1002–7.

54. Papastamelos C, Panitch HB, Allen JL. Chest wall compliance in infants and children with neuromuscular disease. Am J Respir Crit Care Med 1996; 154(4 Pt 1):1045–8.

55. Braun NM, Arora NS, Rochester DF. Respiratory muscle and pulmonary function in polymyositis and other proximal myopathies. Thorax 1983;38(8):616–23.

56. DePalo VA, McCool FD. Respiratory muscle evaluation of the patient with neuromuscular disease. Semin Respir Crit Care Med 2002;23(3):201–9.

57. Black LF, Hyatt RE. Maximal respiratory pressures: normal values and relationship to age and sex. Am Rev Respir Dis 1969;99(5):696–702.

58. Leech JA, Ghezzo H, Stevens D, et al. Respiratory pressures and function in young adults. Am Rev Respir Dis 1983;128(1):17–23.

59. Wilson SH, Cooke NT, Edwards RH, et al. Predicted normal values for maximal respiratory pressures in Caucasian adults and children. Thorax 1984;39(7): 535–8.

60. Koo P, Oyieng'o DO, Gartman EJ, et al. The maximal expiratory-to-inspiratory pressure ratio and supine vital capacity as screening tests for diaphragm dysfunction. Lung 2017;195(1):29–35.

61. Steier J, Kaul S, Seymour J, et al. The value of multiple tests of respiratory muscle strength. Thorax 2007;62(11):975–80.

62. Man WD, Kyroussis D, Fleming TA, et al. Cough gastric pressure and maximum expiratory mouth pressure in humans. Am J Respir Crit Care Med 2003;168(6):714–7.

63. Prigent H, Orlikowski D, Fermanian C, et al. Sniff and Muller manoeuvres to measure diaphragmatic muscle strength. Respir Med 2008;102(12):1737–43.

64. Heritier F, Rahm F, Pasche P, et al. Sniff nasal inspiratory pressure. A noninvasive assessment of inspiratory muscle strength. Am J Respir Crit Care Med 1994;150(6 Pt 1):1678–83.

65. Miller JM, Moxham J, Green M. The maximal sniff in the assessment of diaphragm function in man. Clin Sci (Lond) 1985;69(1):91–6.

66. Laroche CM, Mier AK, Moxham J, et al. The value of sniff esophageal pressures in the assessment of global inspiratory muscle strength. Am Rev Respir Dis 1988;138(3):598–603.

67. Fitting JW, Paillex R, Hirt L, et al. Sniff nasal pressure: a sensitive respiratory test to assess progression of amyotrophic lateral sclerosis. Ann Neurol 1999;46(6):887–93.

68. Hughes PD, Polkey MI, Kyroussis D, et al. Measurement of sniff nasal and diaphragm twitch mouth pressure in patients. Thorax 1998;53(2):96–100.

69. Uldry C, Janssens JP, de Muralt B, et al. Sniff nasal inspiratory pressure in patients with chronic obstructive pulmonary disease. Eur Respir J 1997;10(6):1292–6.

70. Fauroux B, Aubertin G, Cohen E, et al. Sniff nasal inspiratory pressure in children with muscular, chest wall or lung disease. Eur Respir J 2009;33(1):113–7.

71. Kaminska M, Noel F, Petrof BJ. Optimal method for assessment of respiratory muscle strength in neuromuscular disorders using sniff nasal inspiratory pressure (SNIP). PLoS One 2017;12(5):e0177723.

72. Lofaso F, Nicot F, Lejaille M, et al. Sniff nasal inspiratory pressure: what is the optimal number of sniffs? Eur Respir J 2006;27(5):980–2.

73. Wragg S, Aquilina R, Moran J, et al. Comparison of cervical magnetic stimulation and bilateral percutaneous electrical stimulation of the phrenic nerves in normal subjects. Eur Respir J 1994;7(10):1788–92.

74. McCool FD, Leith DE. Pathophysiology of cough. Clin chest Med 1987;8(2):189–95.

75. Sancho J, Servera E, Diaz J, et al. Comparison of peak cough flows measured by pneumotachograph and a portable peak flow meter. Am J Phys Med Rehabil 2004;83(8):608–12.

76. Sancho J, Servera E, Diaz J, et al. Predictors of ineffective cough during a chest infection in patients with stable amyotrophic lateral sclerosis. Am J Respir Crit Care Med 2007;175(12):1266–71.

77. Trebbia G, Lacombe M, Fermanian C, et al. Cough determinants in patients with neuromuscular disease. Respir Physiol Neurobiol 2005;146(2–3):291–300.

78. Kang SW, Kang YS, Sohn HS, et al. Respiratory muscle strength and cough capacity in patients with Duchenne muscular dystrophy. Yonsei Med J 2006;47(2):184–90.

79. Szeinberg A, Tabachnik E, Rashed N, et al. Cough capacity in patients with muscular dystrophy. Chest 1988;94(6):1232–5.

80. Byrd RB, Hyatt RE. Maximal respiratory pressures in chronic obstructive lung disease. Am Rev Respir Dis 1968;98(5):848–56.

81. Polkey MI, Lyall RA, Green M, et al. Expiratory muscle function in amyotrophic lateral sclerosis. Am J Respir Crit Care Med 1998;158(3):734–41.

82. Aiello M, Rampello A, Granella F, et al. Cough efficacy is related to the disability status in patients with multiple sclerosis. Respiration 2008;76(3):311–6.

83. Chaudri MB, Liu C, Hubbard R, et al. Relationship between supramaximal flow during cough and mortality in motor neurone disease. Eur Respir J 2002;19(3):434–8.

84. van Noord JA, Demedts M, Clement J, et al. Effect of rib cage and abdominal restriction on total respiratory resistance and reactance. J Appl Physiol (1985) 1986;61(5):1736–40.

85. van Noord JA, Cauberghs M, Van de Woestijne KP, et al. Total respiratory resistance and reactance in ankylosing spondylitis and kyphoscoliosis. Eur Respir J 1991;4(8):945–51.

86. Wesseling G, Quaedvlieg FC, Wouters EF. Oscillatory mechanics of the respiratory system in neuromuscular disease. Chest 1992;102(6):1752–7.

87. Radulovic M, Spungen AM, Wecht JM, et al. Effects of neostigmine and glycopyrrolate on pulmonary resistance in spinal cord injury. J Rehabil Res Dev 2004;41(1):53–8.

Assessing Diaphragm Function in Chest Wall and Neuromuscular Diseases

Taro Minami, MD[a], Kamran Manzoor, MD[b],
F. Dennis McCool, MD[a],*

KEYWORDS

- Supine vital capacity • Diaphragm ultrasound • Diaphragm CT scan

KEY POINTS

- The diaphragm is one of only a few skeletal muscles that is not amenable to direct examination.
- Traditionally, measures of lung volume, inspiratory muscle strength, and radiographic techniques such as fluoroscopy have been the mainstay of assessing diaphragm function.
- Measurement of transdiaphragmatic pressure has been the "gold standard" of assessing diaphragm function, but this technique is not readily available to clinicians.
- The advent of ultrasound for point-of-care testing has allowed clinicians to become comfortable with this technology and spurred interest in diaphragm ultrasonography.

INTRODUCTION

The deleterious effects of diaphragm dysfunction include potentially life-threatening complications related to diaphragm weakness and paralysis.[1,2] Recently, there has been a heightened awareness of the prevalence of diaphragm weakness and paralysis in a wide range of clinical settings. For example, ventilator-induced diaphragm injury may be present in up to 80% of patients in the intensive care unit and occur as soon as 24 to 36 hours after the institution of mechanical ventilation.[3–5] One of the key tools that has allowed the clinician to detect the presence of diaphragm dysfunction is diaphragm ultrasound. Over the past decade, this diagnostic tool has evolved from a research device to one that has clinical utility.[6–11]

Several disparate disorders can impair diaphragm function. They can be broadly classified into 3 major categories.[12] The first group are those disorders that involve neurons in the central nervous system (polio, amyotrophic lateral sclerosis [ALS]) or peripheral neurons (peripheral neuropathies, Guillain-Barre syndrome, chronic inflammatory demyelinating polyneuropathy or compression of the phrenic nerve by neighboring structures, tumors, and so forth) The second group of disorders are those than impair muscle function, such as the muscular dystrophies, critical-illness polymyopathy, dermatomyositis, and other myopathies. A third group of disorders involve the neuromuscular junction and include myasthenia gravis, Lambert-Eaton syndrome, and botulism.[13] These disorders and others are listed in Table 1 in Franklin Dennis McCool and colleagues' article, "Disorders of the Diaphragm," in this issue. The same general approach can be used to assess diaphragm function for this diverse group of disorders. The workup includes measurement of lung volumes,

Disclosure: None of the authors have any financial interests in subject matter or materials discussed in this article.

[a] The Warren Alpert Medical School of Brown University, Memorial Hospital of Rhode Island, 111 Brewster Street, Pawtucket, RI 02860, USA; [b] The Warren Alpert Medical School of Brown University, 111 Brewster Street, Pawtucket, RI 02860, USA

* Corresponding author.

E-mail address: F_McCool@brown.edu

Clin Chest Med 39 (2018) 335–344
https://doi.org/10.1016/j.ccm.2018.01.013
0272-5231/18/© 2018 Elsevier Inc. All rights reserved.

chestmed.theclinics.com

respiratory pressures, diaphragm ultrasound, and computed tomographic (CT) scanning. Because most patient encounters start with a history and physical examination, pertinent components of the history and physical examination are reviewed first.

HISTORY

A careful history can provide important clues that support or contest the diagnosis of diaphragm dysfunction. Formulation of a pretest probability of the presence or absence of this disorder will enable the clinician to better interpret the results of a test and avoid erroneous conclusions. Often patients with diaphragm dysfunction present with a history of unexplained dyspnea. Enquiring about factors that elicit this symptom can aid in deciding if the dyspnea is due to diaphragm dysfunction. Patients with diaphragm dysfunction often complain of difficulty breathing when lifting objects or bending. Because accessory inspiratory muscles normally are recruited to perform tasks other than breathing, individuals who solely rely on these muscles to breathe will experience dyspnea when they engage in activities that use these muscles. Accordingly, tasks that require raising their arms above their head or lifting objects will trigger dyspnea. Similarly, bending may cause dyspnea. In this instance, displacement of the passive diaphragm into the thoracic cavity limits lung inflation, and activities, such as bending to tie shoelaces or to garden, elicit dyspnea. Orthopnea is another frequent complaint and may initially be mistaken for congestive heart failure. Often these individuals are unable to sleep in a bed and must use a recliner. Some may complain of difficulty breathing when entering a swimming pool.[14] Typically, individuals with diaphragm dysfunction will not become short of breath until the level of water rises to the rib cage. At times, patients will be relatively asymptomatic and will be referred because of an abnormal chest radiograph.

The history may include clues to the cause of diaphragm dysfunction. If the dyspnea is subacute and progressive over a long period of time, there may be an underlying myopathic process. With Parsonage-Turner syndrome (brachial neuritis or neuralgic amyotrophy), dyspnea may be preceded by days or weeks by an episode of sharp neck and shoulder pain with or without upper extremity weakness. A history of neck manipulation or trauma, shoulder manipulation or trauma, percutaneous punctures for central lines, atrial ablation procedures, or exposure to medications or drugs that can produce a neuropathy should be carefully sought. Recently, PD-1 inhibitors have been reported to be associated with muscle weakness.[15]

Inflammatory myopathies may be accompanied by muscle tenderness or rash. If there is a prior history of neuromuscular disease affecting limb or trunk muscles, diaphragm involvement should also be considered. Dyspnea may not be as prominent a symptom in these individuals because their mobility may be severely limited by limb muscle weakness or paralysis. A history of malignancy would increase the possibility of diaphragm weakness because of a paraneoplastic syndrome, such as Lambert-Eaton syndrome. Exposure to chemicals like organophosphates would be important because these are associated with muscle weakness. Family history would be of particular importance when eliciting genetic disorders, such as muscular dystrophies.

PHYSICAL EXAMINATION

Diaphragm dysfunction often results in tachypneic with prominent use of accessory muscles for inspiration.[16] Inspecting the chest wall will often reveal paradoxic inward motion of the abdomen while the rib cage is expanding. This paradoxical motion may be seen with the patient in the seated position but is most pronounced with the patient in the supine position.[2,14] This paradox will not be apparent if someone is fully supported with mechanical ventilation but may be seen once ventilator support is reduced.

A neurologic examination is essential, with the clinician paying particular attention to reflexes. For example, a combination of hyperreflexia and muscle atrophy in a patient with progressive muscle weakness is consistent with ALS, whereas bilateral hyporeflexia with is seen with Guillain-Barre syndrome. If Parsonage-Turner syndrome is suspected, there may be atrophy of the ipsilateral shoulder girdle or upper extremity muscles.

CHEST RADIOGRAPH AND FLUOROSCOPY

The chest radiograph is often one of the first diagnostic tests ordered in the evaluation of dyspnea. With unilateral diaphragm paralysis, the classic finding is an elevated hemidiaphragm. The sensitivity of chest radiography for detecting unilateral diaphragm paralysis is 90%. However, because several other disorders can be associated with an elevated hemidiaphragm, the specific of chest radiography is poor (44%).[1,17] The diaphragm may be elevated because of intrathoracic pathologic condition, including lobar atelectasis, pulmonary or mediastinal masses, prior lung resection, or asymmetrical emphysema. In addition, the diaphragm may be elevated because of intra-abdominal pathologic condition, including ascites, subphrenic abscess, or liver abscess. Insufflation of the abdomen for laparoscopic procedures also can cause an elevated diaphragm. Structural changes of the hemidiaphragm, such as eventration, traumatic diaphragm rupture, Morgagni and Bochdalek hernias, as well as hiatal hernias may cause parts of the diaphragm to be elevated. Finally, the diaphragm may appear to be elevated because the contralateral diaphragm is displaced caudally or there is a subpulmonic effusion. Bilateral diaphragm elevation on chest radiograph may be due to several of the pathologic processes mentioned for unilateral diaphragm paralysis. In addition, if a patient gives a "poor inspiratory effort," both hemidiaphragms will be elevated.[17] Therefore, the chest radiograph is not sensitive or specific for detecting bilateral diaphragm paralysis.

Diaphragm fluoroscopy is a well-accepted means of confirming the diagnosis of unilateral diaphragm paralysis.[18] Fluoroscopy allows for real-time evaluation of the diaphragm during tidal breathing, during deep inspiration, and while the patient performs a "sniff" maneuver. A quick, inspiratory, sniffing effort results in caudal motion of a nonparalyzed hemidiaphragm and paradoxic cephalad motion of an elevated hemidiaphragm if it is paralyzed. False positive results may occur in as many as 6% of individuals without diaphragmatic paralysis during the sniff maneuver.[18] Diaphragm fluoroscopy has limited diagnostic utility with bilateral diaphragmatic paralysis.[14] False positive findings are due to the patient sniffing primarily by elevating the rib cage or using accessory muscles of the neck. This strategy causes paradoxic cephalad motion of the diaphragm in the absence of diaphragm paralysis.[14,18] False negative results may be seen when the abdominal muscles are used to actively exhale, and inspiration is accomplished by passive recoil of the chest wall.[19] In this instance, there is caudal motion of the diaphragm even though it is paralyzed.

LUNG VOLUMES: TOTAL LUNG CAPACITY, VITAL CAPACITY

Once diaphragm dysfunction is suspected, pulmonary function testing is warranted to further support the diagnosis and to give the clinician an idea as to the degree of functional compromise. A restrictive pattern with a reduction in total lung capacity (TLC) and vital capacity (VC) would be consistent with the diagnosis of diaphragm dysfunction but is nonspecific. With unilateral diaphragm paralysis, TLC may be normal or only slightly reduced.[20] However, TLC may be moderately reduced in unilateral paralysis with comorbid conditions such as obesity. By contrast, there is a moderate to severe reduction in TLC and VC with bilateral hemidiaphragm paralysis.[21] The restrictive pattern seen with diaphragm dysfunction may show less of a reduction in residual volume (RV) than the restrictive pattern because of interstitial lung disease; however, this finding cannot reliably distinguish between restriction due to pulmonary parenchymal processes and that due to diaphragm dysfunction.

The change in VC from the seated to supine position (ΔVC-supine) is a more sensitive and specific test for diaphragm dysfunction and is the most common test used to screen for this disorder.[2] Normally, gravitational shifts of the abdominal contents will stretch and displace the passive diaphragm into the thorax. Consequently, there is an increase in RV and a negligible increase in TLC. The net result is a decrease in VC. In addition, blood volume shifts into the thorax will further reduce VC. Therefore, VC may decrease by 8% when a normal individual lies flat. In some individuals, there may be an even greater decline in VC when assuming the supine position with a 19% decline in VC reported as the upper limits of the 95% confidence interval for healthy individuals.[22] Greater reductions in ΔVC-supine suggest the presence of diaphragm paralysis or weakness, making a 20% or greater ΔVC-supine a reasonable cutoff for screening for diaphragm dysfunction with the weakest diaphragm having the greatest decrease in supine VC. A ΔVC-supine between 25% and 50% of the seated VC is associated not only with the degree of diaphragm weakness but also with the presence of orthopnea and the severity of dyspnea.[21] In general, the specificity, sensitivity, positive predictive value, and negative predictive value of a ΔVC-supine greater than 25% are 90%, 79%, 92%, and 75%, respectively, for predicting diaphragm dysfunction. However, individuals with lesser degrees of diaphragm weakness may have a ΔVC-supine that falls within the range of normal. In one series, one-third of patients (5 of 14) with diaphragm dysfunction had a decrease in VC less than 25%.[23,24] A larger study of 76 patients referred for unexplained dyspnea showed on average a 6% decrease in ΔVC-supine in patients without diaphragm dysfunction, a 16% decrease in patients with unilateral paralysis, and a 33% decrease in patients with bilateral diaphragm paralysis.[24] However, there was considerable overlap in ΔVC-supine between the unilateral diaphragm paralysis and normal groups.[24] Thus, the diagnosis of diaphragm dysfunction should not be based solely on this test. However, its high sensitivity makes it a useful test for screening.

INSPIRATORY PRESSURES

Global inspiratory muscle strength and expiratory muscle strength are assessed by measuring maximal static inspiratory and maximal static expiratory pressures (PI_{max} and PE_{max}, respectively).[25] PI_{max} is measured by instructing subjects to breathe to RV and then to forcefully inhale against an occluded mouthpiece for ≥ 3 seconds (maximal Mueller maneuver). PE_{max} is measured by instructing subjects to breathe to TLC and then to forcefully exhale against an occluded mouthpiece for ≥ 3 seconds (maximal expulsive maneuver). Individuals who have difficulty performing a maximal inspiratory effort can be asked to perform a vigorous sniff with one nostril occluded (P_{sniff}). PI_{max} and P_{sniff} reflect the strength of both the diaphragm and the inspiratory muscles of the rib cage. Because the rib cage muscles are weaker and more fatigable than the diaphragm, the value for PI_{max} may be limited by the strength of the rib cage muscles rather than the strength of the diaphragm.[26] Nonetheless, PI_{max} is measured routinely to assess diaphragm strength. Reductions in PI_{max} and P_{sniff} to less than 30% of predicted are consistent with bilateral diaphragm paralysis. PI_{max} and P_{sniff} may be normal or mildly reduced to about 60% of predicted in unilateral diaphragm paralysis.[22,27] With isolated diaphragm weakness, the expiratory muscles retain their strength; and PE_{max} is preserved. If PE_{max} is severely reduced in patients with diaphragm dysfunction (50% predicted or lower), the cause of diaphragm dysfunction likely reflects a more generalized disease process affecting other skeletal muscle groups (eg, muscular dystrophy).[28] With processes that cause isolated diaphragm weakness, the ratio of maximum expiratory pressure (MEP) to maximum inspiratory pressure (MIP) is elevated. In one study, the mean value for MEP/MIP was 2.1 for patients with unilateral diaphragm paralysis, 4.3 for patients with bilateral diaphragm paralysis and 1.5 for a cohort with normal diaphragm function and correlated strongly with ΔVC-supine.[24] MEP/MIP may provide an alternative to ΔVC-supine as a screening test for diaphragm dysfunction when evaluating patients who are unable to tolerate the supine position.

TRANSDIAPHRAGMATIC PRESSURE

The gold standard to assess diaphragm strength is the measurement of transdiaphragmatic pressure (Pdi). This pressure is usually measured during a maneuver in which an individual gives a maximal inspiratory effort. The maximal effort may consist of a maximal static inspiratory effort against an occluded airway (Pdi_{max}) (a maneuver identical to that performed during the measurement of PI_{max}) or during a maximal sniff maneuver (Pdi_{sniff}). A Pdi_{max} greater than 80 cm H_2O in men and greater than 70 cm H_2O in women excludes significant diaphragmatic weakness.[29,30] If an individual is unable to follow instructions or make a maximal effort, Pdi can be measured when the phrenic nerve is either electrically or magnetically stimulated (Pdi twitch).[25] This technique also can be used to separately evaluate the function of each hemidiaphragm. A Pdi twitch greater than 10 cm H_2O with unilateral phrenic nerve stimulation or greater than 20 cm H_2O with bilateral phrenic nerve stimulation excludes significant diaphragm weakness.[31,32] However, irrespective of how the diaphragm is activated (by voluntary or nonvolitional means), it requires placement of catheters in both the lower esophagus and the stomach, thus eliciting some patient discomfort and requiring expertise that may not be available to the clinician.

DIAPHRAGM ULTRASOUND

In contrast to tests used to measure Pdi that are invasive and not readily available to the clinician, diaphragm ultrasound is a useful, noninvasive tool that is available at the bedside or in the clinic. Ultrasound is more accessible, in part, because of the emergence of point of care ultrasound (POCUS)."[33] The availability of relatively low-cost portable ultrasound machines with the capability of providing high-quality images has provided a catalyst to POCUS. As clinicians have developed comfort using ultrasound, more applications have evolved during the past decade, including diaphragm-specific ultrasound.[33] There are 2 general approaches to imaging the diaphragm. The first approach involves visualizing the diaphragm dome and the second approach visualizes the diaphragm muscle at the zone of apposition of the diaphragm to the rib cage (ZOA).[7] Caudal diaphragm motion is best appreciated by visualizing the dome, whereas diaphragm muscle contraction is best visualized by imaging the diaphragm in the ZOA. In addition to diaphragm ultrasound providing a noninvasive means of assessing the diaphragm, it also allows for evaluation of each hemidiaphragm.

The diaphragm dome is easily recognized and is composed of a large central tendon, which is located medially, and the costal diaphragm, whose fibers insert into the central tendon. The crural diaphragm is located posteriorly and makes up a small fraction of the diaphragm dome. The fraction of diaphragm dome attributed to the central tendon ranges from 10% to more than 35%.[34] When imaging the dome, its motion may be due to contraction of the costal diaphragm or displacement of the central tendon, depending on the probe location. To visualize the dome, a 3.5- to 5-MHz phased array probe is placed below the costal margin in the midclavicular line or in the anterior axillary line. The dome is better visualized in the right hemithorax because there is no gastric air and the liver provides an "acoustic window," which allows for the ultrasound waves to penetrate deeper structures such as the diaphragm.[16] The diaphragm appears as a crescentlike echo-dense structure that moves with breathing (**Fig. 1**A). The motion of the diaphragm dome is not uniform. Typically, there is the greater caudal motion of the middle and posterior parts of the diaphragm than of the anterior region. The dome can be visualized in 2 dimensions (B-mode) or as a single point on a time-based plot (M-mode) (**Fig. 1**B). Inspiration and expiration can be clearly identified, and diaphragm excursion can be measured as the distance between end-expiration and end-inspiration. During quiet breathing, the posterior portion of the dome of the diaphragm is displaced anteriorly and caudally. The mean distance displaced is 1.6 cm.[35] With deeper breaths, there is greater motion, averaging 4.8 cm in a group of healthy controls.[36] About two-thirds of the diaphragm movement occurs by the time of midinspiration. A nonfunctioning hemidiaphragm will show no motion at all or move paradoxically cephalad or minimally caudally. Similar to diaphragm fluoroscopy, evaluating diaphragm dome motion has proved useful in the diagnosis of unilateral diaphragm paralysis but is not a reliable means of diagnosing bilateral diaphragm paralysis. In this context, there may be normal caudal displacement of the paralyzed diaphragm because of the rib cage muscles lifting the rib cage and giving the

appearance that the diaphragm is descending. Activation of the rib cage muscles also may lower subdiaphragmatic pressure thereby "sucking" the passive diaphragm caudally. This downward motion will also give a false impression that the diaphragm is functioning normally.

The diaphragm ZOA encircles the lower rib cage and is composed of the costal diaphragm medially and anteriorly and the crural diaphragm posteriorly. Because the central tendon does not extend to the area of the ZOA, one is directly assessing contraction of the diaphragm muscle itself. The ability to directly visualize the muscle, is the major advantage of viewing the diaphragm in the ZOA over viewing the diaphragm dome. The thickness of the diaphragm (tdi) is measured at relaxed end-expiration and again at end-inspiration. When the diaphragm contracts, it thickens, and the change in diaphragm thickness during inspiration (Δtdi) can be measured. This change in thickness is proportional to the degree of diaphragm shortening[7] and is analogous to the strain rate measured during echocardiography. The major advantage of this technique is it allows imaging of the diaphragm muscle as it is activated and alleviates potential errors that may be incurred when assessing motion of the diaphragm dome alone. However, when compared with imaging the dome, it is more difficult and requires more operator skill. A vascular probe in the 5- to 15-MHz range is typically used to visualize the diaphragm in the zone of opposition. The probe is placed in the midaxillary line in the eighth to ninth intercostal space.[16] The higher-frequency probe can be used to visualize the diaphragm in the ZOA because it is more superficial than the dome. Although a high-frequency transducer does not penetrate as deeply as a low-frequency probe, it has the advantage of providing better spatial resolution, enabling one to view the

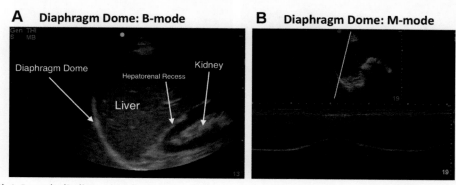

A **Diaphragm Dome: B-mode**

B **Diaphragm Dome: M-mode**

Fig. 1. (*A*) A B-mode (2-dimensional) ultrasound image of the diaphragm dome and its adjacent structures. (*B*) The M-mode I (time based) image depicting a radial placed on the posterior one-third of the diaphragm (*top*). A time base plot (*bottom*) depicts the diaphragm passing through the radial during the respiratory cycle.

diaphragm in more detail. This same resolution cannot be achieved when viewing the dome because it is a deeper structure. Because the ZOA is relatively close to the body surface, the ultrasound depth is usually set to 3 to 6 cm depending on the thickness of the rib cage. Obese or muscular individuals would have a diaphragm that is deeper than a child or someone who is thin. The diaphragm in the ZOA is identified as a structure sandwiched between 2 highly echogenic nearly parallel lines that represent the pleura and the peritoneum. Often a third echogenic line is seen within the diaphragm itself. This is a discontinuous often oblique line that likely represents a neurovascular bundle.[6] Superficial to the echogenic line representing the pleura, other lines can be observed along with rib shadows (**Fig. 2**). Diaphragm thickness (tdi) and its change during inspiration (Δtdi) allow one to assess the contraction of the diaphragm. The more the diaphragm contracts, the more it shortens and thickens. Measuring diaphragm shortening and thickening is analogous to measuring the ejection fraction of the heart. The thicker it is at baseline (tdi at functional residual capacity [FRC]), the more tension it can generate. Diaphragm thickness at FRC is analogous to left ventricular wall thickness. Normal values for diaphragm thickness at end-expiration generally fall between 2.0 and 3.5 mm. The normal value for diaphragm thickening with inspiration (Δtdi%) falls between 20% and 100%. Functional correlates of measurement of Δtdi% and tdi have been reported. Thickness of the relaxed diaphragm at end-expiration (tdi at FRC) is proportional to diaphragm strength and has been used to predict Pdi_{max}.[37,38] Furthermore, increases in diaphragm strength with training or increases in diaphragm strength related to recovery from diaphragm paralysis have been associated with increases in resting diaphragm thickness.[39,40] Finally, changes in diaphragm thickness during inspiration Δtdi% have been related to changes in lung volume over the VC range[7] and have been used to predict extubation outcomes.[41,42]

COMPUTED TOMOGRAPHY, PET, MRI

Additional imaging modalities, including CT, PET, and MRI, play important roles in appraising the structural integrity of the diaphragm and evaluating possible causes of the phrenic nerve injury.

The chest CT provides anatomic details depicting its curvature and the presence of defects, such as hernias and eventration. Coronal and sagittal CT reconstructions are especially helpful. An elevated hemidiaphragm can be readily detected by CT. In the coronal plane, there is greater displacement of the paralyzed hemidiaphragm into the thorax than noted on the posteroanterior chest radiograph because the CT is performed with the patient supine. The CT is especially useful when evaluating the integrity of the diaphragm following blunt or penetrating abdominal trauma. Diaphragm injuries can be graded by CT criteria and may be used to determine if surgical repair is needed. A grade 2 injury is a laceration less than 2 cm, and a grade 5 injury is a laceration greater than 10 cm and a loss of tissue greater than 25 cm[2]. Trauma producing large diaphragm lacerations may allow herniation of the abdominal

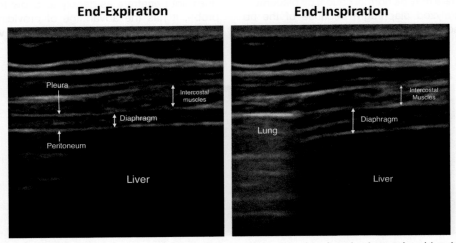

Fig. 2. Right hemidiaphragm ultrasound of the ZOA obtained at relaxed end-expiration and end-inspiration. The pleura and peritoneum, intercostal muscles, and diaphragm are marked. The diaphragm muscle is sandwiched between the pleura and peritoneum. Note the diaphragm thickens during inspiration.

contents and may be detected on chest radiographs or with CT. However, CT has the advantage of detecting concomitant injuries to abdominal viscera or to the lung. When the diaphragm is injured, other organs are involved 50% to 75% of the time.[43,44] Small lacerations will not be appreciated on chest radiographs and may not be detected on standard CT. If suspected, 3-dimensional (3D) reconstruction imaging of the CT may be needed. Other complications associated with diaphragm injury that can be diagnosed using CT include pleural effusion, hemothorax, and atelectasis.

Diaphragmatic hernias can be seen in neonates and adults, and chest CT provides a means of localizing the diaphragm defect and determining whether there is herniation of abdominal contents. Most congenital diaphragmatic hernias (CDH) are evident at birth and are accompanied by respiratory distress or failure. This diaphragm malformation may allow herniation of abdominal contents into the thorax. Strangulation of the herniated contents is life-threatening and requires immediate surgical attention. Often, large diaphragm defects can be seen on prenatal ultrasound, and appropriate arrangements can be made for the care of the newborn with CDH. In contrast to infants, diaphragm hernias in adults are not life-threatening. Morgagni and Bochdalek hernias are typically incidental findings on CT. Morgagni hernias are anteriorly located and mostly involve the right hemidiaphragm with minimal risk of herniation. Bochdalek hernias are larger, are located posteriorly, and can involve either hemidiaphragm. In comparison to Morgagni hernias, herniation of intraabdominal viscera and retroperitoneal structures is more common.[45] The chest CT allows for distinguishing Morgagni and Bochdalek hernias from diaphragm structural defects, such as diaphragm eventration, a condition whereby a portion of the diaphragm is thin and bulges into the thorax but is intact.

Chest CT is also used to evaluate disorders of the chest wall, such as pectus excavatum and scoliosis. With pectus excavatum, the severity of the deformity is assessed using the Haller index. This index is derived as the ratio of the transverse chest diameter to the anteroposterior diameter.[46] A Haller index of 2.5 or less is normal, and an index of more than 3.2 indicates that the pectus deformity is severe and that the individual may be a candidate for surgery. Although restrictive disease is typically mild in pectus excavatum, there is correlation between severity of the pectus deformity and the degree of the restrictive lung disease.[47,48] With kyphoscoliosis, CT can be used to outline the extent of asymmetry in lung volumes between the right and left hemithorax and also to assess displacement and rotation of the heart, an important consideration while considering surgical interventions.[48]

Pathologic condition that may interrupt the course of the phrenic nerve in the neck or thoracic cavity resulting in diaphragm paralysis can be assessed with CT (**Fig. 3**).[49] CT examination of cervical, axillary, or mediastinal areas adjacent to the phrenic nerve may reveal thymic tumors, goiter, lung cancer, lymphoma, thoracic aortic aneurysm, fibrotic changes postradiation or ablation, or pericardial disease, all of which can disrupt the phrenic nerve,[50,51] leading to diaphragm paralysis.[52,53] CT may also detect primary tumors of the phrenic nerve such as neurofibromatosis, although this is rare.[54] This imaging modality is also helpful in evaluating causes of "an elevated hemidiaphragm," which are unrelated to diaphragm paralysis. Such disorders include subdiaphragmatic abscess, subpleural effusion, atelectasis, and pleural thickening.[49]

CT scan of the chest provides in-depth structural details of the diaphragm that is especially useful when searching for diaphragm defects, including diaphragm laceration. It is potentially a tool that can be used to assess intraabdominal pressure from ascites or obesity and

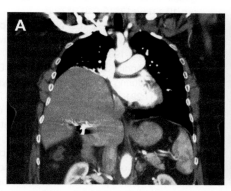
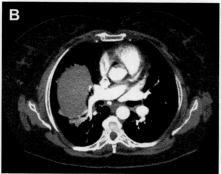

Fig. 3. Elevation of the right hemidiaphragm is demonstrated in (*A*) coronal and (*B*) axial CT images.

to assess diaphragm atrophy or the extent of the eventration (**Fig. 3**).[49,55] With combined PET-CT systems, functional and morphologic imaging is available. However, artifact due to respiratory motion may limit the image acquisition.[56] PET scanning can be used to evaluate the biological behavior and potential response to therapy for various tumors that can involve the diaphragm.[56]

MRI

Although MRI of the cervical spine can play an important role in evaluating potential causes of diaphragm dysfunction, spinal cord lesions, spinal compression, tumor infiltration, transverse myelitis, and syringomyelia (**Fig. 4**) can be detected and are potential sources of diaphragm dysfunction.[49] Although MRI of the chest is not widely used to evaluate diaphragm function, sequential images can be obtained that reveal dynamic changes in the diaphragm during the respiratory cycle. Quantitative diaphragmatic evaluation with MRI provides information regarding diaphragmatic excursion, synchrony, and velocity.[57,58] MRI may potentially be used to assess diaphragm dysfunction in neuromuscular diseases and its response to therapy.[55] MRI compared with CT or fluoroscopy is free of radiation, but it has limited availability, has a high cost, and serves as more of a research tool at this time.

SUMMARY

Diaphragm dysfunction is becoming increasingly recognized in a wide range of disorders.

Measures of lung volumes and inspiratory muscle strength can be helpful in supporting the diagnosis of diaphragm dysfunction but are limited in their specificity. Measures of upright and supine VC provide an adequate means of screening for diaphragm dysfunction. If screening is consistent with diaphragm dysfunction, the diagnosis can be confirmed by measuring Pdi. However, this technique is not readily available to the clinician. Recent advances in diaphragm ultrasound have enabled the clinician to use this technique to confirm the presence or absence of diaphragm dysfunction. The cause of dysfunction can be further evaluated using CT and MRI in appropriate clinical settings. 3D chest CT augments traditional CT in detecting defects of the diaphragm, such as lacerations or hernias. The ubiquitous availability of ultrasound for point-of-care testing will lead to further application of diaphragm ultrasonography.

REFERENCES

1. Dubé BP, Dres M. Diaphragm dysfunction: diagnostic approaches and management strategies. J Clin Med 2016;5(12):113.
2. McCool FD, Tzelepis GE. Dysfunction of the diaphragm. N Engl J Med 2012;366(10):932–42.
3. Hussain SN, Cornachione AS, Guichon C, et al. Prolonged controlled mechanical ventilation in humans triggers myofibrillar contractile dysfunction and myofilament protein loss in the diaphragm. Thorax 2016. https://doi.org/10.1136/thoraxjnl-2015-207559.
4. Dres M, Dubé BP, Mayaux J, et al. Coexistence and impact of limb muscle and diaphragm weakness at time of liberation from mechanical ventilation in medical intensive care unit patients. Am J Respir Crit Care Med 2017. https://doi.org/10.1164/rccm.201602-0367OC.
5. Demoule A, Molinari N, Jung B, et al. Patterns of diaphragm function in critically ill patients receiving prolonged mechanical ventilation: a prospective longitudinal study. Ann Intensive Care 2016. https://doi.org/10.1186/s13613-016-0179-8.
6. Wait JL, Nahormek PA, Yost WT, et al. Diaphragmatic thickness-lung volume relationship in vivo. J Appl Physiol (1985) 1989;67(4):1560–8.
7. Cohn D, Benditt JO, Eveloff S, et al. Diaphragm thickening during inspiration. J Appl Physiol (1985) 1997;83(1):291–6.
8. Gerscovich EO, Cronan M, McGahan JP, et al. Ultrasonographic evaluation of diaphragmatic motion. J Ultrasound Med 2001;20(6):597–604.
9. Lloyd T, Tang YM, Benson MD, et al. Diaphragmatic paralysis: the use of M mode ultrasound for diagnosis in adults. Spinal Cord 2006. https://doi.org/10.1038/sj.sc.3101889.

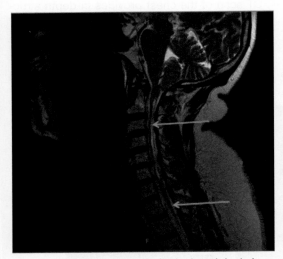

Fig. 4. MRI scan of the cervical spinal cord depicting a syrinx (*arrows*) in a patient with bilateral diaphragm paralysis.

10. He L, Zhang W, Zhang J, et al. Diaphragmatic motion studied by M-mode ultrasonography in combined pulmonary fibrosis and emphysema. Lung 2014;192(4):553–61.
11. Gierada DS, Slone RM, Fleishman MJ. Imaging evaluation of the diaphragm. Chest Surg Clin N Am 1998;8(2):237–80.
12. McCool FD, Mead J. Dyspnea on immersion: mechanisms in patients with bilateral diaphragm paralysis. Am Rev Respir Dis 1989;139(1):275–6.
13. Perrin C, Unterborn JN, Ambrosio CD, et al. Pulmonary complications of chronic neuromuscular diseases and their management. Muscle Nerve 2004; 29(1):5–27.
14. Laghi F, Tobin MJ. Disorders of the respiratory muscles. Am J Respir Crit Care Med 2003; 168(1):10–48.
15. Liewluck T, Kao JC, Mauermann ML. PD-1 inhibitor-associated myopathies: emerging immune-mediated myopathies. J Immunother 2017;1. https://doi.org/10.1097/cji.0000000000000196.
16. McCool FD, Minami T. Ultrasound in the intensive care unit. Springer; 2015. p. 235–48.
17. Chetta A, Rehman AK, Moxham J, et al. Chest radiography cannot predict diaphragm function. Respir Med 2005;99(1):39–44.
18. Alexander C. Diaphragm movements and the diagnosis of diaphragmatic paralysis. Clin Radiol 1966; 17(1):79–83.
19. Davis J, Goldman M, Loh L, et al. Diaphragm function and alveolar hypoventilation. Q J Med 1976; 45(177):87–100.
20. Laroche CM, Mier AK, Moxham J, et al. Diaphragm strength in patients with recent hemidiaphragm paralysis. Thorax 1988;43(3):170–4.
21. Mier-Jedrzejowicz A, Brophy C, Moxham J, et al. Assessment of diaphragm weakness. Am Rev Respir Dis 1988;137(4):877–83.
22. Laroche CM, Carroll N, Moxham J, et al. Clinical significance of severe isolated diaphragm weakness. Am Rev Respir Dis 1988;138(4):862–6.
23. Fromageot C, Lofaso F, Annane D, et al. Supine fall in lung volumes in the assessment of diaphragmatic weakness in neuromuscular disorders. Arch Phys Med Rehabil 2001;82(1):123–8.
24. Koo P, Oyieng'o DO, Gartman EJ, et al. The maximal expiratory-to-inspiratory pressure ratio and supine vital capacity as screening tests for diaphragm dysfunction. Lung 2017;195(1):29–35.
25. American Thoracic Society/European Respiratory Society. ATS/ERS statement on respiratory muscle testing. Am J Respir Crit Care Med 2002;166(4):518–624.
26. Hershenson MB, Kikuchi Y, Tzelepis GE, et al. Preferential fatigue of the rib cage muscles during inspiratory resistive loaded ventilation. J Appl Physiol (1985) 1989;66(2):750–4.
27. Miller JM, Moxham J, Green M. The maximal sniff in the assessment of diaphragm function in man. Clin Sci (Lond) 1985;69(1):91–6.
28. Mills GH, Kyroussis D, Hamnegard CH, et al. Cervical magnetic stimulation of the phrenic nerves in bilateral diaphragm paralysis. Am J Respir Crit Care Med 1997. https://doi.org/10.1164/ajrccm.155.5.9154858.
29. Polkey MI, Green M, Moxham J. Measurement of respiratory muscle strength. Thorax 1995;50(11):1131–5.
30. Steier J, Kaul S, Seymour J, et al. The value of multiple tests of respiratory muscle strength. Thorax 2007. https://doi.org/10.1136/thx.2006.072884.
31. Mier A, Brophy C, Moxham J, et al. Twitch pressures in the assessment of diaphragm weakness. Thorax 1989. https://doi.org/10.1136/thx.44.12.990.
32. Bellemare F, Bigland-Ritchie B. Assessment of human diaphragm strength and activation using phrenic nerve stimulation. Respir Physiol 1984; 58(3):263–77.
33. Moore CL, Copel JA. Point-of-care ultrasonography. N Engl J Med 2011;364(8):749–57.
34. du Plessis M, Ramai D, Shah S, et al. The clinical anatomy of the musculotendinous part of the diaphragm. Surg Radiol Anat 2015. https://doi.org/10.1007/s00276-015-1481-0.
35. Houston JG, Angus RM, Cowan MD, et al. Ultrasound assessment of normal hemidiaphragmatic movement: relation to inspiratory volume. Thorax 1994;49(5):500–3.
36. Harris RS, Giovannetti M, Kim BK. Normal ventilatory movement of the right hemidiaphragm studied by ultrasonography and pneumotachography. Radiology 1983;146(1):141–4.
37. McCool FD, Benditt JO, Conomos P, et al. Variability of diaphragm structure among healthy individuals. Am J Respir Crit Care Med 1997. https://doi.org/10.1164/ajrccm.155.4.9105074.
38. McCool FD, Conomos P, Benditt JO, et al. Maximal inspiratory pressures and dimensions of the diaphragm. Am J Respir Crit Care Med 1997. https://doi.org/10.1164/ajrccm.155.4.9105075.
39. Summerhill EM, El-Sameed YA, Glidden TJ, et al. Monitoring recovery from diaphragm paralysis with ultrasound. Chest 2008;133(3):737–43.
40. DePalo VA, Parker AL, Al-Bilbeisi F, et al. Respiratory muscle strength training with nonrespiratory maneuvers. J Appl Physiol (1985) 2004;96(2):731–4.
41. DiNino E, Gartman EJ, Sethi JM, et al. Diaphragm ultrasound as a predictor of successful extubation from mechanical ventilation. Thorax 2014;69(5):431–5.
42. Blumhof S, Wheeler D, Thomas K, et al. Change in diaphragmatic thickness during the respiratory

cycle predicts extubation success at various levels of pressure support ventilation. Lung 2016. https://doi.org/10.1007/s00408-016-9911-2.

43. Williams M, Carlin AM, Tyburski JG, et al. Predictors of mortality in patients with traumatic diaphragmatic rupture and associated thoracic and/or abdominal injuries. Am Surg 2004;70(2):157–62 [discussion: 162–3].

44. Demetriades D, Kakoyiannis S, Parekh D, et al. Penetrating injuries of the diaphragm. Br J Surg 1988;75(8):824–6.

45. Gedik E, Tuncer MC, Onat S, et al. A review of Morgagni and Bochdalek hernias in adults. Folia Morphol (Warsz) 2011;70(1):5–12.

46. Archer JE, Gardner A, Berryman F, et al. The measurement of the normal thorax using the Haller index methodology at multiple vertebral levels. J Anat 2016. https://doi.org/10.1111/joa.12499.

47. Haller JA Jr, Loughlin GM. Cardiorespiratory function is significantly improved following corrective surgery for severe pectus excavatum: proposed treatment guidelines. J Cardiovasc Surg (Torino) 2000;41(1):125–30.

48. Lawson ML, Mellins RB, Paulson JF, et al. Increasing severity of pectus excavatum is associated with reduced pulmonary function. J Pediatr 2011; 159(2):256–61.e2.

49. Nason LK, Walker CM, McNeeley MF, et al. Imaging of the diaphragm: anatomy and function. Radiographics 2012;32(2):E51–70.

50. Gupta PP, Gupta KB, Yadav R, et al. Diaphragmatic paralysis and hoarseness of voice due to mediastinal tuberculous lymphadenitis. Indian J Tuberc 2004;51:93–6.

51. Akhtar J, Siddiqui MA, Khan NA, et al. Right phrenic nerve palsy: a rare presentation of thoracic aortic aneurysm. Malays J Med Sci 2013;20(4):98–101.

52. Elefteriades J, Singh M, Tang P, et al. Unilateral diaphragm paralysis: etiology, impact, and natural history. J Cardiovasc Surg (Torino) 2008;49(2):289–95.

53. Thornton RH, Solomon SB, Dupuy DE, et al. Phrenic nerve injury resulting from percutaneous ablation of lung malignancy. AJR Am J Roentgenol 2008; 191(2):565–8.

54. Lee KS, Im JG, Kim IY, et al. Tumours involving the intrathoracic vagus and phrenic nerves demonstrated by computed tomography: anatomical features. Clin Radiol 1991;44(5):302–5.

55. Gaeta M, Barca E, Ruggeri P, et al. Late-onset Pompe disease (LOPD): correlations between respiratory muscles CT and MRI features and pulmonary function. Mol Genet Metab 2013;110(3):290–6.

56. Goerres GW, Kamel E, Heidelberg TN, et al. PET-CT image co-registration in the thorax: influence of respiration. Eur J Nucl Med Mol Imaging 2002; 29(3):351–60.

57. Wens SC, Ciet P, Perez-Rovira A, et al. Lung MRI and impairment of diaphragmatic function in Pompe disease. BMC Pulm Med 2015;15(1):54.

58. Kiryu S, Loring SH, Mori Y, et al. Quantitative analysis of the velocity and synchronicity of diaphragmatic motion: dynamic MRI in different postures. Magn Reson Imaging 2006;24(10):1325–32.

Section 2: Disorders

Disorders of the Diaphragm

F. Dennis McCool, MD*, Kamran Manzoor, MD, Taro Minami, MD

KEYWORDS

• Diaphragm dysfunction • Diaphragm ultrasound • Diaphragm eventration

KEY POINTS

- Diaphragm dysfunction can arise from pathologic processes or injuries that affect the central nervous system, phrenic nerve, neuromuscular junction, or muscle itself.
- The difference between upright and supine vital capacity can be used to screen for diaphragm dysfunction.
- A definitive diagnosis can be made by measuring transdiaphragmatic pressure or by ultrasound measurements of diaphragm thickness or diaphragm dome excursion.
- Treatment of diaphragm dysfunction depends on the underlying cause, but may include observation, noninvasive positive pressure ventilation, diaphragm pacing, or surgical interventions such as placation or nerve transfers.

ANATOMY

The diaphragm is a musculotendinous, dome-shaped structure that separates the thorax from the abdomen. It is lined by peritoneum on the abdominal surface and pleura on the intrathoracic surface.[1] It is the major muscle of inspiration and also acts as a barrier to the transmission of abdominal pressure to the thorax (**Fig. 1**). It consists of a muscular component and a central tendon. The muscular component can be subdivided into 2 parts, the costal and crural diaphragm. The costal diaphragm originates anteriorly at the sternum, laterally along the inner surface of the lower 6 ribs and anteromedially along the costal cartilages. The crural diaphragm originates posteriorly along the upper 3 lumbar vertebral bodies and the medial and lateral arcuate ligaments. The region of diaphragm that abuts the lower rib cage constitutes the zone of apposition of the diaphragm to the rib cage. The diaphragm is thicker than the central tendon. In dogs, the thickness of the costal diaphragm is relatively constant from the origin in the chest wall to the insertion in the central tendon. The crural diaphragm is thicker near the central tendon in comparison with its origin.[2]

The muscular component of the diaphragm inserts into the fibrous central tendon, which has a thin but strong aponeurosis. The central tendon of the diaphragm varies in size among individuals. It may comprise less than 10% of the diaphragm to more than 35% of the diaphragm in some individuals and is generally V shaped.[3] The diaphragm and central tendon have several openings that allow for communication between the abdominal and thoracic cavities; the caval hiatus (through the central tendon), aortic hiatus, and esophageal hiatus. These allow for passage of the great vessels, thoracic duct, and esophagus between the abdomen and thorax. The foramen of Morgagni is an anterior parasternal opening that allows for passage of the superior epigastric vessels. The

Disclosure: None of the authors have any financial interests in subject matter or materials discussed in this article.

Division of Pulmonary, Critical Care, and Sleep Medicine, The Warren Alpert Medical School of Brown University, Memorial Hospital of Rhode Island, 111 Brewster Street, Pawtucket, RI 02860, USA
* Corresponding author.
E-mail address: F_McCool@brown.edu

Clin Chest Med 39 (2018) 345–360
https://doi.org/10.1016/j.ccm.2018.01.012
0272-5231/18/© 2018 Elsevier Inc. All rights reserved.

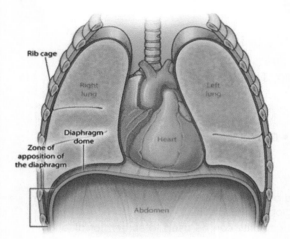

Fig. 1. The zone of apposition of the diaphragm to the rib cage. (*Adapted from* McCool FD, Tzelepis GE. Dysfunction of the diaphragm. N Engl J Med 2012;366:933; with permission.)

phrenic and pericardiophrenic arteries supply blood to the diaphragm. The pericardiophrenic arteries originate above the diaphragm and the phrenic artery originates from the aorta below the diaphragm.

The phrenic nerve innervates the diaphragm. This is primarily a motor nerve that arises from C3, C4, and C5, with most of the motoneurons located at the C4 level. In dogs, there may be more contribution of the rostral spinal phrenic neurons innervating the costal diaphragm. However, the same may not be true in humans. The right main trunk of the phrenic nerve enters the tendon and the left enters the muscle a short distance from the edge of the tendon.[4] Both phrenic nerves divide into 3 branches and sometime up to 5. These 3 to 5 trunks innervate the anterolateral, posteromedial, sternal, and crural portions of the diaphragm. The posterior division innervates the crural diaphragm. The branches then courses within the diaphragm muscle and runs in a plane midway between the pleural and the peritoneal layers. The diameter of the nerve decreases quickly as it branches distally, and it becomes difficult to distinguish nerve from blood vessels.[5] A much smaller accessory phrenic nerve has been described in 20% to 80% of individuals.[6] When present, the accessory phrenic nerve may originate in the spinal cord or the brachial plexus. When the accessory phrenic nerve originates from the brachial plexus, it runs parallel to the phrenic nerve and joins it in at the base of the neck or behind the clavicle. The sensory component of the phrenic nerve provides sensation to the pleura, mediastinum, and upper abdomen.[7] It

also receives input from muscle spindles and tendon organs embedded within the diaphragm muscle fibers. These specialized sensory inputs are involved with detecting changes in diaphragm length and may be important in optimizing sarcomere length–tension relationships.[8]

PHYSIOLOGY

The diaphragm is the major muscle of inspiration, and its action normally accounts for approximately 70% of the inspired tidal volume.[9] When the diaphragm contracts, it moves caudally, increases intraabdominal pressure, and lowers intrapleural pressure. This reduction in pleural pressure results in a decrease in intraalveolar pressure. Once intraalveolar pressure becomes subatmospheric, air moves from atmosphere into the alveoli. ensues. The lower rib cage moves outward when the diaphragm contracts (inflationary), whereas the upper rib cage moves inwards (deflationary). The inflationary movement of the lower rib cage is a consequence of increased intraabdominal pressure in the zone of apposition and to the insertional force of the diaphragm on the lower rib cage (**Fig. 2**). By contrast, the deflationary movement of the upper rib cage is a consequence of the lowering of intrapleural pressure. To prevent the upper rib cage from deflating during inspiration, other inspiratory accessory inspiratory muscles, such as the external intercostals, contract and either stabilize the upper rib cage or cause it to expand.

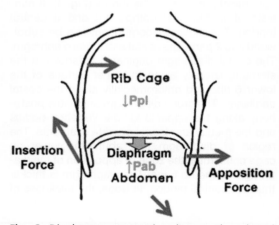

Fig. 2. Diaphragm contraction lowers the pleural pressure (Ppl) and increases abdominal pressure (Pab). The reduction in Ppl causes the upper rib cage to move inwards. The caudal inspiratory motion of the diaphragm causes the lower rib cage to move outwards. This outward displacement is due to diaphragm insertional forces and positive Pab in the zone of apposition.

Because of its critical role in ventilation, the diaphragm is the only skeletal muscle that is continually contracting, even during sleep. The diaphragm is composed of 55% slow twitch (type 1 fibers), which are oxidative and are highly resistant to fatigue; 25% fast twitch glycolytic-oxidative fibers (type 2B), which are relatively resistant to fatigue, and 20% glycolytic fast twitch fibers (type 2A), which are susceptible to fatigue.[10] Therefore, the diaphragm is relatively resistant to fatigue and recovers more quickly from fatigue than other skeletal muscle.[11,12]

There is volitional and automatic control of breathing. The diaphragm is the only skeletal muscle with a "pacemaker." The rhythmic nature of breathing is determined by a respiratory control center located in the brain stem. The rate and depth of breathing are determined by the interaction of pontine and medullary groups of neurons. Inspiration is initiated by groups of neurons located in the ventral respiratory group of the medulla. Efferents project from the ventral respiratory group to the diaphragm and other inspiratory muscles. Afferents from chemoreceptors located in the medulla and, to a lesser extent, in the carotid body project to the respiratory centers in the brainstem to stimulate breathing. The primary stimulus is provided by increasing levels of CO_2 and consequent changes in pH. Typically, ventilation increases by 2 L/min for every mm Hg increase in CO_2. In addition to this automatic control of breathing, there is volitional control.

CLINICAL MANIFESTATIONS OF DIAPHRAGM DYSFUNCTION

The incidence and prevalence of diaphragm paralysis and weakness are unknown. Diaphragmatic weakness or paralysis can involve either one or both hemidiaphragms.[13,14] Individuals with unilateral diaphragmatic paralysis are generally asymptomatic unless there are comorbid conditions such as obesity or underlying lung disease. In this context, patients with unilateral diaphragm paralysis may experience dyspnea in the supine position, dyspnea with exertion, and difficulty sleeping. Individuals with bilateral diaphragm paralysis are generally more symptomatic. They experience more dyspnea and are especially intolerant of the supine position, often to the point where they present with orthopnea. They are dependent on accessory muscles in the neck, rib cage, and shoulder girdle to breathe. Therefore, activities that involve the upper extremities, such as raising the arms above the head, render these muscles less effective for breathing and result in dyspnea. Similarly,

activities that increase the intraabdominal pressure, such as bending or lifting, cause dyspnea by displacing the diaphragm into the thoracic cavity. Immersion in water elicits profound dyspnea because the muscles used to compensate for diaphragm paralysis are rendered ineffective. Nocturnal hypoventilation can be a major problem for individuals with bilateral diaphragm weakness. Normally, during rapid eye movement sleep, the diaphragm is the only functioning inspiratory muscle and the accessory inspiratory muscles are quiescent. Consequently, individuals with weak or paralyzed diaphragms may present with symptoms of hypoventilation, such as frequent nocturnal awakenings, nocturia, vivid nightmares, night sweats, daytime hypersomnolence, depression, and morning headaches.[15–18] This occurs to a lesser extent in individuals with unilateral diaphragm paralysis.

The physical examination is more remarkable in bilateral diaphragm paralysis than unilateral paralysis. Nonspecific abnormalities include a rapid respiratory rate and use of the accessory muscles of inspiration, which can be appreciated by palpation or inspection. More specific to the presence of diaphragm paralysis is the observation of paradoxic inward motion of the abdominal wall during inspiration. This breathing pattern is most noticeable when these individuals are supine and is accompanied by an increase in the respiratory rate. Careful chest wall percussion during inspiration and expiration can detect the absence of diaphragmatic movement.

DIAGNOSIS OF DIAPHRAGM DYSFUNCTION

The presence of unilateral diaphragm paralysis is often suggested by the presence of an elevated hemidiaphragm on a chest radiograph (**Fig. 3**). However, diaphragm eventration, subpulmonic effusion, lobar atelectasis, or a subphrenic abscess can give a similar radiographic appearance. Measurements of lung volumes in the seated position also are nonspecific, demonstrating normal lung volumes or mild restriction. Confirmation of the diagnosis is accomplished by performing a "sniff test." For this test, fluoroscopy or ultrasound imaging is used to evaluate diaphragm motion. When someone with unilateral diaphragm paralysis sniffs vigorously, there is paradoxic (cephalad) movement of the paralyzed hemidiaphragm.

The diagnosis of bilateral diaphragmatic paralysis can be more problematic and requires a high index of suspicion. Chest radiography typically shows low lung volumes accompanied by

UNILATERAL DIAPHRAGM PARALYSIS

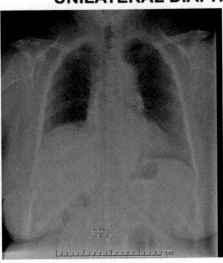
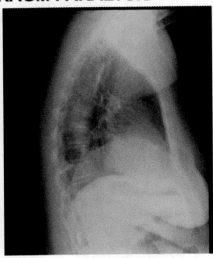

PA   **LATERAL**

Fig. 3. Chest radiographs demonstrating an elevated right hemidiaphragm. This is appreciated on the posteroanterior (PA) view and the lateral view.

elevation of both hemidiaphragms. This finding may be due to a poor inspiratory effort, morbid obesity, or atelectasis. The measurement of lung volumes in the seated position are nonspecific and typically demonstrate moderate to severe restriction with total lung capacity and vital capacity (VC) reduced to a range of 30% to 60% predicted. This degree of restriction may be seen with other pulmonary parenchymal or chest wall processes. Inspiratory muscle strength, as assessed by static maximal inspiratory pressure (MIP), is reduced to 20% to 30% of predicted in individuals with bilateral diaphragmatic paralysis and may be normal in unilateral paralysis. Weakness may be due to a number of processes causing generalized muscle weakness, alterations in diaphragm mechanical advantage, or poor subject performance of the maneuver.

Once suspected, screening for diaphragm dysfunction can be accomplished by measuring the change in VC from the seated to supine position (ΔVC-supine). A reduction in VC of 25% to 50% of the seated VC when assuming the supine position is consistent with diaphragm dysfunction. In general, the greater the reduction in supine VC, the greater the degree of diaphragm weakness.[19,20] The specificity and sensitivity for the presence of diaphragm dysfunction with a 25% or greater decrease in supine VC are 90% and 70%, respectively.[19,21] Calculating the maximal expiratory pressure (MEP) to MIP ratio provides another means of screening for diaphragm dysfunction.[21] Because expiratory muscle

function is often preserved in patients with isolated diaphragm dysfunction and inspiratory strength is decreased, the MEP to MIP ratio will be increased. A MEP/MIP of 1.5 has a sensitivity of 87% when screening for unilateral diaphragm paralysis and a MEP/MIP of 3.0 has a sensitivity of 85% when screening for bilateral diaphragm paralysis. Because this ratio correlates well with the ΔVC-supine and the MEP and MIP are measured with the subject seated, it can be a surrogate for ΔVC-supine for individuals who cannot tolerate the supine position.

Confirming the diagnosis of bilateral diaphragm paralysis can be accomplished by measuring transdiaphragmatic pressure (Pdi). When the diaphragm contracts, it decreases the intrapleural pressure and increases intraabdominal pressure thereby increasing Pdi. Because esophageal pressure (Pes) is a surrogate for pleural pressure and gastric pressure (Pga) is a surrogate for abdominal pressure, Pdi can be assessed by placing small air-filled catheters in the esophagus and stomach and measuring the difference between gastric and Pes (Pdi = Pga − Pes; **Fig. 4**). With diaphragm paralysis, there is no increase in Pdi during inspiration, with vigorous inspiratory efforts against a closed glottis (Pdi_{max} maneuver) or during a maximal sniff (Pdi sniff). Diaphragm dysfunction is present when Pdi sniff is 30 cm H_2O or less, or the ratio of ΔPga/ΔPdi is less than or equal to 0^{19} (**Fig. 5**). A sniff Pdi or Pdi_{max} of greater than 80 cm H_2O in men and greater than 70 cm H_2O in women excludes significant diaphragmatic

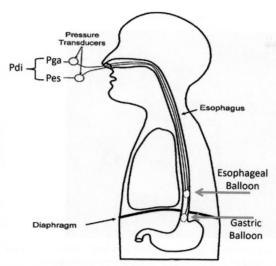

Fig. 4. Esophageal and gastric pressures (Pes and Pga) are measured by placing balloon tipped catheters in the esophagus and stomach. The transdiaphragmatic pressure (Pdi) is the difference between Pga and Pes.

weakness.[22,23] An effort-independent means of assessing diaphragm strength is to measure the Pdi after transcutaneously stimulating the phrenic nerve (twitch Pdi). This measure can be especially useful in cases where the lack of effort is an issue or when diagnosing unilateral diaphragm paralysis. A twitch Pdi of greater than 10 cm H_2O with unilateral phrenic nerve stimulation or greater than 20 cm H_2O with bilateral phrenic nerve stimulation excludes significant weakness of the diaphragm.[23] The Measurements of Pdi_{max} and Pdi twitch are time consuming, difficult to perform, and cause some patient discomfort. Therefore, the measurement of Pdi is not widely incorporated into clinical practice.

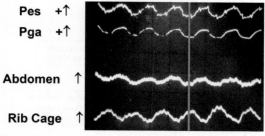

Fig. 5. Tracings of esophageal (Pes), gastric (Pga), rib cage dimensions, and abdominal dimensions in an individual with bilateral diaphragm paralysis. The vertical line represents end-inspiration. Note there is no difference between Pga and Pes and there is paradoxic inward motion of the abdomen during inspiration.

An alternate means of evaluating diaphragm function is the use of transthoracic ultrasound imaging. This technique is less invasive, readily available, and allows for independent assessment of both hemidiaphragms. There are 2 general approaches when using ultrasound imaging, evaluating motion of the diaphragm dome or evaluating diaphragm muscle thickening during inspiration. When the diaphragm contracts, it shortens and thickens. The hallmark for diagnosing diaphragm paralysis with ultrasound imaging is an absence of diaphragm thickening during inspiration. The optimal area for imaging diaphragm thickening is in the zone of apposition of the diaphragm to the rib cage (**Fig. 6**). This area is where the diaphragm abuts the lower rib cage. To visualize the diaphragm in the zone of apposition, the transducer is placed on the skin surface over the lower rib cage in the midaxillary in the coronal plane.[24,25] Diaphragm imaging is further discussed in Taro Minami and colleagues' article, "Assessing Diaphragm Function in Chest Wall and Neuromuscular Diseases," in this issue.

A second ultrasound technique used to evaluate diaphragm function is visualizing motion of the diaphragm dome. This can be accomplished by placing the ultrasound transducer subcostally and aiming the beam in a cephalad direction. Because air is strongly echogenic and will reflect all sound transmitted toward it, the image of the diaphragm dome is comprised of the intensely reflected sound at the interface of the diaphragm and lung and not the diaphragm muscle itself. Normally, the diaphragm dome moves toward the transducer during inspiration.[26–28] A paralyzed diaphragm or hemidiaphragm will not move or will move cephalad rather than toward the transducer. This cephalad motion is exaggerated by having the individual sniff (sniff test). Thus, paradoxic motion of the dome, as documented either with ultrasound or fluoroscopy can be used as a criterion to diagnose unilateral diaphragm paralysis. The sniff test is positive in more than 90% of patients with unilateral paralysis.[29] However, bilateral diaphragm paralysis cannot be confirmed by evaluating the motion of the diaphragm dome. With bilateral paralysis, the diaphragm may move in a normal caudal direction during inspiration. This caudal motion is related to the 2 compensatory strategies that individuals with bilateral paralysis use to breathe.[30] When using the external intercostal muscles to actively inhale or the abdominal muscles to passively inhale, the diaphragm will move caudally because the subdiaphragmatic pressure becomes more negative. Although not helpful in confirming diaphragm paralysis, diaphragm electromyography and phrenic nerve

End - Expiration   Inspiration

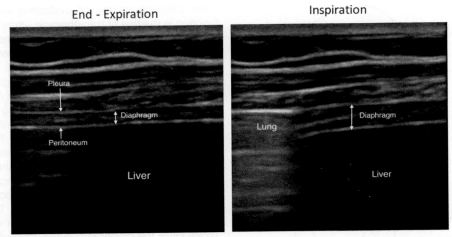

Fig. 6. Diaphragm ultrasound examination of the zone of apposition at end-expiration and end-inspiration in an individual with normal diaphragm function. There is thickening of the normally functioning diaphragm.

conduction studies may be useful to distinguish neuropathy or myopathy.[31]

If the diagnosis of bilateral diaphragmatic paralysis is confirmed, an evaluation for nocturnal hypoventilation should be undertaken. In addition, computed tomography (CT) scan of the chest may be needed to exclude a mediastinal mass, and MRI of the neck may be necessary to evaluate the spinal cord and nerve roots **Fig. 7**. The diagnostic approaches to evaluating unilateral and bilateral diaphragm paralysis are summarized in **Figs. 8** and **9**.

CAUSES OF DIAPHRAGM DYSFUNCTION

A myriad of disorders that involve either the central nervous system, phrenic nerve, neuromuscular junction, or diaphragm muscle itself can cause weakness or paralysis and involve either one or both hemidiaphragms.[18,32–37] A partial list of these disorders is given in **Box 1**.

Central Nervous System Injuries

Injuries to the brain rarely result in diaphragm dysfunction. Cerebrovascular accidents or demyelinating processes involving the brain stem may cause acute or chronic diaphragmatic weakness. This complication is infrequent in multiple sclerosis; typically, the degree of diaphragm weakness seen in multiple sclerosis is not clinically significant.[38] Spinal cord injuries at C1 or C2 cause acute diaphragm paralysis and the immediate

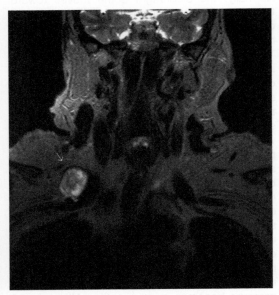

Fig. 7. MRI of the neck revealing a schwannoma (*arrow*) compressing the right phrenic nerve and causing right hemidiaphragm paralysis (same individual as in **Fig. 3**).

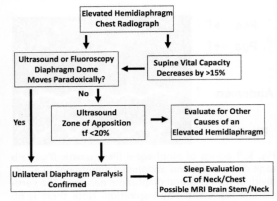

Fig. 8. Algorithm for the evaluation of an elevated hemidiaphragm. CT, computed tomography; tf, thickening fraction.

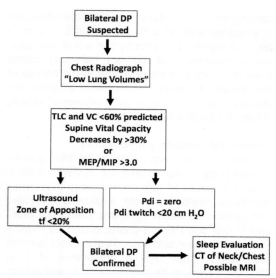

Fig. 9. Algorithm for evaluation of suspected bilateral diaphragm paralysis (DP). CT, computed tomography; MEP, maximal expiratory pressure; MIP, maximal inspiratory pressure; Pdi, transdiaphragmatic pressure; TLC, total lung capacity; VC, vital capacity.

need for ventilator support. Injuries at spinal levels C3 to C5 involve the phrenic nerve roots, resulting in a degree of diaphragm weakness sufficient to require ventilator support. The spinal injury is in part related to spinal cord edema; as the spinal edema resolves, there may be less need for ventilator support.[39] Other diseases that can affect phrenic nerve motor neurons and lead to diaphragm dysfunction include amyotrophic lateral sclerosis, poliomyelitis, syringomyelia, paraneoplastic motor neuropathies (anti-Hu syndrome), and spinal muscular atrophies. Diaphragm dysfunction also can be seen in postpolio syndrome, where there is motor unit degeneration in nerves previously affected by the polio virus decades after the initial polio viral infection.[40]

Phrenic Nerve Injuries

The phrenic nerve traverses a long course from the cervical spine to the diaphragm and is susceptible to injury anywhere along its course. It can be injured directly or severed by trauma, or it can be compressed by adjacent neoplastic processes, anterior or middle mediastinal masses or cervical masses. Tumors of neural origin such as schwannomas may directly involve the phrenic nerve and present as a posterior mediastinal mass. Inflammatory or toxic neuropathies of varied etiologies injure the phrenic nerve and lead to diaphragm dysfunction; a relatively common example is neuralgic amyotrophy (Parsonage

---

Box 1
Causes of diaphragm dysfunction

1. Affecting the nervous system
   a. Central nervous system (brain and/or spinal cord)
      i. Multiple sclerosis
      ii. Stroke
      iii. Arnold-Chiari malformation
      iv. Tetraplegia
      v. Spinal muscular atrophy
      vi. Syringomyelia
      vii. Spinal cord injury
   b. Motor neuron disease
      i. Amyotrophic lateral sclerosis
      ii. Poliomyelitis
   c. Peripheral nervous system
      i. Guillain-Barre syndrome
      ii. Chronic inflammatory demyelinating polyneuropathy
      iii. Neuralgic amyotrophy (Parsonage-Turner syndrome)
      iv. Critical illness polyneuropathy
      v. Phrenic nerve injury (trauma, tumor compression, surgery)
      vi. Idiopathic
2. Affecting muscle
   a. Myopathy
      i. Muscular dystrophies
      ii. Myositis (infectious, inflammatory, metabolic)
      iii. Acid maltase deficiency
      iv. Glucocorticoids
      v. Critical illness polymyopathy
      vi. Disuse atrophy
   b. Mechanical disadvantage
      i. Chronic obstructive pulmonary disease (hyperinflation)
      ii. Asthma (hyperinflation)
      iii. Flail chest (shortened operational length)
3. Affecting neuromuscular junction
   a. Myasthenia gravis
   b. Lambert-Eaton syndrome
   c. Botulism
   d. Organophosphates
   e. Other drugs

Turner syndrome). Neuralgic amyotrophy has been linked to the *SEPT9* gene and may occasionally be an extrahepatic manifestation of hepatitis E. Polyneuropathies such as Guillain-Barre syndrome may cause weakness and should have sequential measurements of VC to monitor the need for mechanical ventilation.[41] Respiratory failure may be impending if the VC drops to 15 mL/kg or less in Guillain-Barre syndrome.[42] Infections such as Lyme disease and those owing to herpes zoster can affect the phrenic nerve. Cervical spine disease can impinge the phrenic nerve. Iatrogenic phrenic injuries can be seen after shoulder or cervical manipulation or internal jugular canalization. Other disorders affecting the phrenic nerves include Charcot-Marie-Tooth disease and chronic inflammatory demyelinating polyneuropathy.

Neuromuscular Junction

Myasthenia gravis, Lambert-Eaton syndrome, and botulism involve the neuromuscular junction and can cause diaphragm paralysis or weakness.[33,41] The pathogenesis of these disorders differs. With myasthenia gravis, antibodies directed against the acetylcholine receptor impair transmission across the neuromuscular junction. With Lambert-Eaton syndrome, antibodies against the presynaptic voltage–gated calcium channels impair signal transmission. The *Clostridium botulinum* toxin (type A) also impairs neuromuscular transmission of acetylcholine.[43] Rarely, aminoglycosides may interfere with neuromuscular transmission.

Myopathies

Diaphragm weakness may be caused by a number of myopathic processes. Duchenne, limb girdle, and Becker muscular dystrophy can be associated with diaphragm weakness and paralysis. Duchenne muscular dystrophy is a relatively common X-linked disorder affecting 1 in 3500 male births.[44] It is caused by a mutation of the dystrophin gene located on chromosome Xp21.[45] This gene encodes dystrophin, which is a 427-kDa protein localized to the sarcolemma, where it forms a dystrophin–glycoprotein complex. In Duchenne muscular dystrophy, muscle degeneration occurs because the absence of dystrophin makes the sarcolemma vulnerable to damage.[46] Weakness manifests in childhood with Duchenne muscular dystrophy. Weakness and respiratory failure may occur at an even younger age in individuals with Ulrich's congenital myopathy and fascio-scapular–humeral dystrophies.[47,48] With Becker dystrophy, dystrophin is present but deficient, causing weakness later in life.[49,50] Other muscular dystrophies such as limb girdle muscular dystrophy and myotonic dystrophy can affect the respiratory muscles, but do not generally cause respiratory impairment until later in the course of the disease. Muscular dystrophies are further discussed in John C. Carter and colleagues' article, "Muscular Dystrophies," in this issue.

Chronic inflammatory myopathies

Dermatomyositis (DM), polymyositis (PM), and inclusion body myositis (IBM) are systemic inflammatory diseases of unknown etiology that cause peripheral skeletal muscle weakness and also can involve the diaphragm, and intercostal muscles.[51] DM and PM are characterized by muscle fiber inflammation and necrosis and affect females more than males with a prevalence of 1 in 100,000.[52] DM can be seen in children and adults, whereas IBM and PM are usually seen in adults with IBM more commonly affecting males. DM involves the perifascicular fibers and blood vessels. The inflammatory process may be due to complement-mediated microangiopathy or related to type 1 interferons. PM involves the muscle fascicles themselves. IBM is characterized by perimysium and perivascular inflammation and the presence of vacuoles. Tau protein and beta-amyloid precursor protein may contribute to muscle injury with IBM.[53,54]

The presence restrictive respiratory disease in patients with PM or DM may be due to respiratory muscle weakness or interstitial lung disease. Respiratory muscle weakness may be found in as many as 75% of individuals if respiratory muscle function is carefully evaluated.[55] Interstitial lung disease may develop in up to 70% of patients with DM or PM.[56] Concomitant interstitial lung disease and diaphragm weakness would worsen the restrictive process.

Muscle biopsy and serology can be used to distinguish among the inflammatory myopathies. Serologic markers that are elevated but nonspecific include creatinine kinase, aldolase, and lactate dehydrogenase. The greatest levels of these markers are typically seen with DM. Serologic markers that are specific for DM and PM include autoantibodies such as anti-Jo-1, antibodies to signal recognition particle (anti-SRP antibodies), and antibodies to Mi-2, a nuclear helicase.[57,58] Type 1 interferon-inducible transcripts may be seen with DM.[59] MRI demonstrates abnormal changes throughout the muscle with IBM, whereas the MRI changes with PM are only noted along fascial planes.[60] The presence of typical inclusion bodies on muscle biopsy is diagnostic of IBM.

Metabolic myopathies

Disordered glycogen metabolism can result in the accumulation of glycogen in skeletal and cardiac muscle. The glycogen storage diseases that are most likely to affect the respiratory system are acid maltase deficiency (type II, Pompe disease) and debranching enzyme deficiency (type III, Forbes-Cori disease). Acid maltase deficiency is due to the deficiency of acid α-glucosidase, an enzyme responsible for the degradation of glycogen polymers to glucose. Deficiency of this enzyme allows the accumulation of glycogen within cardiac and skeletal muscle lysosomes, resulting in myopathy. Although typically involving infants or children, this disease can manifest in adulthood.[61] When the onset of weakness begins after age 1, the disease is less severe and the prognosis is better. Diaphragm involvement may result in a decrease in VC and respiratory failure in the most severe cases.[62] Recombinant acid α-glucosidase enzyme replacement therapy may provide a means of stabilizing pulmonary function.[63,64] Mitochondrial disorders owing to deficiencies of enzymes in the mitochondrial respiratory chain complexes and to defects of phosphorylation–respiration coupling may cause cardiomyopathy or involve the diaphragm. Occasionally, mitochondrial myopathies can cause significant respiratory muscle weakness, resulting in nocturnal hypoventilation and the need for assisted ventilation.[65] Metabolic myopathies that are caused by defects of lipid metabolism (carnitine, palmitoyl transferase deficiency) usually do not cause respiratory disability, but involve other skeletal muscle groups (arms and legs). Other metabolic processes (hypokalemia) can result in diaphragm weakness. Metabolic myopathies are further discussed in Patrick Koo and Jigme M. Sethi's article, "Metabolic Myopathies and the Respiratory System," in this issue.

Critical Illness Neuropathy and Myopathy

Neuromuscular weakness is a common finding in patients who are in the intensive care unit. More than one-half of the patients on mechanical ventilation develop weakness within 24 hours,[66–69] and up to 80% of patients undergoing prolonged mechanical ventilation develop diaphragm weakness.[70] The presence of diaphragm weakness has been assessed by stimulating the phrenic nerve and measuring endotracheal tube pressure. Diaphragm weakness was defined as a twitch pressure endotracheal tube pressure of less than 11 cm H_2O. Potential causes of weakness in this context include Guillain-Barré syndrome, cardiogenic shock, rhabdomyolysis, ventilator-induced diaphragm dysfunction (VIDD), and critical illness neuropathy and myopathy. Myocyte atrophy and necrosis with thick filament (myosin) destruction[71] and vacuolization and phagocytosis of muscle fibers are characteristics of critical illness neuropathy and myopathy.[72]

Diaphragm weakness resulting from critical illness neuropathy and myopathy is associated with poor outcomes, such as increased mortality in the intensive care unit and prolonged duration of mechanical ventilation. Risk factors for developing critical illness neuropathy and myopathy include sepsis, multiorgan failure, total parenteral nutrition, hyperosmolality, renal failure, sedation, denutrition, and the use of medications such as catecholamines, steroids, and neuromuscular blocking agents.[67,73,74] The presence of heightened respiratory loads owing to pneumonia, atelectasis, or bronchospasm in concert with diaphragm weakness will prolong the need for ventilator support. Intensive insulin therapy maintaining serum glucose at 80 to 110 mg/dL may reduce the occurrence of critical illness polyneuropathy.

Ventilator-Induced Diaphragm Dysfunction

VIDD occurs in as many as 80% of mechanically ventilated patients,[75–77] VIDD is associated with atrophy of both fast and slow myofibers and can be manifest after only 24 to 36 hours of mechanical ventilation.[78] Patients with acute infection, systemic inflammation, or on modes of ventilation that promote diaphragm disuse are at risk for developing VIDD.[79] Underlying mechanisms thought to contribute to VIDD include activation of proteolytic pathways involving calpains, caspases, and proteasomes, as well as impaired mitochondrial electron transport function resulting in an increase in reactive oxygen species and oxidative stress.[80]

Individuals undergoing mechanical ventilation with diaphragm weakness are at a greater risk of death than those without weakness.[81] Prompt treatment of infections, avoiding oversedation and neuromuscular blocking agents, minimizing total time patients are ventilated mechanically, and avoiding excessive levels of ventilator support may be key factors to prevent and treat VIDD. Drugs that inhibit proteolytic pathways are under active investigation. The high prevalence of diaphragm dysfunction in mechanically ventilated patients and the poor outcomes they experience highlights the importance of identifying this patient population. To this end, ultrasound examination of the diaphragm has been used to predict extubation success and identify diaphragm atrophy.[82–84] DiNino and colleagues[85] studied diaphragm contraction using ultrasound imaging in 63 patients undergoing mechanical ventilation. They found that thickening of the diaphragm by more than 30% during inspiration (Δtdi% $\geq$30%) was a useful predictor of extubation outcomes when measured during pressure support of 5/5 cm H_2O. The sensitivity, specificity, positive predictive value, and negative predictive value of a Δtdi% of 30% or greater for extubation success was 88%, 71%, 91%, and 63%, respectively, with an area under the receiver operating characteristic curve of 0.79.[85] Sequential measurements of diaphragm thickness using ultrasound imaging have also been used to document diaphragm atrophy and increase in diaphragm thickness with training.[86,87] In a patient with high spinal cord injury, VT and tdi both increased as the diaphragm was electrically stimulated for 33 weeks. VT increased from 220 to 600 mL and tdi increased from 0.18 to 0.34 cm.

DIAPHRAGM EVENTRATION

Eventration refers to a condition where part of the diaphragm is replaced with fibroelastic tissue or where there is localized diaphragm atrophy. Eventration may be noted at birth and is due to failure of the fetal diaphragm to properly develop. In adults, it may be due to phrenic nerve injury or occur for unknown reasons.[88] Eventration can be seen on a chest radiograph as a localized area of diaphragm elevation. The localized nature of the eventration often is best appreciated on the lateral radiograph. The most common area for eventration is the anteromedial portion of the right hemidiaphragm. If the eventration involves an extensive area, the entire hemidiaphragm diaphragm seems to be elevated. Eventration can be distinguished from unilateral paralysis by using ultrasound imaging to demonstrate diaphragm thickening in the zone of apposition or by measuring twitch Pdi while stimulating the phrenic nerve on the side in question.[89]

As with unilateral diaphragm paralysis, eventration involving a hemidiaphragm is usually asymptomatic unless there are comorbid conditions that elicit dyspnea and, at times, chest pain.[90] The differential diagnosis of diaphragm eventration includes unilateral diaphragmatic paralysis, subdiaphragmatic or diaphragmatic masses, and subpulmonic pleural fluid. In the case of a mass, the contour of the diaphragmatic defect is more likely irregular and not necessarily located at the dome.

DIAPHRAGM TUMORS

Diaphragm tumors can be malignant (primary or metastatic), benign (cystic or solid), or owing to endometriosis. Fibrosarcomas and rhabdomyosarcoms of the diaphragm are very rare. Metastatic malignancies that involve the diaphragm with direct extension include primary lung or esophageal cancer and mesothelioma. Malignancies of the pancreas, stomach, or liver also may extend to the diaphragm. Lipomas are the most common benign solid tumor. Cystic lesions involving the diaphragm are bronchogenic or mesothelial cysts. Endometriosis usually presents with pneumothorax at the time of menses. Symptoms may include pleuritic pain, epigastric pain, cough, and dyspnea. Chest radiography may reveal an elevated hemidiaphragm, pleural effusion, or a localized diaphragm hump or diaphragm mass. The solid, cystic, or heterogeneous nature of the mass is better appreciated with CT scanning or ultrasound imaging. CT scans also may aid with determining of the tumor originates in the diaphragm, pleura, or retroperitoneum. The definitive diagnosis is made by obtaining tissue, which may require resection of the mass or CT-guided biopsy. Malignant tumors are resected if possible or may be treated with chemotherapy and radiation. Benign tumors are often resected because there is a concern that they are malignant. Endometriosis is usually treated medically.[91]

DIAPHRAGM TRAUMA

Traumatic injuries to the diaphragm are uncommon with an incidence of less than 1% when there is concurrent abdominal trauma.[92] If present, diaphragm injuries carry a high mortality ($\geq$25%). Diaphragm injury can occur in the setting of either blunt trauma (automobile accidents) or penetrating trauma (gunshot wounds, stabbings). When diaphragm injuries exist, associated injuries to other organs occurs 50% to 75% of the time.[93,94] The left hemidiaphragm seems to be more likely injured during blunt abdominal trauma.[93,94] However, in a porcine model, the right hemidiaphragm is more prone to traumatic rupture than the left.[95] With this model, the combination of the liver, spleen, and stomach may afford more protection to the left hemidiaphragm.

The severity of diaphragm injury ranges from contusion to lacerations, which can be very large with an area more than 25 cm^2. Large lacerations may be accompanied by herniation of abdominal contents seen on chest radiographs. Small lacerations may only be detected with 3-dimensional reconstruction of a CT scan. Intrathoracic complications of diaphragm trauma are common and may be seen on the CT scan. These complications include pleural effusion, hemothorax, and atelectasis. Ultrasound imaging also may be a useful diagnostic tool in evaluating diaphragm injuries.[95,96] Findings such as a discontinuous diaphragm image or herniation of abdominal contents into the thorax are indicative of diaphragm rupture.

A small tear in the diaphragm may not be apparent at the time of injury. However, as the diaphragm tear becomes larger with time, there may be herniation of abdominal contents or the development of symptoms such as chest pain or dyspnea.[97] In this context, the development of symptoms related to diaphragm tears may take days to weeks to develop. Treatment may include observation or surgical intervention. Spontaneous healing may occur in individuals with small tears and a greater proportion of muscle to central tendon, whereas for those with a greater proportion of central tendon, a surgical procedure may be needed.[3,98] Individuals undergoing laparoscopy after abdominal trauma should have the diaphragm inspected and repaired if needed and the timing is appropriate.

DIAPHRAGM HERNIAS

Congenital diaphragmatic hernias occur in approximately 1 in 2500 births in the United States. They form when the diaphragm muscle fails to develop prenatally. Consequently, abdominal viscera may migrate into the thorax. When this occurs in infants, there is hypoplasia of the ipsilateral lung, bronchial structure, and pulmonary arterial tree. The mortality and morbidity of congenital diaphragmatic hernias are related to the severity of lung hypoplasia and pulmonary hypertension, and the presence of associated cardiac anomalies. The diagnosis can be made prenatally with ultrasound examination. Among infants in whom congenital diaphragmatic hernia is not diagnosed in utero, the diagnosis is made by chest radiography or ultrasound imaging soon after birth showing herniation of abdominal contents. Respiratory failure requiring endotracheal intubation may ensue at the time of birth. Occasionally, there may be minimal respiratory distress or symptoms and the diagnosis is made later in life.

Surgical repair is often needed soon after birth. However, the timing of surgery varies and depends whether the infant has stabilized medically and if pulmonary hypertension has resolved. In some instances, extracorporeal membrane oxygenation may be needed to stabilize the infant. Surgical repair consists of closing the diaphragm defect with sutures alone or using a Gore-Tex patch.[99] Occasionally, surgery may need to be repeated later in life. This recurrence may be due to patch-related complications such as infection or to recurrent herniation.[100,101] Recurrent herniation may be more likely to occur in infants with large defects. Other late complications include pectus excavatum and scoliosis. These chest wall disorders are more likely to occur in infants who have had large defects repaired.[102,103] Other complications include gastroesophageal reflux, chronic respiratory disease, pulmonary hypertension, and neurodevelopmental impairment. Repair of congenital and traumatic hernias are reemphasizing the importance of its muscular and tendinous portions.

In contrast with infants, congenital hernias that present in adults are typically found incidentally and are not life threatening. The most common congenital adult hernias are Morgagni and Bochdalek. Bochadalek hernias are present in about 1 in 2200 to 12,500 births and the incidence of Bochadalek's hernia in routine CT scans has been reported to vary from as low as 0.17% to as high as 6.0%. Bochadelek hernia may cause respiratory distress at birth and carry a poor prognosis if large enough. The majority of adults with these hernias are asymptomatic and the hernia is found incidentally. The Morgagni hernias are usually anterior and involve the right hemidiaphragm 90% of the time. There is little risk for herniation, but if it occurs, omental fat usually comprises the herniated content. Bochdalek hernias occur posteriorly and laterally, and can involve either hemidiaphragm. However, they are more commonly are seen on the left. In 1 series, the CT prevalence of asymptomatic Bochdalek hernias in adults was 13%.[104,105] They are generally larger than Morgagni hernias and are more likely to have herniated retroperitoneal structures or intraabdominal viscera. If strangulation of the contents occurs, prompt reduction of the hernia and repair of the diaphragm defect is indicated.[106] Morgagni and Bochdalek hernias can usually be differentiated from diaphragm eventration on the lateral chest radiograph. If the diagnosis is unclear, a CT scan of the thorax is helpful or evaluation with a barium or gastrographin meal and or enema.

TREATMENT AND PROGNOSIS

The natural history of diaphragmatic dysfunction depends largely on its etiology and the rate of progression of underlying disease. In certain neuromuscular diseases (eg, muscular dystrophies) the course of diaphragmatic dysfunction is predictable, whereas in the case of posttraumatic or infectious diaphragmatic paralysis, recovery may occur in some, but not all, cases. The likelihood of spontaneous recovery of diaphragm function occurring depends on the etiology of the dysfunction. The phrenic nerve may be as long as 500 mm and is slow to regenerate. Therefore, diaphragm dysfunction with a brachial plexus neuritis (Parsonage Turner syndrome) or cervical impingement of the phrenic nerve, recovery of diaphragm function may take up to 3 years.[37,107–109] Recovery times may be shorter with diaphragm dysfunction after cardiac surgery, typically recovering within 1 year.[110] Roughly one-half of patients with subacute idiopathic diaphragm dysfunction or with Parsonage Turner syndrome (neuralgic amyotrophy) have full recovery of diaphragm function. Diaphragm dysfunction owing to metabolic myopathies may be improved by correcting electrolyte imbalances (hypokalemia, hypomagnesemia, or hypophosphatemia) or replacing thyroid hormone. Toxic or metabolic disturbances related to diabetes, alcohol, or viral infections may resolve with treatment of the underlying disease. Infectious myopathies owing to parasitic infection may respond to appropriate antimicrobials.

When diaphragm dysfunction persists or progresses, ventilatory support may be needed. The need for noninvasive ventilation may be temporary and only delivered at night, as in cases of diaphragm paralysis after cardiac surgery, or permanent and needed throughout the day as in cases of progressive neuromuscular diseases. Nocturnal hypoventilation may manifest only during rapid eye movement sleep, where there is suppression of intercostal and accessory muscle activity, or may be seen with all stages of sleep.[111] It is most likely to occur in patients with bilateral diaphragm paralysis; however, it can be seen with unilateral paralysis if there is significant weakness (unilateral twitch Pdi <5 cm H_2O).[17] In patients with diaphragmatic weakness owing to a neuromuscular disease who have concomitant weakness of pharyngeal and laryngeal muscles, such as muscular dystrophy or amyotrophic lateral sclerosis, obstructive sleep apnea may also occur.[111]

Noninvasive positive-pressure ventilation can improve both symptoms and physiologic derangements in patients with diaphragm dysfunction by reversing nocturnal hypoventilation. The improvement in ventilation may be related to reducing the work of breathing and resting the diaphragm during periods of mechanical ventilation. Noninvasive positive-pressure ventilation may improve respiratory drive by chronically lowering levels of carbon dioxide and "resetting" chemoreceptors in the medulla such that arterial blood gases normalize. Noninvasive ventilation improves daytime function, quality of life, physical activity, and hemodynamics.[112,113]

Diaphragm plication is a procedure where the flaccid hemidiaphragm is made taut by oversewing the membranous central tendon and the muscular components of the diaphragm thereby immobilizing the flaccid diaphragm and reducing its paradoxic motion. Diaphragm plication may result in up to 20% increases in VC, forced expiratory volume in 1 second, and total lung capacity.[114,115] The indications for this type of surgery are not fully defined. The procedure may be offered to patients with unilateral diaphragm paralysis who are symptomatic (severe dyspnea, cough, or chest pain) and performed with caution in obese individuals and those with neuromuscular diseases.[116] However, a prolonged observation period of several months may be needed to ensure there is no spontaneous recovery of diaphragm function. Prolonged observation may be prudent for patients with diaphragm paralysis after cardiac surgery or other surgical procedures involving the cervical or mediastinal regions, because phrenic nerve function may improve with time.[117] Surgical plication of the paralyzed hemidiaphragm may improve VC, but this intervention has no role in bilateral diaphragm paralysis.

Phrenic nerve pacing has the potential to provide full ventilatory support to ventilator-dependent patients with bilateral diaphragm paralysis and intact phrenic nerves. Candidates for this therapeutic modality are primarily patients with high cervical cord tetraplegia or patients with central hypoventilation. Diaphragm muscle pacing systems differ from phrenic nerve pacers. Electrodes are placed directly in the diaphragm muscle with this technique. This measure can be accomplished laparoscopically and thus is less invasive than placing electrodes on the phrenic nerve. There is continued development diaphragm pacing technology that is further discussed in Anthony F. DiMarco's article, "Diaphragm Pacing," in this issue. Interventions such as sural or intercostal nerve grafting and transfers may provide options in the future to restore diaphragm function.[118]

These techniques have not reached the point of becoming a reliable means of restoring diaphragm function.

SUMMARY

The diaphragm is a dome-shaped structure that separates the thorax from the abdomen. It is the major inspiratory muscle and serves to separate the abdominal contents from the thorax. Disorders of the diaphragm may impair its performance or disrupt its integrity. Impaired performance can result in dyspnea, poor exercise performance, or nocturnal hypoventilation. Its integrity can be impaired locally by eventration. However, with diaphragm hernias or trauma, diaphragm integrity may be diminished to the extent that there is free communication between the thoracic and abdominal cavities. This may lead to herniation of abdominal contents into the thorax, which can be life threatening. Ultrasound examination of the diaphragm zone of apposition provides a noninvasive means of assessing diaphragm dysfunction and CT reconstruction a means of assessing its integrity. Treatment to restore diaphragm function revolves around addressing underlying causes and careful observation because the phrenic nerve may spontaneously recover from injury. VIDD may be avoided by avoiding certain ventilator strategies. Diaphragm plication has a role in selected patients with unilateral paralysis, and phrenic pacing has been beneficial in patients with high cervical spinal cord injuries and central hypoventilation. Sural nerve transplants and diaphragm pacing show promise and are continuing to evolve.

REFERENCES

1. Lessaa TB, de Abreua DK, Bertassoli BM, et al. Diaphragm: a vital respiratory muscle in mammals. Ann Anat 2016;205:122–7.
2. Boriek AM, Aladin M, Rodarte JR. Inferences on passive diaphragm mechanics from gross anatomy. J Appl Physiol 1994;77:2065–70.
3. du Plessis M, Ramai D, Shah S, et al. The clinical anatomy of the musculotendinous part of the diaphragm. Surg Radiol Anat 2015;37:1013–20.
4. Merendino KA. The intradiaphragmatic distribution of the phrenic nerve: surgical significance. Surg Clin North Am 1964;44:1217–26.
5. An X, Yue B, Lee JH, et al. Intramuscular distribution of the phrenic nerve in human diaphragm as shown by Sihler staining. Muscle Nerve 2012;45:522–6.
6. Loukas M, Kinsella CR, Louis RG, et al. Surgical anatomy of the accessory phrenic nerve. Ann Thorac Surg 2006;82:1870–5.
7. Qvist G. Anatomical note. The course and relations of the left phrenic nerve in the neck. J Anat 1977;124:803–5.
8. McCool FD, Brown R, Mayewski RJ, et al. Effects of posture on stimulated ventilation in quadriplegia. Am Rev Respir Dis 1988;138:101–6.
9. Unal O, Arslan H, Uzun K, et al. Evaluation of diaphragmatic movement with MR fluoroscopy in chronic obstructive pulmonary disease. Clin Imaging 2000;24:347–50.
10. Rochester DF. The diaphragm: contractile properties and fatigue. J Clin Invest 1985;75:1397–402.
11. Gandevia SC, Mckenzie DK, Neering IR. Endurance properties of respiratory and limb muscles. Respir Physiol 1983;53:47–61.
12. McKenzie DK, Butler JE, Gandevia SC. Respiratory muscle function and activation in chronic obstructive pulmonary disease. J Appl Physiol 2009;107:621–9.
13. Dubé BP, Dres M. Diaphragm dysfunction: diagnostic approaches and management strategies. J Clin Med 2016;5(12) [pii:E113].
14. Lisboa C, Pare PD, Pertuze J, et al. Inspiratory muscle function in unilateral diaphragmatic paralysis. Am Rev Respir Dis 1986;134(3):488–92.
15. Hart N, Nickol AH, Cramer D, et al. Effect of severe isolated unilateral and bilateral diaphragm weakness on exercise performance. Am J Respir Crit Care Med 2002;165(9):1265–70.
16. Kumar N, Folger WN, Bolton CF. Dyspnea as the predominant manifestation of bilateral phrenic neuropathy. Mayo Clin Proc 2004;79(12):1563–5.
17. Steier J, Jolley CJ, Seymour J, et al. Sleep-disordered breathing in unilateral diaphragm paralysis or severe weakness. Eur Respir J 2008;32(6):1479–87.
18. McCool FD, Tzelepis GE. Dysfunction of the diaphragm. N Engl J Med 2012;366:932–42.
19. Fromageot C, Lofaso F, Annane D, et al. Supine fall in lung volumes in the assessment of diaphragmatic weakness in neuromuscular disorders. Arch Phys Med Rehabil 2001;82:123–8.
20. Mier-Jedrzejowicz A, Brophy C, Moxham J, et al. Assessment of diaphragm weakness. Am Rev Respir Dis 1988;137:877–83.
21. Koo P, Oyieng'o DO, Gartman EJ, et al. The maximal expiratory-to-inspiratory pressure ratio and supine vital capacity as screening tests for diaphragm dysfunction. Lung 2017;195:29–35.
22. Polkey MI, Green M, Moxham J. Measurement of respiratory muscle strength. Thorax 1995;50(11):1131–5.
23. Steier J, Kaul S, Seymour J, et al. The value of multiple tests of respiratory muscle strength. Thorax 2007;62(11):975–80.
24. Wait JL, Nahormek PA, Yost WT, et al. Diaphragmatic thickness–lung volume relationship in vivo. J Appl Physiol 1989;67:1560–8.
25. Cohn D, Benditt JO, Eveloff S. McCool FD diaphragm thickening during inspiration. J Appl Physiol 1997;83:291–6.
26. Gerscovich EO, Cronan M, McGahan JP, et al. Ultrasonographic evaluation of diaphragmatic motion. J Ultrasound Med 2001;20:597–604.
27. Lloyd T, Tang YM, Benson MD, et al. Diaphragmatic paralysis: the use of M mode ultrasound for diagnosis in adults. Spinal Cord 2006;44:505–8.
28. Boussuges A, Gole Y, Blanc P. Diaphragmatic motion studied by M-mode ultrasonography: methods, reproducibility, and normal values. Chest 2009;135:391–400.

29. Gierada DS, Slone RM, Fleishman MJ. Imaging evaluation of the diaphragm. Chest Surg Clin N Am 1998;8:237–80.

30. McCool FD, Mead J. Dyspnea on immersion: mechanisms in patients with bilateral diaphragm paralysis. Am Rev Respir Dis 1989;139(1):275–6.

31. Saadeh PB, Crisafulli CF, Sosner J, et al. Needle electromyography of the diaphragm: a new technique. Muscle Nerve 1993;16(1):15–20.

32. Gibson GJ. Diaphragmatic paresis: pathophysiology, clinical features, and investigation. Thorax 1989;44:960–70.

33. Laroche CM, Carroll N, Moxham J, et al. Clinical significance of severe isolated diaphragm weakness. Am Rev Respir Dis 1988;138:862–6.

34. Laghi F, Tobin MJ. Disorders of the respiratory muscles. Am J Respir Crit Care Med 2003;168(1):10–48.

35. Wilcox PG, Pardy RL. Diaphragmatic weakness and paralysis. Lung 1989;167(6):323–41.

36. Chan CK, Loke J, Virgulto JA, et al. Bilateral diaphragmatic paralysis: clinical spectrum, prognosis, and diagnostic approach. Arch Phys Med Rehabil 1988;69(11):976–9.

37. Hughes PD, Polkey MI, Moxham J, et al. Long-term recovery of diaphragm strength in neuralgic amyotrophy. Eur Respir J 1999;13(2):379–84.

38. Tzelepis GE, McCool FD. Respiratory dysfunction in multiple sclerosis. Respir Med 2015;109(6):671–9.

39. Wicks AB, Menter RR. Long-term outlook in quadriplegic patients with initial ventilator dependency. Chest 1986;90(3):406–10.

40. Dahan V, Kimoff RJ, Petrof BJ, et al. Sleep-disordered breathing in fatigued postpoliomyelitis clinic patients. Arch Phys Med Rehabil 2006;87(10):1352–6.

41. van Doorn PA, Ruts L, Jacobs BC. Clinical features, pathogenesis, and treatment of Guillain-Barre syndrome. Lancet Neurol 2008;7(10):939–50.

42. Cosi V, Versino M. Guillain-Barre syndrome. Neurol Sci 2006;27(Suppl 1):S47–51.

43. Witoonpanich R, Vichayanrat E, Tantisiriwit K, et al. Survival analysis for respiratory failure in patients with food-borne botulism. Clin Toxicol (Phila) 2010;48(3):177–83.

44. Nakamura A, Takeda S. Mammalian models of Duchenne muscular dys-trophy: pathological characteristics and therapeutic applications. J Biomed Biotechnol 2011;11:1–8.

45. Muntoni F, Torelli S, Ferlini A. Dystrophin and mutations: one gene, several proteins, multiple phenotypes. Lancet Neurol 2003;2:731–40.

46. Fairclough RJ, Bareja A, Davies KE. Progress in therapy for Duchenne muscular dystrophy. Exp Physiol 2011;96:1101–13.

47. Gozal D. Pulmonary manifestations of neuromuscular disease with special reference to Duchenne

muscular dystrophy and spinal muscular atrophy. Pediatr Pulmonol 2000;29:141–50.

48. Mercuri E, Yuva Y, Brown SC, et al. Collagen VI involvement in Ullrich syndrome: a clinical, genetic, and immunohistochemical study. Neurology 2002;58:1354–9.

49. Hoffman EP, Brown RH, Kunkel LM. Dystrophin: the protein product of the Duchenne muscular dystrophy locus. Cell 1998;51:919–28.

50. Kornegay JN, Childers MK, Bogan DJ, et al. The paradox of muscle hypertrophy in muscular dystrophy. Phys Med Rehabil Clin N Am 2012;23:149–72.

51. Crestani B. The respiratory system in connective tissue disorders. Allergy 2005;60:715–34.

52. Plotz PH, Dalakas M, Leff RL, et al. Current concepts in the idiopathic inflammatory myopathies: polymyositis, dermatomyositis, and related disorders. Ann Intern Med 1989;111:143–57.

53. Greenberg SA. Inclusion body myositis: review of recent literature. Curr Neurol Neurosci Rep 2009;9:83–9.

54. Salajegheh M, Pinkus JL, Nazareno R, et al. Nature of "Tau" immunoreactivity in normal myonuclei and inclusion body myositis. Muscle Nerve 2009;40:520–8.

55. Teixeira A, Cherin P, Demoule A, et al. Diaphragmatic dysfunction in patients with idiopathic inflammatory myopathies. Neuromuscul Disord 2005;15:32–9.

56. Watanabe K, Handa T, Tanizawa K, et al. Detection of antisynthetase syndrome in patients with idiopathic interstitial pneumonias. Respir Med 2011;105(8):1238–47.

57. Mammen AL. Dermatomyositis and polymyositis: clinical presentation, autoantibodies, and pathogenesis. Ann N Y Acad Sci 2010;1184:134.

58. Gunawardena H, Betteridge ZE, McHugh NJ. Myositis-specific autoantibodies: their clinical and pathogenic significance in disease expression. Rheumatology (Oxford) 2009;48:607–12.

59. Greenberg SA. Dermatomyositis and type 1 interferons. Curr Rheumatol Rep 2010;12:198–203.

60. Dion E, Cherin P, Payan C, et al. Magnetic resonance imaging criteria for distinguishing between inclusion body myositis and polymyositis. J Rheumatol 2002;29:1897–906.

61. Winkel LP, Hagemans ML, van Doorn PA, et al. The natural course of non-classic Pompe's disease: a review of 225 published cases. J Neurol 2005;252:875–84.

62. Prigent H, Orlikowski D, Laforêt P, et al. Supine volume drop and diaphragmatic function in adults with Pompe disease. Eur Respir J 2012;39(6):1545–6.

63. de Vries JM, van der Beek NA, Hop WC, et al. Effect of enzyme therapy and prognostic factors in 69 adults with Pompe disease: an open-label

single-center study. Orphanet J Rare Dis 2012; 26(7):73.

64. Toscano A, Schoser B. Enzyme replacement therapy in late-onset Pompe disease: a systematic literature review. J Neurol 2013;260(4):951–9.

65. van Adel BA, Tarnopolsky MA. Metabolic myopathies: update 2009. J Clin Neuromuscul Dis 2009; 10:97–121.

66. Chawla J, Gruener G. Management of critical illness polyneuropathy and myopathy. Neurol Clin 2010;28(4):961–77.

67. De Jonghe B, Lacherade JC, Durand MC, et al. Critical illness neuromuscular syndromes. Neurol Clin 2008;26:507–20.

68. Demoule A, Jung B, Prodanovic H, et al. Diaphragm dysfunction on admission to the intensive care unit. Prevalence, risk factors, and prognostic impact—a prospective study. Am J Respir Crit Care Med 2013;188:213–9.

69. Laghi F, Cattapan SE, Jubran A, et al. Is weaning failure caused by low-frequency fatigue of the diaphragm? Am J Respir Crit Care Med 2003;167: 120–7.

70. Dres M, Goligher EC, Heunks LMA, et al. Critical illness-associated diaphragm weakness. Intensive Care Med 2017;43:1441–52.

71. Amaya-Villar R, Garnacho-Montero J, Garcia-Garmendia JL, et al. Steroid-induced myopathy in patients intubated due to exacerbation of chronic obstructive pulmonary disease. Intensive Care Med 2005;31:157–61.

72. Helliwell TR, Coakley JH, Wagenmakers AJ, et al. Necrotizing myopathy in critically-ill patients. J Pathol 1991;64:307–14.

73. de Letter MA, Schmitz PI, Visser LH, et al. Risk factors for the development of polyneuropathy and myopathy in critically ill patients. Crit Care Med 2001;29:2281–6.

74. Deem S. Intensive-care-unit-acquired muscle weakness. Respir Care 2006;51:1042–52.

75. Hussain SN, Cornachione AS, Guichon C, et al. Prolonged controlled mechanical ventilation in humans triggers myofibrillar contractile dysfunction and myofilament protein loss in the diaphragm. Thorax 2016;71(5):436–45.

76. Dres M, Dube BP, Mayaux J, et al. Coexistence and impact of limb muscle and diaphragm weakness at time of liberation from mechanical ventilation in medical intensive care unit patients. Am J Respir Crit Care Med 2017;195(3):57–66.

77. Demoule A, Molinari N, Jung B, et al. Patterns of diaphragm function in critically ill patients receiving prolonged mechanical ventilation: a prospective longitudinal study. Ann Intensive Care 2016;6(1):75.

78. Jaber S, Petrof BJ, Jung B, et al. Rapidly progressive diaphragmatic weakness and injury during mechanical ventilation in humans. Am J Respir Crit Care Med 2011;183(3):364–71.

79. Supinski GS, Morris PE, Dhar S, et al. Diaphragm dysfunction in critical illness. Chest 2017;152: 1140–50.

80. Nelson WB, Smuder AJ, Hudson MB, et al. Crosstalk between the calpain and caspase-3 proteolytic systems in the diaphragm during prolonged mechanical ventilation. Crit Care Med 2012;40(6): 1857–63.

81. Supinski GS, Westgate P, Callahan LA. Correlation of maximal inspiratory pressure to transdiaphragmatic twitch pressure in intensive care unit patients. Crit Care 2016;20:77.

82. Grosu HB, Lee YI, Lee J, et al. Diaphragm muscle thinning in patients who are mechanically ventilated. Chest 2012;142:1455–60.

83. Umbrello M, Formenti P. Ultrasonographic assessment of diaphragm function in critically ill subjects. Respir Care 2016;61(4):542–55.

84. Blumhof S, Wheeler D, Thomas K, et al. Change in diaphragmatic thickness during the respiratory cycle predicts extubation success at various levels of pressure support ventilation. Lung 2016;194(4): 519–25.

85. DiNino EK, Gartman EJ, Sethi JM, et al. Diaphragm ultrasound as a predictor of successful extubation from mechanical ventilation. Thorax 2014;69:423–7.

86. Ayas NT, McCool FD, Gore R, et al. Prevention of diaphragm atrophy with brief periods of electrical stimulation. Am J Respir Crit Care Med 1999;159: 2018–20.

87. DePalo VD, Parker AL, Al-Bilbeisi F, et al. Respiratory muscle strength training with non-respiratory maneuvers. J Appl Physiol 2004;96(2):731–4.

88. Maish MS. The diaphragm. Surg Clin North Am 2010;90:955–68.

89. Zoumot Z, Jordan S, Hopkinson NS, et al. Twitch transdiaphragmatic pressure morphology can distinguish diaphragm paralysis from a diaphragm defect. Am J Respir Crit Care Med 2013;188:e3.

90. Groth SS, Andrade RS. Diaphragmatic eventration. Thorac Surg Clin 2009;19:511–9.

91. Olafsson G, Rausing A, Holen O. Primary tumors of the diaphragm. Chest 1971;59(5):568–70.

92. Fair KA, Gordon NT, Barbosa RR, et al. Traumatic diaphragmatic injury in the American College of Surgeons National Trauma Data Bank: a new examination of a rare diagnosis. Am J Surg 2015; 209:864.

93. Williams M, Carlin AM, Tyburski JG, et al. Predictors of mortality in patients with traumatic diaphragmatic rupture and associated thoracic and/or abdominal injuries. Am Surg 2004;70:157–62.

94. Demetriades D, Kakoyiannis S, Parekh D, et al. Penetrating injuries of the diaphragm. Br J Surg 1988;75:824–6.

95. Zierold D, Perlstein J, Weidman ER, et al. Penetrating trauma to the diaphragm: natural history and ultrasonographic characteristics of untreated injury in a pig model. Arch Surg 2001;136:32–7.

96. Panda A, Kumar A, Gamanagatti S, et al. Traumatic diaphragmatic injury: a review of CT signs and the difference between blunt and penetrating injury. Diagn Interv Radiol 2014;20:121–8.

97. Feliciano DV, Cruse PA, Mattox KL, et al. Delayed diagnosis of injuries to the diaphragm after penetrating wounds. J Trauma 1988;28:1135–44.

98. Schnitzer JJ, Kikiros CS, Short BL, et al. Experience with abdominal wall closure for patients with congenital diaphragmatic hernia repaired on ECMO. J Pediatr Surg 1995;30:19–22.

99. Laje P, Hedrick HL, Flake AW, et al. Delayed abdominal closure after congenital diaphragmatic hernia repair. J Pediatr Surg 2016;51:240–3.

100. Putnam LR, Gupta V, Tsao K, et al. Factors associated with early recurrence after congenital diaphragmatic hernia repair. J Pediatr Surg 2017;52: 928–32.

101. Al-Iede MM, Karpelowsky J, Fitzgerald DA. Recurrent diaphragmatic hernia: modifiable and non-modifiable risk factors. Pediatr Pulmonol 2016;51: 394–401.

102. Jancelewicz T, Chiang M, Oliveira C, et al. Late surgical outcomes among congenital diaphragmatic hernia (CDH) patients: why long-term follow-up with surgeons is recommended. J Pediatr Surg 2013;48:935–41.

103. Trachsel D, Selvadurai H, Bohn D, et al. Long-term pulmonary morbidity in survivors of congenital diaphragmatic hernia. Pediatr Pulmonol 2005;39: 433–9.

104. Mullins ME, Stein J, Saini SS, et al. Prevalence of incidental Bochdalek's hernia in a large adult population. Am J Roentgenol 2001;177:363–6.

105. Gale ME. Bochdalek hernia: prevalence and CT characteristics. Radiology 1985;156:449–52.

106. Giannoulis K, Sutton R. Bochdalek hernia presenting in adult life: report of an unusual case and review of the literature. Ann Gastroenterol 2004; 17(1):109–12.

107. Lahrmann H, Grisold W, Authier FJ, et al. Neuralgic amyotrophy with phrenic nerve involvement. Muscle Nerve 1999;22(4):437–42.

108. Oo T, Watt JW, Soni BM, et al. Delayed diaphragm recovery in 12 patients after high cervical spinal cord injury. A retrospective review of the diaphragm status of 107 patients ventilated after acute spinal cord injury. Spinal Cord 1999;37(2): 117–22.

109. Summerhill EM, El-Sameed YA, Glidden TJ, et al. Monitoring recovery from diaphragm paralysis with ultrasound. Chest 2008;133(3):737–43.

110. Efthimiou J, Butler J, Woodham C, et al. Diaphragm paralysis following cardiac surgery: role of phrenic nerve cold injury. Ann Thorac Surg 1991;52(4): 1005–8.

111. Bourke SC, Gibson GJ. Sleep and breathing in neuromuscular disease. Eur Respir J 2002;19(6): 1194–201.

112. Shneerson JM, Simonds AK. Noninvasive ventilation for chest wall and neuromuscular disorders. Eur Respir J 2002;20:480–7.

113. Simonds AK, Muntoni F, Heather S, et al. Impact of nasal ventilation on survival in hypercapnic Duchenne muscular dystrophy. Thorax 1998;53: 949–52.

114. Freeman RK, Van WJ, Vyverberg A, et al. Long-term follow-up of the functional and physiologic results of diaphragm plication in adults with unilateral diaphragm paralysis. Ann Thorac Surg 2009;88(4):1112–7.

115. Mouroux J, Venissac N, Leo F, et al. Surgical treatment of diaphragmatic eventration using video-assisted thoracic surgery: a prospective study. Ann Thorac Surg 2005;79(1):308–12.

116. Groth SS, Andrade RS. Diaphragm plication for eventration or paralysis: a review of the literature. Ann Thorac Surg 2010;89(6):S2146–50.

117. Gayan-Ramirez G, Gosselin N, Troosters T, et al. Functional recovery of diaphragm paralysis: a long-term follow-up study. Respir Med 2008; 102(5):690–8.

118. Kaufman MR, Elkwood AI, Colicchio AR, et al. Functional restoration of diaphragmatic paralysis: an evaluation of phrenic nerve reconstruction. Ann Thorac Surg 2014;97(1):260–6.

Disorders of the Chest Wall
Clinical Manifestations

Mazen O. Al-Qadi, MD

KEYWORDS

- Chest wall • Rib cage • Kyphoscoliosis • Ankylosing spondylitis • Flail chest • Pectus excavatum

KEY POINTS

- Chest wall disorders impair breathing without affecting the lungs themselves.
- Restrictive defect is the physiologic hallmark of chest wall disorders.
- Chest wall disorders decrease total lung capacity (TLC) to variable degrees; deformities of the thoracic cage with no (or minimal) spinal involvement have modest effect on respiratory efficiency.

INTRODUCTION

Chest wall disorders comprise a group of diseases and deformities that affect the rib cage (thoracic spine, ribs, sternum), respiratory muscles (diaphragm, intercostal muscles), and abdomen. These disorders may impair breathing without affecting the lungs themselves. The physiologic hallmark of these disorders is restriction caused by a poorly distensible chest wall. The reduced chest wall compliance places an elastic load on the respiratory muscles, which increases the work of breathing and predisposes these individuals to fatigue of the respiratory muscles. The respiratory system adapts to increased elastic load by intrinsic (muscular training) and/or extrinsic (increased central drive) mechanisms.[1] This article focuses on disorders that affect the bony parts of chest wall (ie, spine and rib cage). The most common disorder that affects the abdomen (obesity) is discussed elsewhere in this issue (See Imran H. Iftikhars' article, "Obesity Hypoventilation Syndrome," in this issue), as is the pathophysiology of disorders affecting the chest wall (See George E. Tzelepis' article, "Chest Wall Diseases: Respiratory Pathophysiology," in this issue).

ANATOMY AND MECHANICS OF THE THORACIC CAGE

Knowledge of the normal structure and function of the thorax in relation to the spine is essential in understanding chest wall disorders. The anterolateral rib cage is comprised of the sternum and 10 pairs of ribs attached at the costosternal junctions. The posterior boundary of the rib cage consists of the thoracic spine and 12 pairs of ribs articulated at the costovertebral junctions (**Fig. 1**). The diaphragm forms the inferior boundary. The costosternal and costovertebral junctions represent true synovial joints with synovial spaces that facilitate expansion of the chest wall during inspiration. Mobility of the upper thoracic cage is somehow limited because the true ribs (one through seven) are attached anteriorly to the sternum and posteriorly to the spine. The lower rib cage is more mobile because the false ribs (8–10) are attached to the long costal cartilages. The greatest mobility is at the lower part of the rib cage at the level of floating ribs (11 and 12), which are not attached to the sternum at all. Therefore, inspiration normally results in cephalad motion of the upper ribs and greater lateral motion of the lower rib cage.

Disclosure Statement: Nothing to disclose (no funding sources).
Section of Pulmonary, Critical Care, and Sleep Medicine, Yale-New Haven Hospital, Yale University School of Medicine, 20 York Street, New Haven, CT 06510, USA
E-mail address: mazen.al-qadi@ynhh.org

Clin Chest Med 39 (2018) 361–375
https://doi.org/10.1016/j.ccm.2018.01.010

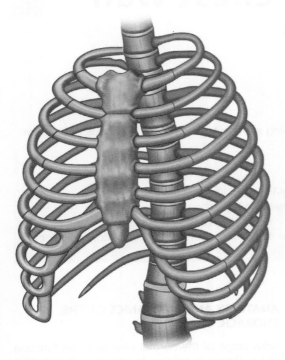

Fig. 1. Normal anatomy of the thoracic cage.

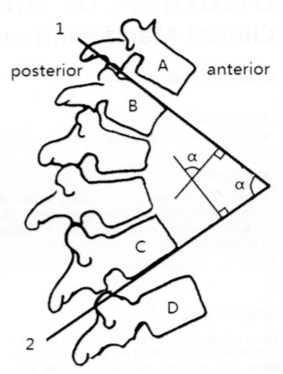

Fig. 2. Measurement of the Cobb angle on standing radiograph at the intersection of the line parallel to the end plate of the superior end vertebra and the line parallel to the end plate of the inferior end vertebra. (*From* Lin N, Li Y, Bebawy JF, et al. Abdominal circumference but not the degree of lumbar flexion affects the accuracy of lumbar interspace identification by Tuffier's line palpation method: an observational study. BMC Anesthesiol 2015;15:9; with permission.)

KYPHOSCOLIOSIS

The term scoliosis describes lateral deformation of the spine in the coronal plane with an angle of spinal curvature greater than 10° (Cobb angle) (**Fig. 2**). Scoliosis can affect the thoracic, lumbar, or thoracolumbar vertebrae. Kyphosis represents excessive forward curvature and commonly complicates scoliosis. The reported prevalence of kyphoscoliosis (KS) varies considerably. This variation reflects inconsistency in defining scoliosis and differences in studied populations. Nevertheless, KS is the most common spinal deformity, affecting 4% of the population worldwide. The prevalence of clinically significant scoliosis that is severe enough to impair chest mechanics (>100°) or result in alveolar hypoventilation (>120°) is 1 in 10,000 people.[2]

KS affects females more than males (female-to-male ratio of 3–4:1) and is primary (idiopathic) in more than 80% of patients. Less commonly it is secondary to neuromuscular disease (dysfunction of the central or peripheral nervous system) or caused by congenital defects (failure of vertebral formation or segmentation, impaired osseous development), or related to trauma or tumors (**Box 1**).[3] The prevalence of KS is higher in first-degree relatives of patients with scoliosis.[4,5]

Pulmonary Function

KS is the leading cause of respiratory failure among all chest wall disorders.[6] Scoliosis starts with vertebral rotation in the axial plane, causing displacement of the ribs in the posterior and outward direction. This leads to unequal load on the ventral and dorsal aspects of the vertebral column and subsequent lateral curvature to counterbalance the primary curve.

Lung volumes have been extensively studied in KS. In 1854, Schneevogt[7] reported a significant reduction in vital capacity (VC). This finding was confirmed by several other investigators.[8,9] The reduction in VC was most notable when the dorsal spine was affected and is worse in patients with Cobb angle greater than 100°.[10] Later, several studies demonstrated reduction in total lung capacity (TLC) in those patients.[11] The reduction in VC generally is proportional to the reduction in TLC. Residual volume (RV) is usually

Box 1
Causes of kyphoscoliosis

Primary (idiopathic) kyphoscoliosis

  Infantile (from birth up to 3 years of age)

  Juvenile (3–10 years of age)

  Adolescent (children older than 10 years of age)

Secondary kyphoscoliosis

  Neuropathic or myopathic (cerebral palsy, poliomyelitis, spinocerebellar degeneration, Duchenne dystrophy syringomyelia, meningocele, Chiari malformation)

  Developmental (achondroplasia, neurofibromatosis, osteogenesis imperfecta)

  Connective tissue diseases (Ehlers-Danlos syndrome, Marfan syndrome, Morquio syndrome)

  Tumors (osteoma, osteoblastoma)

Congenital

  Osteogenic (hemivertebrae, fused vertebrae)

normal or modestly reduced.[12] As a result, the RV/TLC ratio is increased and sometimes misinterpreted as evidence of obstructive pathology. Obstructive physiology (expiratory flow limitation and increased airway resistance), however, may occur if the deformed spine causes bronchial torsion.[13] Functional residual capacity is the lung volume at which the outward elastic recoil of the chest wall is balanced by the inward recoil of the lung. In KS, chest wall deformation leads to alteration in this equilibrium point, which can be 15% less than predicted functional residual capacity.

Patients with KS may also have respiratory muscle weakness as demonstrated by impaired maximal inspiratory (PI_{max}) and expiratory pressures (PE_{max}). Cooper and colleagues[14] studied patients with mild-to-moderate (angle <60°) idiopathic KS and found that PI_{max} was decreased, whereas PE_{max} was normal. Preserved functions of expiratory muscles suggest that inspiratory muscles are also intact and that the reduced PI_{max} likely signifies mechanical disadvantage of the inspiratory muscles. With severe idiopathic KS, PI_{max} is markedly diminished, and patients with such severe deformity have low transdiaphragmatic pressures with more negative esophageal pressures, suggesting active recruitment of accessory muscles of breathing.[8] In contrast to idiopathic KS, secondary (paralytic) KS is associated with greater

reduction in PI_{max} and PE_{max} because of primary muscle weakness and greater restrictive impairment.

Mild to moderate KS may result in mild hypoxemia without hypercapnia. This results from ventilation–perfusion (V/Q) mismatching.[15] Asymmetry between the right and left lungs contributes to V/Q mismatching because the lung on the convex side is better ventilated than the lung on the concave side.[16] Spinal rotation accompanied by lateral displacement of the ribs and sternum further distort the lungs. Lung compression (on the convex side) is greater with a more cephalad curve. As the spinal deformity progresses, alveolar hypoventilation and hypercapnia develop. This is in part caused by a rapid shallow breathing pattern that increases the ratio of dead space to tidal volume (V_D/V_T) with normal or only slightly elevated (14–25 mm Hg) alveolar-arterial gradient.[17] Pulmonary shunt (caused by atelectasis) and diffusion limitation may also contribute to hypoxemia and a widened alveolar-arterial gradient with severe spinal deformities.

Exercise capacity is usually maintained in mild KS; however, physical deconditioning is not uncommon in moderate to severe disease and may result in some physical limitation.[18] Additionally, the V_T is reduced in proportion to VC during exercise.[19] Ineffective ventilation is found in more severe deformities, where rapid shallow breathing is adopted to reduce the work per breath and pressure needed to inhale. Finally, cardiac performance is compromised because thoracic distortion may impede stroke volume during exercise.

Clinical Manifestations and Diagnosis

The course and prognosis of KS largely depend on the cause, pattern of deformity, and age of onset. Progression of the spinal deformity depends the cause of scoliosis, location and size of the scoliotic segment, and bone maturity. Severe deformities can cause significant cardiopulmonary insufficiency. Cobb angles greater than 50° at the thoracic apex that develop before bone maturity have the greatest probability to progress later in life, typically at rate of 0.75° to 2.00° per year,[20,21] whereas curvatures with Cobb angles less than 30° to 40° at the time of skeletal maturity rarely progress in adulthood.[22,23] Early onset KS (before the age of 8) can result in rapid decline in pulmonary functions, the development of pulmonary hypertension, and respiratory failure.[24,25] By contrast patients with idiopathic KS that arises around puberty have an overall good prognosis.

The severity of deformity in idiopathic KS correlates with impaired chest mechanics and may predict respiratory symptoms; patients with a Cobb angle less than 70° are usually asymptomatic. With angles between 70° and 100°, patients may not have symptoms in youth, but may become symptomatic in middle age as the deformity progresses. Restrictive defects are usually seen in patients with angles of 90° or greater. Exercise intolerance and exertional dyspnea are some of the early respiratory manifestations of KS. Those patients have significant reduction in oxyhemoglobin saturation with exercise and distance walked compared with normal subjects.[26] When the curvature measures greater than 120°, exertional shortness of breath ensues and they may develop respiratory failure. Notably, patients with KS secondary to neuromuscular dysfunction (ie, paralytic KS) may develop symptoms with much less spinal deformity (they are more symptomatic at a given Cobb angle than those with idiopathic KS). Several factors (other than the Cobb angle) may predict respiratory insufficiency. These include age of onset, spinal rotation, loss of thoracic kyphosis, and the level of the curvature.

Chronic sagittal vertebral imbalance results in paraspinous muscle fatigue and may cause radicular back pain. Chronic back pain is seen in 50% to 61% of patients with KS but rarely causes significant disability.[27,28] In addition, prolonged standing worsens symptoms, which negatively impacts activities of daily living. Relaxation of extensor spinal muscles is achieved by resting in the recumbent position. Moreover, perception of poor image may significantly impact the psychological status of those patients.

Treatment

Management of KS depends on several factors, including patient's age, Cobb angle, rate of progression of the deformity, functional status, and degree of symptoms. Therapeutic modalities should focus on relieving symptoms, allowing maximum growth of the spine and thoracic cage, and arresting the deformity (before skeletal maturity) to levels less than 30° to 40°.

Nonsurgical treatment
Patients with mild to moderate disease (angle <50°) and those who are poor candidates for operative interventions are treated conservatively with medications to relieve pain (eg, nonsteroidal anti-inflammatory drugs, neuromodulars [eg, gabapentin], tricyclic antidepressants, or opioids), physical therapy, and regular exercises to enhance physical fitness. Rigid orthotic braces provide truncal stability and may slow the

progression of the deformity. Braces may be effective in patients at risk for progression, especially children (older than 3 years of age) with curves less than 40° and considerable time to maturity.[29] In a multicenter, randomized trial, bracing significantly reduced the curve progression compared with watchful waiting.[30] It should be noted that braces are most beneficial when used for at least 12 hours per day. Many patients are advised to use them 18 to 20 hours per day; however, this is rarely achieved because the brace is poorly tolerated by some patients.[31]

Supplemental oxygen is indicated when patients develop hypoxemia. However, in the presence of alveolar hypoventilation, addition of positive pressure ventilation is preferred over oxygen alone.[32] The long-term use of noninvasive positive pressure ventilation (NIPPV) increases alveolar ventilation, improves the ventilatory response to carbon dioxide, reduces symptoms, improves pulmonary function and gas exchange, reduces pulmonary artery pressures, and lessens mortality.[33–36]

NIPPV is recommended in patients with scoliosis who have features of cor pulmonale and any of the following: (1) daytime $Paco_2$ greater than 45 mm Hg, (2) VC less than 50% of predicted, (3) PI_{max} less than 60 cm H_2O, and (4) arterial oxygen saturation less than 88% to 90% for greater than 5 minutes or greater than 10% of the total recorded time.[37] Historically, volume-targeted ventilation was used in those patients. However, pressure- and volume-targeted modes have been shown to be equally effective.[38–40] Ventilators with sensitive triggering system (ie, short response time) should be used to match the breathing pattern (high respiratory frequency) seen in KS and optimize synchrony. In patients with KS secondary to poliomyelitis, early initiation of NIPPV in the presence of nocturnal hypoventilation (with normal daytime $Paco_2$) may delay the progression of postpoliomyelitis syndrome.[41]

Surgical treatment
Patients with skeletal immaturity who have severe deformities (angle >45°), and those with curves 40° to 45° accompanied by significant physical or functional limitations, may be candidates for surgical repair. Patients with skeletal maturity and impaired functional performance, progression greater than 10° in 1 year, sagittal imbalance, and neurologic symptoms (eg, radicular pain) refractory to medications may also be considered for surgery.[42,43] Surgical procedures include fixation of the facet joints (with screws), internal spinal fixation with rods, and spinal fusion. Failure of early techniques using facet screws led to the

development of hook-and-rod construct, and later dual "growing" rods that allow for intermittent lengthening of the construct. Currently, the most widely used surgical technique to correct KS involves internal fixation with stainless-steel rods. Spinal fusion is required in many patients to maintain a straight alignment. This is usually avoided in children younger than 10 years of age to allow for growth of the spine.[44] Loss of spinal flexibility caused by sagittal flattening is a major concern of spinal fusion, especially if fusion extends into the lumbar spine, but occurs less frequently with modern segmental instrumentation.

The effect of these surgical modalities on pulmonary functions is controversial. Surgery violates chest mechanics and may cause decline in pulmonary functions in the early postoperative period, with delay in return of these functions up to 1 year postoperatively.[45] Despite this, a meta-analysis of five trials found small but statistically significant improvement in mean VC (from 2% to 11%) after Harrington instrumentation.[46]

ANKYLOSING SPONDYLITIS

Ankylosing spondylitis (AS) is a chronic deforming autoinflammatory disorder that primarily affects the axial skeleton. The disease affects 0.02% to 1.4% of the general population and 20% of HLA-B27-positive people.[47–49] Genetic predisposition plays a major role in the pathogenesis of AS with heritability (HLA-B27 positivity) in more than 90% of cases.[50] Overexpression of tumor necrosis factor (TNF)-α independent of B or T cells activation,[51,52] and upregulation of the genes encoding the proinflammatory interleukin-17, have been implicated in the pathogenesis of AS.[53] Men are affected more commonly and have more severe disease than women. Although the spine is affected primarily by AS, other organ systems can be involved, including the respiratory (chest wall, lung parenchyma), eyes (uveitis), cardiovascular (aortitis, aortic valve regurgitation, conduction disturbances), and kidneys (glomerular disease).

Pulmonary Function

Inflammation of the sternocostal, intervertebral, and costovertebral joints and adjacent tendons (enthesitis) leads to progressive fibrosis, ossification, and stiffness (fusion) of the thorax. In the early stages of AS, inflammation involves the axial skeleton that starts from the sacroiliac joint and spreads upward. This leads to impaired spine mobility and back pain.[54] The anterior chest wall is affected at later stages; inflammation starts in the first sternocostal articulation and spreads

downward, causing immobility of the affected articulations.[55] Involvement of the sternoclavicular and manubriosternal joints may also limit the mobility of chest wall by causing pain rather than mechanically.[55] Together, these changes reduce rib cage compliance and favor lung inflation via the abdomen rather than the rib cage.[56,57] This explains why there is less contribution of the rib cage to resting tidal breathing than normal (56% in AS compared with 75% in normal subjects) and the shifted distribution of ventilation from apical to basal lung regions.[58,59] The unequal ventilation may also predispose apical regions to recurrent infections and contribute to the predilection of these areas to inflammation and fibrosis in AS.[60,61] In contrast to the chest wall, elastance of the lungs is not reduced unless parenchymal lung disease is present.[54,62] Coexisting KS is present in approximately half of AS patients and adds more mechanical load on the respiratory system.[63] As the disease progresses, the chest wall becomes more rigid and fixed in an inspiratory position causing an increased RV and RV/TLC ratio[64]

Early studies of pulmonary functions in AS have shown an average TLC of 89% of predicted in mild AS, whereas patients with advanced disease may have TLC of 60% of predicted.[62,65,66] In general, VC and TLC are mildly reduced, and the degree of restriction correlates with disease severity and mobility of the rib cage.[56,67–70] Inconsistencies among studies, in part, is attributed to whether the investigators corrected for the patient's height or not (the height used in some studies was the actual height rather than the height corrected for spinal deformity). Respiratory muscle weakness is thought to be caused by intercostal muscle atrophy secondary to chronic immobilization of the rib cage.[71] Although reduced pressures (PI$_{max}$ and PE$_{max}$) correlate with limited chest expansion and disease duration, the functional status of these patients is not affected. Alternatively, respiratory muscle weakness may result from vertebral fractures with concomitant spinal cord injuries (especially cervical spine). Such injuries can occur with simple trauma (eg, slipping or falls from low heights).[72,73]

Clinical Manifestations and Diagnosis

Symptoms of AS typically start in the second decade of life. Chronic back pain caused by sacroiliitis is the hallmark of AS and is seen in more than two-thirds of patients.[74] The pain is worse in the early morning after a period of immobilization and is often associated with morning stiffness and constitutional symptoms, such as fever, weight loss, and malaise. In addition, peripheral arthritis and enthesitis (inflammation at the bony insertions of joint capsules) are very common and manifest as swelling, pain, and tenderness of the joints and surrounding tissues. Often, symptoms of AS are present for years before the diagnosis is made.[75]

AS also may affect the tracheobronchial tree and lung parenchyma (apical fibrobollous disease).[76–79] Therefore, parenchymal disease may contribute to a restrictive defect seen on pulmonary function tests. Thoracic rigidity and straightening of the spine impairs chest expansion and can result in pain on inspiration in 40% of patients.[80–82] A progressive decline in exercise capacity occurs as the disease progresses. A study of 100 patients with AS found that female gender, the presence of anterior uveitis, and a fused "bamboo" spine correlated with significant disability and loss of work.[83] Dyspnea may occur in patients with rib cage restriction or with parenchymal lung disease, which may progress to cystic or cavitary disease, fibrosis, or bronchiectasis. Fungal and mycobacterial infections occur in approximately one-third of AS patients.[84] As a result, cough, sputum production, or hemoptysis is seen.[85] Cases of acute respiratory failure have been reported caused by spontaneous pneumothorax or upper airway obstruction as a result of cricoarytenoid arthritis.[85,86]

Palpation of the chest wall may reveal tenderness of the affected (eg, costochondral, manubriosternal) joints and indicate active synovitis. Additionally, assessment of chest expansion (at the level of the fourth intercostal space) is an important part of the physical examination and should be routinely performed. Thus, young patients with unexplained chronic back pain and limited chest wall expansion (<2.5 cm) should be evaluated for AS.

Treatment

Physiotherapy and rehabilitation are important aspects of AS management. Regular chest wall expansion and postural training exercises should be encouraged. Analgesics are frequently used to treat pain and facilitate participation in physiotherapy programs. Nonsteroidal anti-inflammatory drugs are particularly useful for the dual analgesic and anti-inflammatory properties.[87] In the absence of contraindications, nonsteroidal anti-inflammatory drugs are considered first-line therapy for AS. Patients with high disease activity are offered TNF-α inhibitors. These agents have been shown to improve symptoms, axial inflammation, and chest expansion in AS.[88,89] Several agents of this class are currently available, including infliximab, etanercept, adalimumab, certolizumab, and golimumab. TNF-α inhibitors should be avoided in patients with advanced heart failure, and patients receiving theses agents require careful monitoring for reactivation of mycobacterial infection.[90] More recently, the US Food and Drug Administration has approved secukinumab, an anti-interleukin-17A monoclonal antibody, for the treatment of AS.[91] Occasionally, vertebral osteotomy is performed to correct spinal deformities.[92]

FLAIL CHEST

Rib fractures commonly complicate blunt thoracic trauma and account for 35% to 40% of all thoracic injuries.[93] Although seat belts are life-saving in motor vehicle accidents, their use has been linked to the development of rib fractures. Approximately 10% to 25% of rib injuries result in flail chest.[94] This condition occurs when three or more ribs are fractured in multiple sites causing disruption of the integrity of the chest wall. As a result, a segment of the chest wall moves (paradoxically) inward during inspiration and outward during expiration.[95] Overall, flail injury is associated with mortality rates of 33%.[96] A recent retrospective study that used the National Trauma Data Bank for more than 200 trauma centers in North America revealed that 82% of patients with flail chest injuries required intensive care unit admission and 59% needed mechanical ventilation.[93]

Flail chest injury requires severe kinetic force to the torso (eg, motor vehicle accidents, aggressive cardiopulmonary resuscitation, work-related crush injuries, falls from height, and assaults). This often results in simultaneous injuries to viscera and major blood vessels.[97] Low-velocity trauma may be sufficient to cause flail injury in elderly individuals with underlying osteoporosis and low muscle mass or patients with an absent sternum (eg, congenital absence of sternum or total sternectomy). Blunt injury to the chest causes compression injury to the ribs if the force exceeds the strength of the rib cage. Frequently, ribs break at 60° rotation from the sternum and posteriorly.[98] Anatomically, flail segments are classified into four types: (1) anterolateral (rib injury that involves the anterior rib angle), (2) posterolateral flail (rib fracture lies in the posterior rib angle), (3) sternal flail (costochondral junctions are disrupted bilaterally), and (4) vertebral flail (complete bony disruption of posterior ribs at the vertebral articulations bilaterally). Vertebral flail is exceedingly rare and unlikely to cause paradoxic movement because of splinting of the paraspinal muscles. Early after the injury, paradoxic movement of the flail segment is limited by the surrounding intact chest wall structures (ie, splinting of the muscles). However, the underlying pulmonary contusion, atelectasis, and retained secretions increases the lung stiffness. Consequently, more negative intrathoracic pressure is generated during inspiration, and the flail segment becomes prominent. The presence of positive pressure ventilation, therefore, may conceal the paradoxic movement.

Clinical Manifestations and Diagnosis

The diagnosis of flail chest is clinical. Visualization of the paradoxic movement of part of the chest wall during the respiratory cycle in the spontaneously breathing patient is diagnostic. Chest wall pain and dyspnea are common in patients who sustain chest injury but are nonspecific. Certain physical examination findings should raise the suspicion for the presence of rib fractures; these include localized tenderness, bruises, and crepitus. Additionally, palpation of the chest wall should include careful assessment for the symmetry of expansion. This is more sensitive than inspection alone, especially in patients requiring mechanical ventilation. Nevertheless, the diagnosis of flail chest is delayed for several days after injury in up to 22% of patients.[99] Imaging studies of the chest are required in patients who sustained blunt thoracic trauma. Chest radiograph may reveal fractures of the ribs at multiple sites and suggest the diagnosis of flail chest in 70% of patients, but is less likely to suggest mechanical instability of the ribs. Computed tomography of the chest with three-dimensional reconstruction is more sensitive in detecting rib fractures and is helpful in evaluating associated injuries or abnormalities (eg, pulmonary contusions).[100]

Several factors contribute to the gas exchange abnormalities seen in flail chest. Severe pain impairs normal inspiration and cough. Therefore, areas with V/Q inequality are created. Specifically, pulmonary shunt is increased because of retained secretions, atelectasis, and underlying pulmonary contusion, resulting in hypoxemia. Ventilatory failure and hypercapnia occur less frequently than hypoxemia. Pain (alters recruitment of respiratory muscle), splinting, and respiratory muscle dysfunction often decrease V_T, causing increased V_D/V_T and diminished minute ventilation.[101] The previously postulated pendelluft phenomenon where deoxygenated air flows back and forth between the two hemithoraces is minimal (<2% of V_T).[102] Finally, associated pleuropulmonary complications (eg, pneumothorax, contusion) may play a role in V/Q mismatch.

Treatment

The management of flail chest has evolved significantly in the last few decades. Stabilization of the flail segment is of paramount importance to restore chest wall integrity. Previously, interventions to achieve this included external splinting ("sandbagging") and internal stabilization using positive pressure ventilation ("internal pneumatic stabilization"). Positive pressure ventilation (noninvasively or via tracheal intubation) maintains positive pleural pressure and provides further stabilization of the floating segment. However, it should be offered to patients with respiratory compromise or gas exchange abnormalities and not solely for internal stabilization.[103] Additionally, adequate pain control and aggressive pulmonary toilet are crucial. Analgesia facilitates chest physiotherapy and allows patients to breathe deeply and cough effectively. Oral and parenteral analgesics are used to alleviate pain in patients with flail chest. Often, more invasive measures are needed for this purpose. Thoracic epidural analgesia is an effective modality and has been suggested in patients with refractory pain. Furthermore, thoracic paravertebral block is considered if thoracic epidural analgesia is contraindicated.[104]

Surgical fixation with open reduction and internal fixation of the flail ribs is another method of achieving mechanical stability of the flail segment. Although this modality remains controversial, it has gained some popularity recently. Several randomized controlled trials compared outcomes of flail injuries treated with surgical fixation with conservative therapy (internal pneumatic stabilization with positive pressure ventilation or external stabilization with strapping). Significant reduction in the length of stay, days on mechanical ventilation, and rates of pneumonia was observed with surgical fixation, but no mortality benefit was found.[105–107] Similar results were seen in a recent systematic review comparing operative management of flail segment with conservative management.[108] Surgical fixation was also associated with improvement in pulmonary function at 2 months in one study.[106] Currently accepted indications for surgical intervention in flail chest include (1) the presence of significant respiratory compromise requiring ventilation, (2) inability to wean off mechanical ventilation, (3) abnormal pulmonary function (with or without mechanical ventilatory support), and (4) presence of significant chest wall deformity or parenchymal injury caused by displaced rib fractures. Notably, deformities of the chest wall are minimized even with surgical fixation of one fracture per rib.[109] Timing of surgical fixation is poorly defined, but generally preferred within the first 3 to 5 days of injury.

PECTUS EXCAVATUM

The thoracic cage can be affected by a group of congenital deformities. Pectus excavatum (PE) accounts for more than 90% of all chest wall deformities and is characterized by central depression of the sternum, producing a funnel-shaped chest (**Fig. 3**). Consequently, the anteroposterior distance of the thoracic cage is diminished. Reduction in the sternovertebral distance may result in displacement of the heart with possible compression of the right ventricle.[110] The estimated incidence of PE is 1 in 400 to 1 in 1000 live births, with a 3:1 male-to-female ratio.[111] Other less common congenital defects that affect the anterior chest wall include pectus carinatum (outward protrusion of the sternum and ribs), Poland syndrome (unilateral absence of the pectoralis muscles with deformity of the costal cartilages of the upper ribs), and cleft sternum (sternal defect caused by failure of fusion of the two sternal halves).

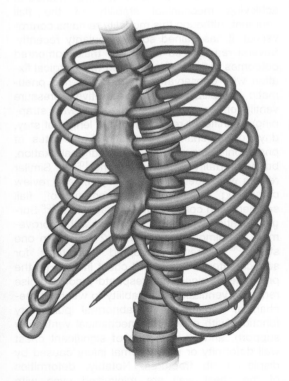

Fig. 3. Morphology of pectus excavatum.

Although different hypotheses exist, the exact mechanism responsible for PE is still unclear. PE is familial in 43% of patients, and is associated with collagen vascular diseases, such as Marfan syndrome and Ehler-Danlos syndrome.[112] Furthermore, scoliosis is commonly associated with PE (26%) and is associated with other anomalies (eg, mitral valve prolapse).[113,114] It is believed that abnormal growth of the sternocostal cartilage is related to upregulation of various genes, such as transforming growth factor-β, collagen, and fibrillin, causing abnormal collagen cross-linking within the cartilage. As a result, there is inward displacement of the sternum.[115,116] Alternatively, posterior tethering of the sternum to the diaphragm may contribute to the development of PE, and this may explain acquired PE seen after repair of congenital diaphragmatic hernias.[117] PE may not always be the primary process; increased inspiratory work caused by chronic upper airway abnormalities in infancy (eg, chronic upper airway obstruction or laryngomalacia) may produce paradoxic movement of the sternum and affect the growth of the chest wall.[118] Occasionally, overgrowth may result in outward displacement of the sternal body, causing the opposite geometric deformity (ie, pectus carinatum).

Pulmonary Function

The cardiopulmonary functions of patients with PE have been evaluated extensively. In 1982, Castile and colleagues[119] studied seven patients with mild to moderate PE, of whom five patients were symptomatic (on exercise only). No significant restrictive defect, abnormalities in lung compliance, or flow-volume configurations were found. Additionally, oxygen uptake during exercise was normal in those patients. Patients with more severe deformities showed normal oxygen uptake at low workloads but had increased oxygen uptake at maximal effort. Lawson and colleagues[120,121] more recently demonstrated (mostly in patients with Haller index >4.3) approximately 15% to 20% reduction in forced expiratory volume in 1 second and forced expiratory flow, with 1.4 times increased likelihood of restrictive pattern for each unit increase in the Haller index.

Restricted growth of the lung caused by smaller thoracic cavity seems intuitive. However, normal lung volumes are often reported. Koumbourlis and colleagues[122] reported that restriction was found in only 5% of PE patients, whereas 41% of had an obstructive pattern. Evidence of air-trapping (increased RV/TLC ratio) was seen not only in patients with restriction but also with normal or obstructive patterns. This suggests that altered chest wall mechanics in PE may impair lung emptying and places the respiratory muscles at a mechanical disadvantage as evident by the impaired maximal inspiratory and expiratory pressures (PI_{max} and PE_{max}).[123] The increased RV (implies decreased VC) would explain, at least in part, the reduced forced vital capacity seen in PE.

The mild restriction seen on pulmonary function tests does not fully explain the associated symptoms. Therefore, other mechanisms may play a role in these symptoms, especially lack of endurance with exercise. First, focal chest wall motion abnormalities at the area of the depressed sternum have been described and associated with an increased abdominal contribution to breathing. This may reduce the efficiency of breathing, particularly on exertion.[124] Second, subtle cardiac abnormalities may not produce symptoms at rest but impair exercise fitness. For example, compression of the right ventricle by the depressed sternum can impair cardiac filling and output. Other right ventricular abnormalities have been described (using two-dimensional echocardiography and cardiac magnetic resonance) in PE patients and include significant narrowing of the right ventricular outflow tract diameter and reduced right ventricular ejection fraction. These right ventricle abnormalities improved significantly after surgical repair of the pectus deformity.[125–128]

Clinical Manifestations and Diagnosis

PE is commonly classified based on the shape (deep and localized cup-shaped vs wide and shallow saucer-shaped), symmetry, and degree of deformity (based on sternovertebral distance). Notably, the asymmetric type is associated with more reduction in pulmonary functions compared with the symmetric type.[129] Most patients with mild-to-moderate PE are asymptomatic, whereas patients with more severe deformities may have nonspecific symptoms. Exercise intolerance, lack of endurance, and exertional shortness of breath are the most common symptoms, although chest pain and palpitation have been reported.[112] Psychological disturbances and concerns over appearance are not uncommon. Mycobacterial infection is more common in PE patients than the general population.[130,131] Moreover, depression of the sternum may affect the trachea and airways, leading to compression and deformation. The clinical significance of these observations remains unclear.

The diagnosis of PE is made clinically mostly shortly after birth. Occasionally, the deformity is mild and may not become apparent until later in adolescence. Imaging studies (eg, chest computed tomography scan) are helpful in quantifying the severity of PE and detecting associated thoracic or spinal deformities, especially KS. In 1987, Haller and colleagues[132] evaluated the ratio of transverse dimension of the chest (from inner rib to inner rib) to the sternovertebral distance (measured at the area of greatest deformity) in patients with PE. A ratio (or pectus index) of 3.25 was predictive of need for surgical repair of PE. The pectus index is now widely referred to as the Haller index (**Fig. 4**) and is calculated with two-view chest radiographs.[133] Further evaluation of the cardiopulmonary function (pulmonary function resting, echocardiogram, cardiopulmonary exercise testing) is often needed in symptomatic patients.

Treatment

Most PE patients do not require surgical intervention. However, repair may be indicated in symptomatic patients with significant deformity (Haller index >3.5) and cardiopulmonary compromise. Ideally, reducing the length of the elongated costal cartilage (by resection) is needed to restore the normal geometry of the chest wall. The modified Ravitch open surgical repair is one method to achieve this goal. Preserving the perichondrium may result in regrowth of the costal cartilage in a more anatomic fashion.[134,135] The procedure involves bilateral resection of the deformed costal cartilages (**Fig. 5**A). Then, a wedge-shaped resection is made in the sternum at the area of posterior angulation, and the distal sternum is aligned with the manubrium anteriorly (**Fig. 5**B). Often, the sternum is supported posteriorly with a metal strut that is attached to the ribs laterally and left in place for several months (**Fig. 5**C).

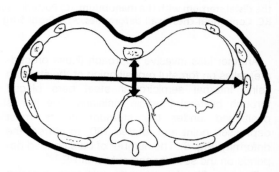

Fig. 4. The Haller "pectus" index. (*From* Williams AM, Crabbe DC. Pectus deformities of the anterior chest wall. Paediatr Respir Rev 2003;4(3):240; with permission.)

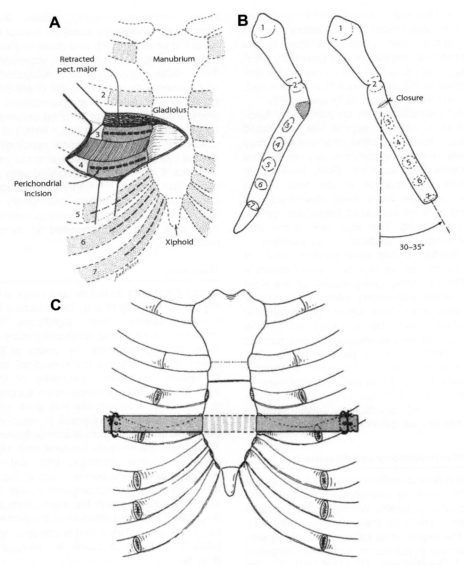

Fig. 5. Open surgical (modified Ravitch) repair of pectus excavatum deformity. (*A*) Resection of the deformed costal cartilages. (*B*) Wedge resection of the sternum at the area of posterior angulation, and alignment of the distal sternum with the manubrium. (*C*) Posterior support of the sternum with a metal strut. (*From* Stanberger RC. Congenital chest wall deformities. Ann Probl Surg 1996;33(6):497; with permission.)

Another less invasive approach (Nuss procedure) relies on forceful repositioning of the sternum using internal semicircular steel bars placed through bilateral thoracic incisions. The bar is positioned under the sternum at its most depressed point and rotated 180° to correct the deformity (**Fig. 6**). The number of bars needed depends on the severity and extent of PE.[135]

The benefits of surgery on pulmonary function are uncertain. A study of 138 patients with PE demonstrated reduction in VC at 2 months after surgical repair; recovery to the preoperative baseline was noted within 1 year after surgery. However, no improvement beyond baseline was reported at 42 months after surgery.[136] Similar findings were reported by Haller and Loughlin[137] who compared pulmonary functions in 36 PE patients with 10 normal control subjects. Notably, surgery was associated with improved exercise tolerance and oxygen pulse (a surrogate for stroke volume). Another study indicated that improvement in pulmonary function was only noted in patients who had surgical repair at age 11 years or older.[119,120]

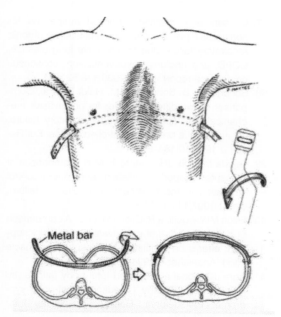

Fig. 6. The minimally invasive Nuss procedure. (*From* Elias JA. Fishman's pulmonary diseases and disorders [Chapter 92]. 4th edition. New York: McGraw-Hill Companies; 2008; with permission.)

SUMMARY

Chest wall deformities impair the rib cage expansion and result in restrictive defect (reduced TLC) to variable degrees primarily caused by reduced chest wall compliance and to a lesser degree, reduction in lung compliance. The degree of respiratory symptoms and impairment of pulmonary functions depend on the severity of deformity, the underlying cause, and coexisting weakness of respiratory muscles. KS is the most common and leading cause of respiratory insufficiency among rib cage deformities. Stiffness of the chest wall is greatest in individuals with KS and is only slightly increased in PE and AS. In general, these disorders result in chronic ventilator failure; however, flail chest causes acute respiratory failure. Supplemental oxygen and NIPPV are used to treat gas exchange abnormalities. Surgical interventions may be needed in patients with severe KS and some patients with flail chest and PE.

REFERENCES

1. Tardif C, Sohier B, Derenne JP. Control of breathing in chest wall diseases. Monaldi Arch Chest Dis 1993;48(1):83–6.
2. Bergofsky EH. Respiratory failure in disorders of the thoracic cage. Am Rev Respir Dis 1979;119: 643–69.
3. Arlet V, Reddi V. Adolescent idiopathic scoliosis. Neurosurg Clin N Am 2007;18(2):255–9.
4. Wynne-Davies R. Familial (idiopathic) scoliosis: a family survey. J Bone Joint Surg Br 1968;50: 24–30.
5. Riseborough EJ, Wynne-Davies R. A genetic survey of idiopathic scoliosis in Boston, Massachusetts. J Bone Joint Surg Am 1973;55:974–82.
6. Kafer ER. Idiopathic scoliosis. Mechanical properties of the respiratory system and the ventilatory response to carbon dioxide. J Clin Invest 1975; 55:1153–63.
7. Schneevogt GEV. Z Rationielle AMed 1854;5:9.
8. Lisboa C, Moreno R, Fava M, et al. Inspiratory muscle function in patients with severe kyphoscoliosis. Am Rev Respir Dis 1985;132:48–52.
9. Weber B, Smith JP, Briscoe WA, et al. Pulmonary function in asymptomatic adolescents with idiopathic scoliosis. Am Rev Respir Dis 1975;111: 389–97.
10. Flagstad AE, Kollman S. Vital capacity and muscle study in one hundred patients with scoliosis. J Bone Jt Surg 1928;10:724–34.
11. Chapman EM, Dill DB, Graybiel A. The decrease in functional capacity of the lungs and heart resulting from deformities of the chest. Medicine 1939;18: 167–202.
12. Iticovici HN, Lyons HA. Ventilatory and lung volume determinations in patients with chest deformities. Am J Med Sci 1956;232(3):265–75.
13. Al-Kattan K, Simonds A, Chung KF, et al. KS and bronchial torsion. Chest 1997;111(4):1134–7.
14. Cooper DM, Rojas JV, Mellins RB, et al. Respiratory mechanics in adolescents with idiopathic scoliosis. Am Rev Respir Dis 1984;130(1):16–22.
15. Redding G, Song K, Inscore S, et al. Lung function asymmetry in children with congenital and infantile scoliosis. Spine J 2008;8(4):639–44.
16. Bake B, Bjure J, Kasalichy J, et al. Regional pulmonary ventilation and perfusion distribution in patients with untreated idiopathic scoliosis. Thorax 1972;27(6):703–12.
17. Bergofsky EH, Turino GM, Fishman AP. Cardiorespiratory failure in kyphoscoliosis. Medicine (Baltimore) 1959;38:263–317.
18. Kesten S, Garnkel SK, Wright T, et al. Impaired exercise capacity in adults with moderate scoliosis. Chest 1991;99:663–6.
19. Kearon C, Viviani GR, Killian KJ. Factors influencing work capacity in adolescent idiopathic thoracic scoliosis. Am Rev Respir Dis 1993;148: 295–303.
20. Picault C, deMauroy JC, Mouilleseaux B, et al. Natural history of idiopathic scoliosis in girls and boys. Spine 1981;11:777–8.
21. Bunnell WP. The natural history of idiopathic scoliosis before skeletal maturity. Spine 1986;11:773.

22. Weinstein SL, Zavala DC, Ponseti IV. Idiopathic scoliosis: long-term follow-up and prognosis in untreated patients. J Bone Joint Surg Am 1981;63: 702–12.

23. Weinstein SL, Ponseti IV. Curve progression in idiopathic scoliosis. J Bone Joint Surg Am 1983;65:447.

24. Nachemson A. A long term follow-up study of non-treated scoliosis. Acta Orthop Scand 1968; 39:466–76.

25. Branthwaite MA. Cardiorespiratory consequences of unfused idiopathic scoliosis patients. Br J Dis Chest 1986;80:360–9.

26. Alves VL, Avanzi O. Objective assessment of the cardiorespiratory function of adolescents with idiopathic scoliosis through the six-minute walk test. Spine (Phila Pa 1976) 2009;34(25):E926–9.

27. Weinstein SL, Dolan LA, Spratt KF, et al. Health and function of patients with untreated idiopathic scoliosis: a 50-year natural history study. JAMA 2003; 289:559–67.

28. Deyo RA, Mirza SK, Martin BI. Back pain prevalence and visit rates: estimates from US national surveys, 2002. Spine 2006;31:2724–7.

29. Nachemson AL, Peterson LE. Effectiveness of treatment with a brace in girls who have adolescent idiopathic scoliosis: a prospective, controlled study based on data from the Brace Study of the Scoliosis Research Society. J Bone Joint Surg Am 1995;77:815–22.

30. Weinstein SL, Dolan LA, Wright JG, et al. Effects of bracing in adolescents with idiopathic scoliosis. N Engl J Med 2013;369(16):1512.

31. Morton A, Riddle R, Buchanan R, et al. Accuracy in the prediction and estimation of adherence to brace wear before and during treatment of adolescent idiopathic scoliosis. J Pediatr Orthop 2008;28: 336–41.

32. Mesa J, Celli B, Riesco J, et al. Noninvasive positive pressure ventilation and not oxygen may prevent overt ventilatory failure in patients with chest wall diseases. Chest 1997;112:207–13.

33. Gonzalez C, Ferris G, Diaz J, et al. Kyphoscoliotic ventilatory insufficiency: effects of long-term intermittent positive-pressure ventilation. Chest 2003; 124(3):857–62.

34. Goldstein R. Hypoventilation: neuromuscular and chest wall disorders. Clin Chest Med 1992;13: 507–21.

35. Schlenker E, Feldmeyer F, Hoster M, et al. Effect of noninvasive ventilation on pulmonary artery pressure in patients with severe kyphoscoliosis. Med Klin (Munich) 1997;92(Suppl 1):40–4.

36. Buyse B, Meersseman W, Demedts M. Treatment of chronic respiratory failure in kyphoscoliosis: oxygen or ventilation? Eur Respir J 2003;22: 525–8.

37. Consensus Conference. Clinical indications for noninvasive positive pressure ventilation in chronic respiratory failure due to restrictive lung disease, COPD, and nocturnal hypoventilation: consensus conference report. Chest 1999;116:521–34.

38. Schonhofer B, Sonneborn M, Haidl P, et al. Comparison of two different modes for noninvasive mechanical ventilation in chronic respiratory failure: volume versus pressure controlled device. Eur Respir J 1997;10:184–91.

39. Tejeda M, Boix JH, Alvarez F, et al. Comparison of pressure support ventilation and assist-control ventilation in the treatment of respiratory failure. Chest 1997;111:1322–5.

40. Elliott MW, Aquilina R, Green M, et al. A comparison of different modes of non-invasive ventilatory support: effects on ventilation and inspiratory muscle effort. Anaesthesia 1994;49:279–83.

41. Agre JC. Local muscle and total body fatigue. In: Halstead LS, Grimby C, editors. Post-polio syndrome. Philadelphia: Hanley and Belfus Inc.; 1994. p. 35–67.

42. Drummond DS. A perspective on recent trends for scoliosis correction. Clin Orthop Relat Res 1991; 264:90–102.

43. Potter BK, Lenke LG, Kuklo TR. Prevention and management of iatrogenic flatback deformity. J Bone Joint Surg Am 2004;86A:1793–808.

44. Akbarnia BA, Breakwell LM, Marks DS, et al. Dual growing rod technique followed for three to eleven years until final fusion: the effect of frequency of lengthening. Spine (Phila Pa 1976) 2008;33: 984–90.

45. Yaszay B, Jazayeri R, Lonner B. The effect of surgical approaches on pulmonary function in adolescent idiopathic scoliosis. J Spinal Disord Tech 2009;22(4):278–83.

46. Kinnear WJ, Johnston ID. Does Harrington instrumentation improve pulmonary function in adolescents with idiopathic scoliosis? A meta-analysis. Spine (Phila Pa 1976) 1993; 18(11):1556–9.

47. Gran JT, Husby G, Hordvik M. Prevalence of ankylosing spondylitis in males and females in a young middle-aged population of Tromso, northern Norway. Ann Rheum Dis 1985;44:359–67.

48. Braun J, Bollow M, Remlinger G, et al. Prevalence of spondylarthropathies in HLA-B27 positive and negative blood donors. Arthritis Rheum 1998; 41(1):58–67.

49. Dean LE, Jones GT, Macdonald AG, et al. Global prevalence of ankylosing spondylitis. Rheumatology 2014;53:650–7.

50. Brown MA, Kennedy LG, MacGregor AJ, et al. Susceptibility to ankylosing spondylitis in twins: the role of genes, HLA, and the environment. Arthritis Rheum 1997;40:1823–8.

51. Kontoyiannis D, Pasparakis M, Pizarro TT, et al. Impaired on/off regulation of TNF biosynthesis in mice lacking TNF AU-rich elements: implications for joint and gut-associated immunopathologies. Immunity 1999;10:387–98.

52. Jacques P, Lambrecht S, Verheugen E, et al. Proof of concept: enthesitis and new bone formation in spondyloarthritis are driven by mechanical strain and stromal cells. Ann Rheum Dis 2014;73:437–45.

53. Diveu C, McGeachy MJ, Cua DJ. Cytokines that regulate autoimmunity. Curr Opin Immunol 2008; 20:663–8.

54. Romagnoli I, Gigliotti F, Galarducci A, et al. Chest wall kinematics and respiratory muscle action in ankylosing spondylitis patients. Eur Respir J 2004;24:453–60.

55. Fournie B, Boutes A, Dromer C, et al. Prospective study of anterior chest wall involvement in ankylosing spondylitis and psoriatic arthritis. Rev Rhum Engl Ed 1997;64:22–5.

56. van Noord JA, Cauberghs M, Van de Woestijne KP, et al. Total respiratory resistance and reactance in ankylosing spondylitis and kyphoscoliosis. Eur Respir J 1991;4:945–51.

57. Tzelepis GE, Kalliakosta G, Tzioufas AG, et al. Thoracoabdominal motion in ankylosing spondylitis: association with standardised clinical measures and response to therapy. Ann Rheum Dis 2009;68:966–71.

58. Sackner MA, Silva G, Banks JM, et al. Distribution of ventilation during diaphragmatic breathing in obstructive lung disease. Am Rev Respir Dis 1974;109(3):331–7.

59. Grimby G, Fugl-Meyer A, Blomstrand A. Partitioning of the contribution of the rib cage and abdomen to ventilation in ankylosing spondylitis. Thorax 1974;29:129.

60. Stewart RM, Ridyard JB, Pearson JD. Regional lung function in ankylosing spondylitis. Thorax 1976;31(4):433–7.

61. Hamilton KA. Pulmonary disease manifestations of ankylosing spondyloarthritis. Ann Intern Med 1949; 31:216–27.

62. Trvais DM, Cook CD, Julian DJ, et al. The lungs in rheumatoid spondylitis, gas exchange and lung mechanics in a form of restrictive lung disease. Am J Med 1960;29:623–32.

63. Vosse D, van der Heijde D, Landewe R, et al. Determinants of hyperkyphosis in patients with ankylosing spondylitis. Ann Rheum Dis 2006;65: 770–4.

64. Hunninghake GW, Fauci AS. Pulmonary involvement in the collagen vascular diseases. Am Rev Respir Dis 1979;119:471–503.

65. Rogan MD, Needham CD, McDonald I. Effect of ankylosing spondylitis on ventilatory function. Clin Sci 1955;14(1):91–6.

66. Sharp JT, Sweeny SK, Henry JP, et al. Lung and thoracic complications in ankylosing spondylitis. J Lab Clin Med 1964;63:254–63.

67. Renzetti AD Jr, Nicholas W, Dutton RE Jr, et al. Some effects of ankylosing spondylitis on pulmonary gas exchange. N Engl J Med 1960;262: 215–8.

68. Franssen MJAM, van Herwaarden CLA, van de Putte LBA, et al. Lung function in patients with ankylosing spondylitis. A study of the influence of disease activity and treatment with nonsteroidal anti- inflammatory drugs. J Rheumatol 1986;13: 936–40.

69. Vanderschueren D, Decramer M, Van den Daele P, et al. Pulmonary function and maximal transrespiratory pressures in ankylosing spondylitis. Ann Rheum Dis 1989;48:632–5.

70. Fisher LR, Cawley MI, Holgate ST. Relation between chest expansion, pulmonary function, and exercise tolerance in patients with ankylosing spondylitis. Ann Rheum Dis 1990;49:921–5.

71. Sahin G, Calikoglu M, Ozge C, et al. Respiratory muscle strength but not BASFI score relates to diminished chest expansion in ankylosing spondylitis. Clin Rheumatol 2004;23:199–202.

72. Murray GC, Persellin RH. Cervical fracture complicating ankylosing spondylitis: a report of eight cases and review of the literature. Am J Med 1981;70(5):1033–41.

73. Thumbikat P, Hariharan RP, Ravichandran G, et al. Spinal cord injury in patients with ankylosing spondylitis: a 10-year review. Spine (Phila Pa 1976) 2007;32:2989–95.

74. van den Berg R, de Hooge M, Rudwaleit M, et al. ASAS modification of the Berlin algorithm for diagnosing axial spondyloarthritis: results from the SPondyloArthritis Caught Early (SPACE)-cohort and from the Assessment of Spondylo Arthritis International Society (ASAS)-cohort. Ann Rheum Dis 2013;72:1646–53.

75. Feldtkeller E, Khan MA, van der Heijde D, et al. Age at disease onset and diagnosis delay in HLA-B27 negative vs. positive patients with ankylosing spondylitis. Rheumatol Int 2003;23:61–6.

76. Campbell AH, McDonald CB. Upper lobe fibrosis associated with ankylosing spondylitis. Br J Dis Chest 1965;59:90–101.

77. Rosenow EC III, Strimlan CV, Muhm JR, et al. Pleuropulmonary manifestations of ankylosing spondylitis. Mayo Clin Proc 1977;52:641–9.

78. Davies D. Ankylosing spondylitis and lung fibrosis. Q J Med 1972;41:395–417.

79. Boushea DK, Sundstrom WR. The pleuropulmonary manifestations of ankylosing spondylitis. Semin Arthritis Rheum 1989;18:277–81.

80. Wendling D, Prati C, Demattei C, et al. Anterior chest wall pain in recent inflammatory back pain

suggestive of spondyloarthritis. data from the DE-SIR cohort. J Rheumatol 2013;40:1148–52.

81. Gupta SM, Johnston WH. Apical pulmonary disease in ankylosing spondylitis. N Z Med J 1978; 88:186–8.

82. Mercieca C, van der Horst-Bruinsma IE, Borg AA. Pulmonary, renal and neurological comorbidities in patients with ankylosing spondylitis; implications for clinical practice. Curr Rheumatol Rep 2014;16:434.

83. Gran JT, Skomsvoll JF. The outcome of ankylosing spondylitis: a study of 100 patients. Br J Rheumatol 1997;36:766–71.

84. Rumancik WM, Firooznia H, Davis MS, et al. Fibrobullous disease of the upper lobes: an extraskeletal manifestation of ankylosing spondylitis. J Comput Tomogr 1984;8:225–9.

85. Tanoue LT. Pulmonary involvement in collagen vascular disease: a review of the pulmonary manifestations of the Marfan syndrome, ankylosing spondylitis, Sjogren's syndrome and relapsing polychondritis. J Thorac Imaging 1992;7:62–77.

86. Libby DM, Schley WS, Smith JP. Cricoarytenoid arthritis in ankylosing spondylitis. A cause of acute respiratory failure and cor pulmonale. Chest 1981; 80(5):641–2.

87. McVeigh CM, Cairns AP. Diagnosis and management of ankylosing spondylitis. BMJ 2006; 333(7568):581–5.

88. Marzo-Ortega H, McGonagle D, O'Connor P, et al. Efficacy of etanercept in the treatment of the entheseal pathology in resistant spondylarthropathy: a clinical and magnetic resonance imaging study. Arthritis Rheum 2001;44(9):2112–7.

89. Gorman JD, Sack KE, Davis JC Jr. Treatment of ankylosing spondylitis by inhibition of tumor necrosis factor alpha. N Engl J Med 2002;346: 1349–56.

90. Fouque-Aubert A, Jette-Paulin L, Combescure C, et al. Serious infections in patients with ankylosing spondylitis with and without TNF. Ann Rheum Dis 2010;69(10):1756–61.

91. Baeten D, Sieper J, Braun J, et al. Secukinumab, an interleukin-17A inhibitor, in ankylosing spondylitis. N Engl J Med 2015;373(26):2534–48.

92. Albert GW, Menezes AH. Ankylosing spondylitis of the craniovertebral junction: a single surgeon's. J Neurosurg Spine 2011;14(4):429–36.

93. Dehghan N, de Mestral C, McKee MD, et al. Flail chest injuries: a review of outcomes and treatment practices from the national trauma Data Bank. J Trauma Acute Care Surg 2014;76:462–8.

94. LoCicero J, Mattox KL. Epidemiology of chest trauma. Surg Clin North Am 1989;69:15–9.

95. Bastos R, Calhoon JH, Baisden CE. Flail chest and pulmonary contusion. Semin Thorac Cardiovasc Surg 2008;20:39–45.

96. Lafferty PM, Anavian J, Will RE, et al. Operative treatment of chest wall injuries: indications, technique, and outcomes. J Bone Joint Surg Am 2011;93:97–110.

97. Battle CE, Evans PA. Predictors of mortality in patients with flail chest: a systematic review. Emerg Med J 2015;32(12):961–5.

98. Kleinman PK, Schlesinger AE. Mechanical factors associated with posterior rib fractures: laboratory and case studies. Pediatr Radiol 1997;27:87–91.

99. Landercasper J, Cogbill TH, Strutt PJ. Delayed diagnosis of flail chest. Crit Care Med 1990;57: 780–4.

100. Erickson U, Johansson L, Nylen O, et al. Radiographic findings in pulmonary insufficiency following non-penetrating trauma of the chest. Scand J Thorac Cardiovasc Surg 1972;6:278–86.

101. Tzelepis GE, McCool FD, Hoppin FG Jr. Chest wall distortion in patients with flail chest. Am Rev Respir Dis 1989;140:31–7.

102. Shinozuka N, Sato J, Kohchi A, et al. Pendelluft is not the major contributor to respiratory insufficiency in dogs with flail chest: a mathematical analysis. J Anesth 1995;9:252–9.

103. Shackford SR, Virgilio RW, Peters RM. Selective use of ventilator therapy in flail chest injury. J Thorac Cardiovasc Surg 1981;81(2):194–201.

104. Simon B, Ebert J, Bokhari F, et al. Management of pulmonary contusion and flail chest: an Eastern Association for the Surgery of Trauma practice management guideline. J Trauma Acute Care Surg 2012;73:S351–61.

105. Tanaka H, Yukioka T, Yamaguti Y, et al. Surgical stabilization of internal pneumatic stabilization? A prospective randomized study of management of severe flail chest patients. J Trauma 2002;52(4): 727–32.

106. Granetzny A, Abd El-Aal M, Emam E, et al. Surgical versus conservative treatment of flail chest. evaluation of the pulmonary status. Interact Cardiovasc Thorac Surg 2005;4(6):583–7.

107. Marasco SF, Davies AR, Cooper J, et al. Prospective randomized controlled trial of operative rib fixation in traumatic flail chest. J Am Coll Surg 2013; 216(5):924–32.

108. Schuurmans J, Goslings JC, Schepers T. Operative management versus non-operative management of rib fractures in flail chest injuries: a systematic review. Eur J Trauma Emerg Surg 2016;43(2):163–8.

109. Marasco S, Liew S, Edwards E, et al. Analysis of bone healing in flail chest injury: do we need to fix both fractures per rib? J Trauma Acute Care Surg 2014;77:452–8.

110. Malek MH, Berger DE, Housh TJ, et al. Cardiovascular function following surgical repair of pectus excavatum: a metaanalysis. Chest 2006;130: 506–16.

111. Chung CS, Myrianthopoulos NC. Factors affecting risks of congenital malformations. I. Analysis of epidemiologic factors in congenital malformation. Report from the collaborative perinatal project. Birth Defects Orig Artic Ser 1975;11(10):1–22.

112. Kelly RE Jr, Shamberger RC, Mellins RB, et al. Prospective multicenter study of surgical correction of pectus excavatum: design, peri operative complications, pain, and baseline pulmonary function facilitated by internet-based data collection. J Am Coll Surg 2007;205(2):205–16.

113. Waters P, Welch K, Micheli LJ, et al. Scoliosis in children with pectus excavatum and pectus carinatum. J Pediatr Orthop 1989;9(5):551–6.

114. Shamberger RC, Welch KJ. Cardiopulmonary function in pectus excavatum. Surg Gynecol Obstet 1988;166(4):383–91.

115. Prozorovskaya NN, Kozlov EA, Voronov AV, et al. Characterization of costal cartilage collagen in funnel chest. Biomed Sci 1991;2:576–80.

116. Creswick HA, Stacey MW, Kelly RE, et al. Family study of the inheritance of pectus excavatum. J Pediatr Surg 2006;41:1699–703.

117. Nobuhara KK, Lund DP, Mitchell J, et al. Long-term outlook for survivors of congenital diaphragmatic hernia. Clin Perinatol 1996;23:873–87.

118. Schaerer D, Virbalas J, Willis E, et al. Pectus excavatum in children with laryngomalacia. Int J Pediatr Otorhinolaryngol 2013;77:1721.

119. Castile RG, Staats BA, Westbrook PR. Symptomatic pectus deformities of the chest. Am Rev Respir Dis 1982;126:564–8.

120. Lawson ML, Mellins R, Tabangin M, et al. Impact of pectus excavatum on pulmonary function before and after repair with the Nuss procedure. J Pediatr Surg 2005;40(1):174–80.

121. Lawson ML, Mellins RB, Paulson JF, et al. Increasing severity of pectus excavatum is associated with reduced pulmonary function. J Pediatr 2011;159(2):256–61.

122. Koumbourlis AC, Stolar CJ. Lung growth and function in children and adolescents with idiopathic pectus excavatum. Pediatr Pulmonol 2004;38:339–43.

123. Koumbourlis AC, Stolar CJ. Respiratory muscle strength and air-trapping in pectus excavatum. Pediatr Res 2004;55:A3418.

124. Redlinger RE, Kelly RE, Nuss D, et al. Regional chest wall motion dysfunction in patients with pectus excavatum demonstrated via optoelectronic plethysmography. J Pediatr Surg 2011;46(6):1172–6.

125. Mocchegiani R, Badano L, Lestuzzi C, et al. Relation of right ventricular morphology and function in pectus excavatum to the severity of the chest wall deformity. Am J Cardiol 1995;76(12):941–6.

126. Töpper A, Polleichtner S, Zagrosek A, et al. Impact of surgical correction of pectus excavatum on cardiac function: insights on the right ventricle. A cardiovascular magnetic resonance study. Interact Cardiovasc Thorac Surg 2016;22(1):38–46.

127. Saleh RS, Finn JP, Fenchel M, et al. Cardiovascular magnetic resonance in patients with pectus excavatum compared with normal controls. J Cardiovasc Magn Reson 2010;12:73.

128. Chao CJ, Jaroszewski DE, Kumar PN, et al. Surgical repair of pectus excavatum relieves right heart chamber compression and improves cardiac output in adult patients: an intraoperative transesophageal echocardiographic study. Am J Surg 2015;210(6):1118–24 [discussion: 1124–5].

129. Jeong JY, Ahn JH, Kim SY, et al. Pulmonary function before and after the Nuss procedure in adolescents with pectus excavatum: correlation with morphological subtypes. J Cardiothorac Surg 2015;10:37.

130. Iseman MD, Buschman DL, Ackerson LM. Pectus excavatum and scoliosis. Thoracic anomalies associated with pulmonary disease caused by Mycobacterium avium complex. Am Rev Respir Dis 1991;144:914–6.

131. Kamiyama M, Usui N, Tani G, et al. Airway deformation in patients demonstrating pectus excavatum with an improvement after the Nuss procedure. Pediatr Surg Int 2011;27(1):61–6.

132. Haller JA Jr, Kramer SS, Lietman SA. Use of CT scans in selection of patients for pectus excavatum surgery: a preliminary report. J Pediatr Surg 1987;22:904–6.

133. Khanna G, Jaju A, Don S, et al. Comparison of Haller index values calculated with chest radiographs versus CT for pectus excavatum evaluation. Pediatr Radiol 2010 Nov;40(11):1763–7.

134. Ravitch MM. The operative treatment of pectus excavatum. Ann Surg 1949;129(4):429–44.

135. Elsayed HH, Hassaballa AS, Abdel Hady SM, et al. Choosing between the modified Ravitch and Nuss procedures for pectus excavatum: considering the patients's perspective. Ann R Coll Surg Engl 2016;98(8):581–5.

136. Kaguraoka H, Ohnuki T, Itaoka T, et al. Degree of severity of pectus excavatum and pulmonary function in preoperative and postoperative periods. J Thorac Cardiovasc Surg 1992;104(5):1483–8.

137. Haller JA Jr, Loughlin GM. Cardiorespiratory function is significantly improved following corrective surgery for severe pectus excavatum. Proposed treatment guidelines. J Cardiovasc Surg (Torino) 2000;41(1):125–30.

Muscular Dystrophies

John C. Carter, MD[a], Daniel W. Sheehan, PhD, MD[b], Andre Prochoroff, MD[c], David J. Birnkrant, MD[d],*

KEYWORDS

- Muscular dystrophy • Duchenne muscular dystrophy • Limb girdle muscular dystrophy
- Facioscapulohumeral muscular dystrophy • Respiratory failure • Cardiomyopathy

KEY POINTS

- The muscular dystrophies are a heterogeneous group of disorders defined by dystrophic pathologic features on muscle biopsy.
- Clinically, muscular dystrophies are characterized by progressive muscle weakness affecting skeletal muscles, although significant variability exists in the genetic and biochemical features, the distribution of affected musculature, degree of respiratory and cardiac compromise, and the involvement of other organ systems, such as the eyes and central nervous system.
- There is variability, even among patients with the same disorder and genetic mutations, in age of onset, severity, progression, prognosis, and thus optimal management.

INTRODUCTION

The muscular dystrophies are a heterogeneous group of disorders defined by dystrophic pathologic features on muscle biopsy. Clinically, they are characterized by progressive muscle weakness affecting skeletal muscles, although significant variability exists in the genetic and biochemical features, the distribution of affected musculature, degree of respiratory and cardiac compromise, and the involvement of other organ systems such as the eyes and central nervous system. There is also variability, even among patients with the same disorder and genetic mutations, in age of onset, severity, progression, prognosis, and thus optimal management.

This article provides an introduction to the taxonomy, basic genetics, clinical profile, natural history, and fundamentals of management of the muscular dystrophies. Pulmonologists are likely to encounter patients with muscular dystrophy across a variety of settings, including in the clinic, in the intensive care unit, and as part of multidisciplinary programs specializing in the care of neuromuscular disorders.

Substantial progress in the care of patients with muscular dystrophy has been made in recent years, driven by international collaboration, a growing understanding of the underlying genetic processes, and clinical consensus guidelines. Implementation of standards of care can improve anticipatory guidance, can promote proactive management, and has been shown to improve survival. Implementation of standards of care is also needed to provide stable baselines for assessment of the clinical effects of new treatments. Prevention of respiratory complications via anticipatory therapy with lung volume recruitment, assisted coughing and noninvasive ventilation, is a critically important component of the multidisciplinary care of patients with muscular dystrophy. Duchenne muscular dystrophy (DMD),

[a] Division of Pulmonary, Critical Care and Sleep Medicine, MetroHealth Medical Center, Case Western Reserve University School of Medicine, 2500 MetroHealth Drive, Cleveland, OH 44019, USA; [b] Division of Pediatric Pulmonology, John R. Oishei Children's Hospital, University at Buffalo, 955 Main Street, Buffalo, NY 14203, USA; [c] Division of Pediatric Neurology, MetroHealth Medical Center, Case Western Reserve University School of Medicine, 2500 MetroHealth Drive, Cleveland, OH 44019, USA; [d] Division of Pediatric Pulmonology, MetroHealth Medical Center, Case Western Reserve University School of Medicine, 2500 MetroHealth Drive, Cleveland, OH 44019, USA
* Corresponding author.
E-mail address: dbirnkrant@metrohealth.org

Clin Chest Med 39 (2018) 377–389
https://doi.org/10.1016/j.ccm.2018.01.004

the most common inherited muscle disease of childhood, is used as a model because it is by far the best studied muscular dystrophy. This article includes the latest recommendations for the respiratory management of DMD, adapted from the updated Centers for Disease Control and Prevention (CDC)-sponsored care considerations, recently published in *Lancet Neurology*.[1]

EPIDEMIOLOGY

The muscular dystrophies as individual disorders are relatively rare, but as a group represent a sizable fraction of patients with neuromuscular disease encountered in both the outpatient and the inpatient setting. DMD, the most common inherited muscle disease in childhood, is found in roughly 8.3 per 100,000 boys, whereas its cousin Becker muscular dystrophy occurs in roughly 7.3 per 100,000.[2] In adults, myotonic dystrophy is the most common form, affecting roughly 10.6 per 100,000 people, followed by facioscapulohumeral dystrophy, which affects an estimated 3 per 100,000 people.[3] The prevalence of congenital muscular dystrophies varies significantly by region. Ullrich congenital muscular dystrophy is the most common form of congenital muscular dystrophy globally,[4] although Fukuyama muscular dystrophy is the most common type in Japan due to a recessive founder mutation.[5]

CLINICAL MANIFESTATIONS

Historically, muscular dystrophies have been classified based on the age of onset, principal pattern of muscle involvement, and other clinical features. Subtypes were defined based on inheritance and the underlying genetic defect, if known. It has subsequently become clear that a wide variety of genetic defects may result in similar phenotypes,[6,7] and conversely, that substantial phenotypic variability exists among patients with the same pathogenic genotype.[8,9] This discordance highlights the importance of regular screening and monitoring of patients with muscular dystrophy, particularly for progressive changes in pulmonary and/or cardiac function. Second, it highlights the need for additional definition of subphenotypes for better anticipatory guidance, prognosis, and evaluation of therapies in both clinical and research settings.

The onset of symptoms and signs in muscular dystrophies varies from birth to adulthood (**Table 1**). The congenital muscular dystrophies typically present with signs at birth or within the first few months of life. DMD and many of the limb girdle muscular dystrophies present in early childhood or adolescence, often after independent

ambulation has been achieved. Other limb girdle muscular dystrophies, as well as myotonic dystrophy and facioscapulohumeral muscular dystrophy, characteristically manifest in adulthood. Skeletal muscle weakness characterizes all muscular dystrophies, although the distribution, degree, and progressive nature of weakness differ among disorders. In most of the congenital muscular dystrophies, ambulation is never achieved. In childhood-onset forms, such as DMD, ambulation is achieved but is typically lost before adolescence. In later-onset limb girdle muscular dystrophies and facioscapulohumeral dystrophy, ambulation may be preserved throughout adulthood, with the need for wheelchair assistance developing much later. In myotonic dystrophy, motor function varies significantly, ranging from severely affected infants with congenital myotonia and significant respiratory compromise to minimally affected adults with preserved ambulation and minimal respiratory impairment. Additional features in the muscular dystrophies, such as muscle atrophy or compensatory hypertrophy, joint contractures, myotonia, degree of respiratory involvement, and cardiac abnormalities, are also variable.

Respiratory impairment is common in patients with muscular dystrophy. Although the degree and onset of impairment are variable, respiratory impairment generally develops after the loss of ambulation, related to generalized inspiratory weakness or selective diaphragmatic weakness. Weakness of the expiratory muscles and of the muscles involved in coughing and swallowing results in impaired airway clearance and secretion management, necessitating lung recruitment maneuvers and assisted coughing. Respiratory impairment typically begins as nocturnal hypoventilation, which may precede daytime respiratory compromise by months or years in slowly progressive conditions.[10–12] Respiratory complications are a frequent cause of morbidity and mortality in patients with muscular dystrophy, including atelectasis, mucus plugging, pneumonia, bulbar dysfunction, dyspnea, and respiratory failure.[13] Evaluation and management of respiratory impairment are discussed later.

DUCHENNE MUSCULAR DYSTROPHY

As the most common inherited muscle disease of childhood, DMD is the most studied muscular dystrophy with regard to respiratory issues and represents an important prototype for the respiratory management of the muscular dystrophies. Boys with DMD typically present to medical attention in early childhood, due to weakness, clumsiness,

Table 1
Overview of muscular dystrophies

Muscular Dystrophy	Pathogenetic Factors			Clinical Characteristics						
	Inheritance	Gene(s)	Affected Protein(s)	Distribution of Weakness	Natural History	Motor Function	Respiratory Impairment	Cardiomyopathy	CK Levels	Other Findings
Early onset										
Congenital muscular dystrophy with merosin deficiency	AR	LAMA2	Laminin alpha2 chain of merosin	Primarily upper limbs	Slowly progressive	Ambulation generally not achieved	Frequent	Not common	High	White matter changes on MRI
Dystroglycanopathies (Waker-Warburg, Fukuyama muscular dystrophy, muscle-eye-brain disease)	AR	Multiple	Dystroglycan and glycosyl-transferase enzymes	Primarily upper limbs	Slowly progressive	Ambulation generally not achieved	Frequent	Not common	High	Structural brain anomalies
Ullrich muscular dystrophy	AR	COL6A1, COL6A2, COL6A3	Collagen VI subunits	Primarily axial and limb muscles	Progressive	Early ambulation achieved in about half of patients but typically lost by teenage years	Frequent; usually early	Not common	Normal or slight elevation	Rigid spine, laxity of distal joints
SEPN1 myopathy (muscular dystrophy with rigid spine syndrome)	AR	SEPN1	Selenoprotein N1	Axial > Limb muscles	Respiratory progression more so than motor progression	Ambulation typically achieved	Frequent; usually early	Not common	Normal or slight elevation	Rigid spine, scoliosis
Childhood and young-adult onset										
DMD	X-linked R	DMD	Dystrophin	Proximal > distal muscles	Progressive	Ambulation typically achieved, but lost around adolescence	Frequent	Common	High	Cognitive and neurobehavioral problems
Becker muscular dystrophy	X-linked R	DMD	Dystrophin	Proximal > distal muscles	Significant variability but slower than DMD	Ambulation typically achieved	Not common	Common	High	Milder than DMD
Emery-Dreifuss muscular dystrophy	Variable depending on type (X-linked R, AD, AR)	EMD, FHL1, LMNA, SYNE1, SYNE2	Emerin, Lamin A/C, Nesprin	Scapuloperoneal pattern	Slowly progressive	Ambulation typically achieved	Typically in adulthood	Common, with conduction defects	Moderate to high	Rigid spine, associated with Dunnigan-type lipodystrophy, insulin resistance

(continued on next page)

Table 1
(continued)

Muscular Dystrophy	Pathogenetic Factors			Clinical Characteristics						
	Inheritance	Gene(s)	Affected Protein(s)	Distribution of Weakness	Natural History	Motor Function	Respiratory Impairment	Cardiomyopathy	CK Levels	Other Findings
Limb girdle muscular dystrophies	AR > AD	Multiple	Sarcoglycan, Dystroglycan, Telethonin, Titin, and so forth	Variable, mostly proximal > distal	Progressive in adulthood	Ambulation typically achieved, sometimes lost in early adulthood or middle age	Common in sarcoglycan deficiencies, variable in dystrogly-canopathies, uncommon in dysferlin and titin deficiency	Variable (common in sarcoglycan deficiency, dystrogly-canopathy), tends to track with respiratory impairment	Usually high	Intellectual disabilities
Facioscapulohumeral dystrophy	AD	DUX4, SMCHD1	Subtelomeric chromatin rearrangement	Facial, shoulder, scapular, arm weakness	Slowly progressive	Ambulation typically achieved	Rare	Rare	Normal or slight elevation	Hearing loss, retinal degeneration
Myotonic dystrophy	AD, trinucleotide repeat disorder with anticipation	DMPK, CNBP	Myotonic dystrophy protein kinase	Distal weakness	Slowly progressive in early adulthood or middle age, may be earlier in type 1	Ambulation typically achieved	Not common; sleep-disordered breathing common	Common, with conduction defects	Normal or slight elevation	Myotonia, cataracts, intellectual disabilities, insulin resistance, hypersomnolence, circadian abnormalities
Adult onset										
Other limb girdle muscular dystrophies	AR > AD	ANO5, MYOT, CAV3	Anoctamin, myotilin, caveolin	Variable	Slowly progressive in adulthood	Independent ambulation achieved and often maintained	Rare	Rare except for caveolin deficiency	High	Cramps, muscle rippling

toe-walking, or trouble climbing stairs, along with typical physical features (such as the Gowers sign and/or calf muscle pseudohypertrophy). Ideally, they obtain early referral to a neuromuscular specialist who can assume responsibility for coordination of care.[14] Deletion-duplication analysis of the *DMD* gene will detect roughly 70% of cases, with gene sequencing detecting the remaining 25% to 30% due to point mutations or smaller deletions/duplications.[15,16] A muscle biopsy specimen showing the absence of dystrophin protein makes a definitive diagnosis if genetic testing is negative, but the need for muscle biopsy has greatly diminished thanks to the sensitivity of contemporary genetic techniques.

Upon diagnosis, prompt involvement in a multidisciplinary management program is indicated. Such programs are generally coordinated by a neuromuscular specialist and include representatives from neurology, rehabilitation medicine, pulmonology, cardiology, gastroenterology/nutrition, endocrinology/bone health, genetics, orthopedics, psychology/mental health, occupational and physical therapy, social work, nursing, and other specialties as needed. The comprehensive update of the CDC-sponsored care considerations for DMD[1] is a useful resource regarding contemporary multidisciplinary assessment and management. Glucocorticoids are a mainstay of treatment in DMD and are associated with prolonged ambulatory ability, improved respiratory function, improved upper limb strength,[17] and delayed need for scoliosis surgery.[18] Initiation of glucocorticoid therapy early, before loss of ambulation, has proven to be beneficial,[19,20] and studies of glucocorticoid therapy in younger boys (less than the age of 30 months) are ongoing. However, controversy exists regarding the optimal type and dose of glucocorticoid,[21] and blinded trials of prednisone versus deflazacort are currently underway.[22] Complications of glucocorticoid therapy such as weight gain and resultant sleep-disordered breathing[12] need to be monitored.

Novel therapies in development for DMD include mutation-specific treatments such as ataluren (approved in Europe and induces read-through of a stop codon in the dystrophin gene),[23] eteplirsen (approved in the United States and induces exon 51 skipping),[24] as well as other compounds targeting mitochondrial function, anti-inflammatory and vasodilatory agents, antioxidants, and utrophin molecular regulators.[25] At least one novel compound targeting oxidative phosphorylation aimed at improving mitochondrial function (idebenone) has demonstrated efficacy in reducing loss of respiratory function (assessed via peak expiratory flow) in DMD.[26] The rapid expansion of the therapeutic armamentarium highlights the importance of studies delineating the natural history of DMD, and definition of clinically meaningful pulmonary outcome measures.[27]

Respiratory Care in Duchenne Muscular Dystrophy

Anticipatory respiratory management has been shown to prolong survival, improve quality of life, and reduce respiratory complications in DMD.[28–32] The updated CDC-sponsored care considerations was recently published,[1] and a related specialty article is expected soon. The new guidelines update the 2010 version of the care considerations. Meanwhile, pulmonary management guidelines can be found in the 2010 care considerations and the related specialty article.[33,34] The authors refer the reader to those guidelines for additional details. Recommendations are divided according to the stage of disease progression. **Fig. 1**, reproduced from the latest care considerations, provides an overview of respiratory assessments and interventions. All of the specific assessment and treatment recommendations found in the later sections are from the updated CDC care considerations article.

In the ambulatory stage, spirometry should be initiated at the age of 5 to 6 years, with serial measurement of forced vital capacity (FVC) yearly (see **Fig. 1**). During this stage, FVC increases with somatic growth until plateauing around the age at which ambulation is lost, followed by a progressive decline in FVC over time (**Fig. 2**).[35,36] Significant variability exists among individuals in terms of the age at which FVC plateaus, the level of the peak FVC, and the rate of subsequent FVC decline.[8,36,37] Polysomnography with capnography should be considered as well for boys with symptoms of sleep-disordered breathing, particularly those with glucocorticoid-related weight gain.[12] Prevention of respiratory illness with routine vaccinations is also indicated, including annual inactivated influenza vaccine and administration of 23-valent pneumococcal immunization according to standard schedules.[38]

In the early nonambulatory stage, which tends to begin in mid adolescence, respiratory function plateaus and subsequently declines. Seated FVC, peak cough flow, maximum inspiratory and expiratory pressures (MIPs/MEPs), and pulse oximetry should be measured at least every 6 months[33] (see **Fig. 1**). If the necessary equipment is available, blood carbon dioxide levels should be monitored via end-tidal or transcutaneous capnography every 6 months, or when Spo_2 is less than 95% while the patient is awake and in room air. Respiratory

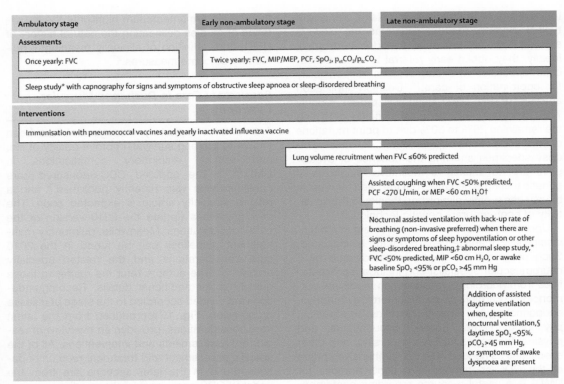

Fig. 1. Recommended assessments and interventions in DMD. DMD, duchenne muscular dystrophy; FVC, forced vital capacity; MEP, maximum expiratory pressure; MIP, maximum inspiratory pressure; PCF, peak cough flow; petCO2, end-tidal partial pressure of CO_2; ptcCO2, transcutaneous partial pressure of CO_2; SpO2, blood oxygen saturation by pulse oximetry. * See text for definitions of sleep study results. † All specified threshold values of PCF, MEP, and MIP apply to older teenage and adult patients. ‡ Fatigue, dyspnoea, morning or continuous head-aches, frequent nocturnal awakenings or difficult arousal, hypersomnolence, difficulty concentrating, awaken-ings with dyspnoea and tachycardia, or frequent nightmares. § We strongly endorse the use of non-invasive methods of assisted ventilation instead of tracheostomy to optimise patient quality of life; indications for trache-ostomy include patient preference, inability of patient to use non-invasive ventilation successfully, three failed extubation attempts during a critical illness despite optimum use of non-invasive ventilation and mechanically assisted coughing, or failure of non-invasive methods of cough assistance to prevent aspiration of secretions into the lungs due to weak bulbar muscles. (*From* Birnkrant DJ, Bushby K, Bann CM, et al. Diagnosis and manage-ment of Duchenne muscular dystrophy, an update, part 2: respiratory, cardiac, bone health, and orthopedic man-agement. Lancet Neurol, 2018;17(4):347–61; with permission.)

interventions such as lung volume recruitment become important during this stage, as chest wall compliance begins to decrease with falling vital ca-pacities. When FVC is ≤60% predicted, lung vol-ume recruitment should be undertaken via manual bag ventilation or mechanical in-exsufflation once or twice daily.[39–41] For patients undergoing surgery for scoliosis or other indications, guidelines for use of assisted coughing devices and/or noninvasive ventilation should be followed.[42]

In the late nonambulatory stage, ineffective cough and hypoventilation are common, increasing the likelihood of pneumonia, atelectasis, and respiratory failure, particularly with respiratory tract infections.[33] Manual and mechanically assisted coughing is indicated when FVC is <50%

predicted, peak cough flow is <270 L/min, or when MEP is <60 cm H_2O[43,44] (see **Fig. 1**). During respiratory infections, assisted coughing should be undertaken more frequently. Early and judicious use of antibiotics is also recommended when pa-tients manifest signs of pneumonia.[33]

Boys with DMD are at high risk for sleep-disordered breathing. The principal phenotype of sleep-disordered breathing in young patients is obstructive sleep apnea (OSA), and nocturnal hypoventilation at older ages,[45] although there is considerable overlap given variable progression of muscle weakness, obesity, steroid use, and other factors. Central sleep apnea may also be pre-sent in up to 33% of patients with DMD,[12] although it can be challenging to differentiate central from

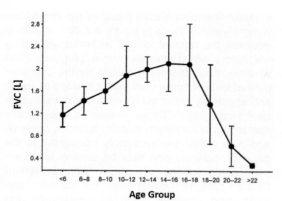

Fig. 2. FVC in DMD increases with age and somatic growth until plateauing at the age at which ambulation is lost (typically in adolescence), with a subsequent more rapid decline. (*Adapted from* Mayer OH, Finkel RS, Rummey C, et al. Characterization of pulmonary function in Duchenne muscular dystrophy. Pediatr Pulmonol 2015;50(5):491; with permission.)

obstructive events in the setting of poor respiratory excursion due to decreased muscle strength.

With progressive muscle weakness, DMD patients develop nocturnal, sleep-related hypoventilation, followed by daytime hypoventilation while they are awake. The use of assisted ventilation to treat hypoventilation has been a key contributor to increased lifespan for patients with DMD.[28,45] In one study, nocturnal hypoventilation was associated with an FVC less than 1820 mL and daytime hypercapnia with an FVC less than 680 mL.[46] However, spirometry levels are imperfect predictors of hypoventilation,[12,45] and in other studies, FVC and forced expiratory volume in 1 second (FEV-1) were only marginally specific for hypoventilation and not predictive of OSA severity as defined by the apnea-hypopnea index (AHI).[46,47] Furthermore, typical symptoms of sleep-disordered breathing (snoring, sleep disturbance, daytime headaches, lethargy, or sleepiness) may be helpful if present but are not reliably associated with either hypoventilation or OSA in DMD.[45]

With regard to specific treatment recommendations, nocturnally assisted ventilation is indicated for patients with DMD who have symptoms of hypoventilation (fatigue, dyspnea, morning or continuous headaches, frequent nocturnal awakenings or difficult arousal, hypersomnolence, difficulty concentrating, awakenings with dyspnea and tachycardia, and/or frequent nightmares). For patients who are asymptomatic, additional indications for nocturnal ventilation are as follows: an FVC <50% predicted; absolute value of MIP less than 60 cm water pressure; or when the individual is awake and, because of daytime hypoventilation,

any of the following is present: end-tidal CO_2 or transcutaneous P_{CO_2} is >45 mm Hg; the arterial, venous, or capillary blood P_{CO_2} is >45 mm Hg; or baseline Sp_{O_2} is less than 95% in room air.[12,46,48,49]

Nocturnally assisted ventilation is also indicated in patients with abnormal sleep studies. These studies include overnight oximetry, combination oximetry-capnography, and polysomnography with capnography (the latter being preferred whenever possible). Symptomatic patients should have sleep studies as often as annually, if the necessary equipment and personnel are available. Nocturnally assisted ventilation is indicated if a sleep study results show any of the following: end-tidal or transcutaneous CO_2 greater than 50 mm Hg for $\geq$2% of sleep time, a sleep-related increase in end-tidal or transcutaneous CO_2 of 10 mm Hg above the awake baseline for $\geq$2% of sleep time, $Sp_{O_2} \leq$88% for $\geq$2% of sleep time or for at least 5 minutes continuously,[46,50] or an AHI $\geq$5 events per hour.[33,46,50–52]

Instead of continuous positive airway pressure, bilevel positive airway pressure is first-line therapy for boys with DMD who have OSA due to their inevitable need for assisted ventilation to treat hypoventilation. Hypoxemia in patients with DMD is typically due to hypoventilation, atelectasis, pneumonia, or some combination thereof.[44] Thus, supplemental oxygen should not be used alone; however, in conjunction with assisted ventilation and assisted coughing, oxygen therapy can be safe. Blood CO_2 levels should be measured when possible to determine adequacy of ventilatory support.

Daytime assisted ventilation typically comes about as a natural extension of nocturnal ventilation, as the patient becomes increasingly symptomatic with dyspnea, fatigue, and/or difficulty concentrating.[53] Daytime awake hypercapnia and hypoxemia *despite the use of nocturnal ventilation* (Sp_{O_2} <95% in room air or P_{CO_2} >45 mm Hg) are indications for diurnal-assisted ventilation, which can be accomplished in several ways (eg, via mouthpiece or "sip" ventilation using a portable volume ventilator, or via nasal bilevel ventilation depending on patient and clinician preferences). Noninvasive ventilation can be used safely and effectively up to 24 hours per day.[54] The use of invasive ventilation via tracheostomy involves some controversy, with practices depending on local standards of care, availability of home nursing or other skilled support, the ability of the patient to use noninvasive ventilation, and patient preference. Although the use of noninvasive ventilation up to 24 h/d is strongly recommended,[33] exclusive use of noninvasive ventilation can be challenging for very weak patients, especially during periods of acute illness, when they may require endotracheal intubation (assuming there is no advance directive to the contrary). Other indications for tracheostomy include the following: 3 failed extubation attempts during a critical illness despite optimal use of noninvasive ventilation and mechanically assisted coughing,[55] or failure of noninvasive methods of cough assistance to prevent aspiration of secretions into the lungs due to weak bulbar muscles.

A PULMONOLOGIST'S PERSPECTIVE ON PROLONGED SURVIVAL AND THE RESPIRATORY COMPLICATIONS OF DUCHENNE MUSCULAR DYSTROPHY

This time is transformative in neuromuscular respiratory medicine, involving a new optimism about the potential benefits of emerging therapies.[56] Using DMD as the model, multidisciplinary therapies (including respiratory, cardiac, and nutritional support, and the widespread use of glucocorticoids) have caused expected survival to increase from approximately 20 years of age to 30 years of age and longer.[57,58] However, prolonged survival has also created a new set of contemporary challenges related to previously unknown medical complications, and the need to consider nonmedical issues that have a profound effect on the quality of life of patients and their families.[59] Pulmonologists and other respiratory clinicians often find themselves at the center of this group of problematic contemporary issues. In addition, prolonged survival has unmasked the variability of cardiopulmonary function over time in individual patients, including patients with identical dystrophin genotypes, prompting ongoing studies of the prevalence, implications, and possible causes of cardiopulmonary phenotypic variability.

IMPLICATIONS AND FUTURE DIRECTIONS
Implications of Prolonged Survival: Complex Medical Decision Making

Medical complications related to prolonged survival can include the need for gastrostomy tube feeding in patients with severe dysphagia[60] and unexpected complications, like nephrolithiasis.[61] As a result, pulmonologists are often asked to help manage the respiratory support and anesthetic techniques when patients with advanced DMD undergo high-risk procedures, such as gastrostomy placement and lithotripsy; relevant guidelines are available.[42] As implied in the recommendations section earlier, prolonged survival has also resulted in patients living with 24-h/d assisted ventilation for extended periods of time.[62] Thus, respiratory clinicians need to consider the best mode of ventilation for these patients (tracheostomy vs noninvasive), the best

equipment and interfaces (nasal vs sip ventilation; volume ventilators vs pressure support or bilevel devices), the risks of 24-h/d ventilation (including respiratory arrest due to mucus plugging), and whether resources are available for the unprecedented level of home care that is needed to safely and effectively enact such an intensive respiratory treatment plan.[34] Those resources are usually sparse; home nursing availability is usually minimal, and care duties are commonly consigned to the patient's parents, who may be dealing with their own complications of aging. With advanced DMD, patients commonly experience life-threatening illnesses, such as pneumonia and advanced heart failure due to cardiomyopathy. Patients must decide if they are willing to undergo repeated hospitalizations, critical care, intubation, resuscitation, and other potentially risky, painful, intrusive, and/or invasive therapies involving difficult and complex risk/benefit decisions.[63] Patients must also decide if they wish to participate in trials of new and emerging therapies for DMD, with pulmonary function a key outcome measure. Multiple new therapies are now in the clinical pipeline,[56] and a "competition" of sorts is occurring for subject recruitment, because the pool of DMD patients is relatively small. These decisions involve the risk of the new therapies themselves as well as the "opportunity cost" that occurs when patients choose to initiate a particular emerging therapy to the exclusion of others, without knowing which therapy might be most efficacious. Pulmonologists and other respiratory professionals are involved in all of the medical issues discussed earlier and often find themselves to be the front-line consultants to DMD patients and their families with regard to this contemporary group of complex, stressful, high-stakes medical decisions.

Implications of Prolonged Survival: Care Transitions

As they age, severe respiratory and cardiac issues become the main determinants of patient survival, and the medical care of young adult DMD patients generally shifts out of the multidisciplinary pediatric environment to technologically based specialists in adult care venues. This shift results in care fragmentation, with the adult medicine pulmonologist, intensivist, and cardiologist becoming the key medical providers. These providers may be more accustomed to caring for a geriatric population than for young adults with DMD. In addition, a significant proportion of patients with DMD has mild intellectual disability and/or psychological diagnoses, such as autism spectrum disorder or attention deficit disorder, complicating their ability to make informed, autonomous medical decisions.[64] The environment of adult medicine care venues, especially intensive care units, can thus be traumatic for DMD patients and their families. These dilemmas highlight the critical need for actively managed, beneficial, and humane transitions of care between pediatric and adult medical care providers and care venues.[65] Strategies that ease the transition between these 2 medical environments include care coordination by a primary, designated neuromuscular specialist; attention to the psychosocial needs of younger patients in adult medicine hospital wards and intensive care units; and the involvement of palliative and end-of-life care providers before the onset of life-threatening illnesses.[66] A recent examination of the authors' own muscular dystrophy clinic showed that almost three-quarters of the DMD patients are now aged 18 years or older. There is a great need to create pediatric to adult care transitions that maximize patient survival while optimizing patient autonomy, functionality, dignity, and quality of life.

Implications of Prolonged Survival: Cardiopulmonary Phenotypic Variability

The key role of the respiratory system in patient survival, coupled with the emergence of new molecular and genetic therapies, has increased the urgency to understand the natural history of DMD pulmonary function and to develop clinically meaningful, validated pulmonary outcome measures, the current "gold standard" for which is FVC.[27] With prolonged survival, patterns of DMD pulmonary function over time have become more evident. These patterns define pulmonary phenotypes. As discussed earlier, it is generally the case that the absolute value of FVC increases over time, during the ambulatory stage of DMD; FVC peaks and plateaus near the age at loss of ambulation, and then, FVC progressively declines during the patient's remaining lifespan.[35] However, this model trajectory is likely an oversimplification; in reality, a high prevalence of cardiopulmonary phenotypic variability has become apparent, including the unreliability of genotype-phenotype correlations.[37,67,68] Elucidation of the different subtypes of phenotypic variability has become a significant area of inquiry, with implications for predicting patient prognosis and for the evaluation and design of new DMD therapies. One type of phenotypic variability is illustrated by the variable pulmonary and cardiac function observed among patients with identical dystrophin genotypes, including brothers with DMD (**Fig. 3**).[8] Another type of cardiopulmonary phenotypic variability is a "phenotypic disconnect," presenting in an individual as discordant heart (cardiac muscle) function and lung (respiratory skeletal muscle) function. For example, prolonged survivors of DMD seem to have unexpectedly good heart function despite profound respiratory muscle weakness, that is, a surprisingly beneficial cardiac phenotype coupled with a detrimental pulmonary phenotype. Conversely, DMD patients who experience early death have unexpectedly poor heart function coupled with preserved respiratory muscle strength—a detrimental cardiac phenotype coupled with a beneficial pulmonary phenotype.[32] In the authors' recent study, DMD patients who were alive and had a deletion of exon 44 as their dystrophin mutation were equally likely to manifest either combination: good heart/bad lung, or bad heart/good lung (ie, there was no correlation between dystrophin genotype and cardiopulmonary phenotype).[69] The implications of cardiopulmonary phenotypic variability are profound; for example,

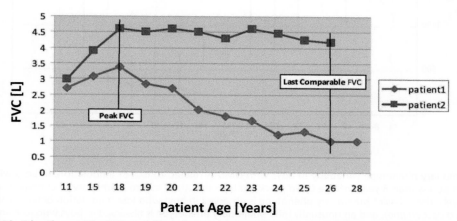

Fig. 3. FVC in 2 brothers with DMD and discordant pulmonary function. (*From* Birnkrant DJ, Ashwath ML, Noritz GH, et al. Cardiac and pulmonary function variability in Duchenne/Becker muscular dystrophy: an initial report. J Child Neurol 2010;25(9):1111; with permission.)

prognostic predictions become unreliable when a patient's genotype does not accurately predict his cardiopulmonary function over time. Moreover, because phenotypic variability appears to be common, evaluating the effect of therapies on the cardiac and pulmonary systems may require knowledge of each individual patient's natural history of cardiac and pulmonary function over time. For example, if the presence of unexpectedly beneficial cardiac phenotypes is common, as shown in the authors' study of prolonged survivors,[69] this could confound the evaluation of new therapies. Aggregate data may be inaccurate because of the frequency of "outliers" with good cardiac function. Prolonged patient survival could be attributed to a new therapy when in fact a significant subset of subjects in the study is simply expressing their beneficial cardiac phenotypes.

These issues illustrate the potential value of nongenotypic predictors of DMD pulmonary phenotypes. For example, in one recent study,[37] a typical pulmonary phenotype was predicted by loss of ambulation between 8 and 11 years of age, whereas loss of ambulation at less than 8 years of age was associated with an unusually severe pulmonary phenotype, and loss of ambulation at greater than 11 years of age was correlated with an unusually mild phenotype (**Fig. 4**). If validated with larger studies, age at loss of ambulation could be used to predict a patient's pulmonary course over time, allowing clinicians to accurately predict a patient's pulmonary prognosis and to accurately assess the pulmonary effect of new and existing DMD therapies.

Finally, cardiopulmonary phenotypic variability has suggested a strategy for creating new DMD therapies. It appears that in the prolonged survivors of DMD who manifest unexpectedly good cardiac function, the mechanism of their cardiopulmonary phenotypic disconnect (good heart function, bad lung function) may be the presence of beneficial modifier genes that selectively change the phenotypic expression of cardiac but not respiratory (skeletal) muscle.[32,70,71] These patients have poor lung function, but their respiratory failure is compensated with 24 h/d assisted ventilation; thus, cardiac function appears to be the main determinant of their survival. This important phenotypic disconnect suggests that amplifying beneficial cardiac modifier genes or blocking detrimental cardiac modifiers is a potential strategy for creating new DMD therapies that prolong patient survival.[32]

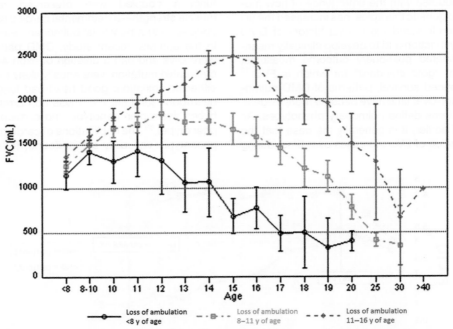

Fig. 4. Pulmonary phenotype variability in boys with DMD is related to loss of ambulation. In boys with loss of ambulation at less than 8 years of age (*solid black line*), an unusually severe pulmonary phenotype is observed. Comparatively, the "classic" pulmonary phenotype is observed in boys who lose ambulation between ages 8 and 11 years (*red dashed line*), and an unusually mild pulmonary phenotype is observed in boys who lose ambulation at greater than 11 years of age (*blue dashed line*). (*From* Humbertclaude V, Hamroun D, Bezzou K, et al. Motor and respiratory heterogeneity in Duchenne patients: implication for clinical trials. Eur J Paediatr Neurol 2012;16(2):155; with permission.)

SUMMARY

The muscular dystrophies are a varied and complex group of neuromuscular conditions with significant genetic and phenotypic heterogeneity as well as unique respiratory and other medical needs. DMD, the best studied of the muscular dystrophies, has provided an important body of evidence in support of multidisciplinary care teams for patients with neuromuscular disorders, a structured approach to respiratory assessment and therapy, the necessity to define and evaluate meaningful pulmonary outcome measures, and the recognition that cardiopulmonary phenotypic variability has significant implications for patient prognosis, the evaluation of current therapies, and the design of future therapies.

REFERENCES

1. Birnkrant DJ, Bushby K, Bann CM, et al. Diagnosis and management of Duchenne muscular dystrophy, an update, part 2: respiratory, cardiac, bone health, and orthopedic management. Lancet Neurol 2018; 17(4):347–61.
2. Mercuri E, Muntoni F. Muscular dystrophies. Lancet 2013;381(9869):845–60.
3. Tawil R, Van Der Maarel SM. Facioscapulohumeral muscular dystrophy. Muscle Nerve 2006;34(1):1–15.
4. Graziano A, Bianco F, D'Amico A, et al. Prevalence of congenital muscular dystrophy in Italy: a population study. Neurology 2015;84(9):904–11.
5. Matsumoto H, Hayashi YK, Kim DS, et al. Congenital muscular dystrophy with glycosylation defects of alpha-dystroglycan in Japan. Neuromuscul Disord 2005;15(5):342–8.
6. Mercuri E, Muntoni F. The ever-expanding spectrum of congenital muscular dystrophies. Ann Neurol 2012;72(1):9–17.
7. van Reeuwijk J, Maugenre S, van den Elzen C, et al. The expanding phenotype of POMT1 mutations: from Walker-Warburg syndrome to congenital muscular dystrophy, microcephaly, and mental retardation. Hum Mutat 2006;27(5):453–9.
8. Birnkrant DJ, Ashwath ML, Noritz GH, et al. Cardiac and pulmonary function variability in Duchenne/Becker muscular dystrophy: an initial report. J Child Neurol 2010;25(9):1110–5.
9. Bertrand AT, Chikhaoui K, Yaou RB, et al. Clinical and genetic heterogeneity in laminopathies. Biochem Soc Trans 2011;39(6):1687–92.
10. LoMauro A, D'Angelo MG, Aliverti A. Sleep disordered breathing in Duchenne muscular dystrophy. Curr Neurol Neurosci Rep 2017;17(5):44.
11. Della Marca G, Frusciante R, Dittoni S, et al. Sleep disordered breathing in facioscapulohumeral muscular dystrophy. J Neurol Sci 2009;285(1–2): 54–8.
12. Sawnani H, Thampratankul L, Szczesniak RD, et al. Sleep disordered breathing in young boys with Duchenne muscular dystrophy. J Pediatr 2015; 166(3):640–5.e1.
13. Tzeng AC, Bach JR. Prevention of pulmonary morbidity for patients with neuromuscular disease. Chest 2000;118(5):1390–6.
14. Ciafaloni E, Fox DJ, Pandya S, et al. Delayed diagnosis in Duchenne muscular dystrophy: data from the Muscular Dystrophy Surveillance, Tracking, And Research Network (MD STARnet). J Pediatr 2009;155(3):380–5.
15. Ankala A, da Silva C, Gualandi F, et al. A comprehensive genomic approach for neuromuscular diseases gives a high diagnostic yield. Ann Neurol 2015;77(2):206–14.
16. Sansovic I, Barisic I, Dumic K. Improved detection of deletions and duplications in the DMD gene using the multiplex ligation-dependent probe amplification (MLPA) method. Biochem Genet 2013;51(3–4):189–201.
17. Gloss D, Moxley RT 3rd, Ashwal S, et al. Practice guideline update summary: corticosteroid treatment of Duchenne muscular dystrophy: report of the guideline development subcommittee of the American Academy of Neurology. Neurology 2016;86(5):465–72.
18. Lebel DE, Corston JA, McAdam LC, et al. Glucocorticoid treatment for the prevention of scoliosis in children with Duchenne muscular dystrophy: long-term follow-up. J Bone Joint Surg Am 2013;95(12):1057–61.
19. Merlini L, Gennari M, Malaspina E, et al. Early corticosteroid treatment in 4 Duchenne muscular dystrophy patients: 14-year follow-up. Muscle Nerve 2012; 45(6):796–802.
20. Lamb MM, West NA, Ouyang L, et al. Corticosteroid treatment and growth patterns in ambulatory males with Duchenne muscular dystrophy. J Pediatr 2016; 173:207–13.e3.
21. Griggs RC, Herr BE, Reha A, et al. Corticosteroids in Duchenne muscular dystrophy: major variations in practice. Muscle Nerve 2013;48(1):27–31.
22. Guglieri M, Bushby K, McDermott MP, et al. Developing standardized corticosteroid treatment for Duchenne muscular dystrophy. Contemp Clin Trials 2017;58:34–9.
23. Bushby K, Finkel R, Wong B, et al. Ataluren treatment of patients with nonsense mutation dystrophinopathy. Muscle Nerve 2014;50(4):477–87.
24. Mendell JR, Goemans N, Lowes LP, et al. Longitudinal effect of eteplirsen versus historical control on ambulation in Duchenne muscular dystrophy. Ann Neurol 2016;79(2):257–71.
25. Malik V, Rodino-Klapac LR, Mendell JR. Emerging drugs for Duchenne muscular dystrophy. Expert Opin Emerg Drugs 2012;17(2):261–77.

26. Buyse GM, Voit T, Schara U, et al. Efficacy of idebenone on respiratory function in patients with Duchenne muscular dystrophy not using glucocorticoids (DELOS): a double-blind randomised placebo-controlled phase 3 trial. Lancet 2015;385(9979):1748–57.

27. Finder J, Mayer OH, Sheehan D, et al. Pulmonary endpoints in Duchenne muscular dystrophy. A workshop summary. Am J Respir Crit Care Med 2017; 196(4):512–9.

28. Gomez-Merino E, Bach JR. Duchenne muscular dystrophy: prolongation of life by noninvasive ventilation and mechanically assisted coughing. Am J Phys Med Rehabil 2002;81(6):411–5.

29. Bach JR, Martinez D. Duchenne muscular dystrophy: continuous noninvasive ventilatory support prolongs survival. Respir Care 2011;56(6):744–50.

30. Eagle M, Baudouin SV, Chandler C, et al. Survival in Duchenne muscular dystrophy: improvements in life expectancy since 1967 and the impact of home nocturnal ventilation. Neuromuscul Disord 2002; 12(10):926–9.

31. Ishikawa Y, Miura T, Ishikawa Y, et al. Duchenne muscular dystrophy: survival by cardio-respiratory interventions. Neuromuscul Disord 2011;21(1):47–51.

32. Birnkrant DJ, Ararat E, Mhanna MJ. Cardiac phenotype determines survival in Duchenne muscular dystrophy. Pediatr Pulmonol 2016;51(1):70–6.

33. Bushby K, Finkel R, Birnkrant DJ, et al. Diagnosis and management of Duchenne muscular dystrophy, part 2: implementation of multidisciplinary care. Lancet Neurol 2010;9(2):177–89.

34. Birnkrant DJ, Bushby KM, Amin RS, et al. The respiratory management of patients with Duchenne muscular dystrophy: a DMD care considerations working group specialty article. Pediatr Pulmonol 2010;45(8):739–48.

35. Rideau Y, Jankowski LW, Grellet J. Respiratory function in the muscular dystrophies. Muscle Nerve 1981;4(2):155–64.

36. Mayer OH, Finkel RS, Rummey C, et al. Characterization of pulmonary function in Duchenne muscular dystrophy. Pediatr Pulmonol 2015;50(5):487–94.

37. Humbertclaude V, Hamroun D, Bezzou K, et al. Motor and respiratory heterogeneity in Duchenne patients: implication for clinical trials. Eur J Paediatr Neurol 2012;16(2):149–60.

38. National Center for Immunization and Respiratory Diseases. Pneumococcal vaccination: information for healthcare professionals. 2017. Available at: https://www.cdc.gov/vaccines/vpd/pneumo/hcp/index.html. Accessed November 26, 2017.

39. Chiou M, Bach JR, Jethani L, et al. Active lung volume recruitment to preserve vital capacity in Duchenne muscular dystrophy. J Rehabil Med 2017;49(1):49–53.

40. Stehling F, Bouikidis A, Schara U, et al. Mechanical insufflation/exsufflation improves vital capacity in neuromuscular disorders. Chron Respir Dis 2015; 12(1):31–5.

41. McKim DA, Katz SL, Barrowman N, et al. Lung volume recruitment slows pulmonary function decline in Duchenne muscular dystrophy. Arch Phys Med Rehabil 2012;93(7):1117–22.

42. Birnkrant DJ, Panitch HB, Benditt JO, et al. American College of Chest Physicians consensus statement on the respiratory and related management of patients with Duchenne muscular dystrophy undergoing anesthesia or sedation. Chest 2007; 132(6):1977–86.

43. LoMauro A, Romei M, D'Angelo MG, et al. Determinants of cough efficiency in Duchenne muscular dystrophy. Pediatr Pulmonol 2014; 49(4):357–65.

44. Szeinberg A, Tabachnik E, Rashed N, et al. Cough capacity in patients with muscular dystrophy. Chest 1988;94(6):1232–5.

45. Suresh S, Wales P, Dakin C, et al. Sleep-related breathing disorder in Duchenne muscular dystrophy: disease spectrum in the paediatric population. J Paediatr Child Health 2005;41(9–10):500–3.

46. Hukins CA, Hillman DR. Daytime predictors of sleep hypoventilation in Duchenne muscular dystrophy. Am J Respir Crit Care Med 2000;161(1):166–70.

47. Smith PE, Calverley PM, Edwards RH. Hypoxemia during sleep in Duchenne muscular dystrophy. Am Rev Respir Dis 1988;137(4):884–8.

48. Mendoza M, Gelinas DF, Moore DH, et al. A comparison of maximal inspiratory pressure and forced vital capacity as potential criteria for initiating non-invasive ventilation in amyotrophic lateral sclerosis. Amyotroph Lateral Scler 2007; 8(2):106–11.

49. Clinical indications for noninvasive positive pressure ventilation in chronic respiratory failure due to restrictive lung disease, COPD, and nocturnal hypoventilation–a consensus conference report. Chest 1999;116(2):521–34.

50. Hamada S, Ishikawa Y, Aoyagi T, et al. Indicators for ventilator use in Duchenne muscular dystrophy. Respir Med 2011;105(4):625–9.

51. Bersanini C, Khirani S, Ramirez A, et al. Nocturnal hypoxaemia and hypercapnia in children with neuromuscular disorders. Eur Respir J 2012;39(5):1206–12.

52. Amaddeo A, Moreau J, Frapin A, et al. Long term continuous positive airway pressure (CPAP) and noninvasive ventilation (NIV) in children: initiation criteria in real life. Pediatr Pulmonol 2016;51(9): 968–74.

53. Toussaint M, Steens M, Soudon P. Lung function accurately predicts hypercapnia in patients with Duchenne muscular dystrophy. Chest 2007;131(2): 368–75.

54. McKim DA, Griller N, LeBlanc C, et al. Twenty-four hour noninvasive ventilation in Duchenne muscular

dystrophy: a safe alternative to tracheostomy. Can Respir J 2013;20(1):e5–9.

55. Bach JR, Gonçalves MR, Hamdani I, et al. Extubation of patients with neuromuscular weakness: a new management paradigm. Chest 2010;137(5): 1033–9.

56. Shimizu-Motohashi Y, Miyatake S, Komaki H, et al. Recent advances in innovative therapeutic approaches for Duchenne muscular dystrophy: from discovery to clinical trials. Am J Transl Res 2016; 8(6):2471–89.

57. Saito T, Kawai M, Kimura E, et al. Study of Duchenne muscular dystrophy long-term survivors aged 40 years and older living in specialized institutions in Japan. Neuromuscul Disord 2017;27(2):107–14.

58. Passamano L, Taglia A, Palladino A, et al. Improvement of survival in Duchenne muscular dystrophy: retrospective analysis of 835 patients. Acta Myol 2012;31(2):121–5.

59. Birnkrant DJ. New challenges in the management of prolonged survivors of pediatric neuromuscular diseases: a pulmonologist's perspective. Pediatr Pulmonol 2006;41:1113–7.

60. Birnkrant DJ, Ferguson RD, Martin JE, et al. Noninvasive ventilation during gastrostomy tube placement in patients with severe Duchenne muscular dystrophy: case reports and review of the literature. Pediatr Pulmonol 2006;41(2):188–93.

61. Shumyatcher Y, Shah TA, Noritz GH, et al. Symptomatic nephrolithiasis in prolonged survivors of Duchenne muscular dystrophy. Neuromuscul Disord 2008;18(7):561–4.

62. Bach JR, Gonçalves MR, Hon A, et al. Changing trends in the management of end-stage neuromuscular respiratory muscle failure: recommendations of an international consensus. Am J Phys Med Rehabil 2013;92(3):267–77.

63. Birnkrant DJ, Noritz GH. Is there a role for palliative care in progressive pediatric neuromuscular diseases? The answer is "Yes! J Palliat Care 2008;24(4):265–9.

64. Snow WM, Anderson JE, Jakobson LS. Neuropsychological and neurobehavioral functioning in Duchenne muscular dystrophy: a review. Neurosci Biobehav Rev 2013;37(5):743–52.

65. Schrans DG, Abbott D, Peay HL, et al. Transition in Duchenne muscular dystrophy: an expert meeting report and description of transition needs in an emergent patient population: (Parent Project Muscular Dystrophy Transition Expert Meeting 17-18 June 2011, Amsterdam, The Netherlands). Neuromuscul Disord 2013;23(3):283–6.

66. Arias R, Andrews J, Pandya S, et al. Palliative care services in families of males with Duchenne muscular dystrophy. Muscle Nerve 2011;44(1):93–101.

67. Desguerre I, Christov C, Mayer M, et al. Clinical heterogeneity of Duchenne muscular dystrophy (DMD): definition of sub-phenotypes and predictive criteria by long-term follow-up. PLoS One 2009;4(2):e4347.

68. Pettygrove S, Lu Z, Andrews JG, et al. Sibling concordance for clinical features of Duchenne and Becker muscular dystrophies. Muscle Nerve 2014; 49(6):814–21.

69. Jin JB, MS, Birnkrant DJ. Cardiopulmonary phenotypic disconnects are common in Duchenne muscular dystrophy. Chest 2017;152(4):A844.

70. Barp A, Bello L, Politano L, et al. Genetic modifiers of Duchenne muscular dystrophy and dilated cardiomyopathy. PLoS One 2015;10(10):e0141240.

71. Hightower RM, Alexander MS. Genetic modifiers of Duchenne and facioscapulohumeral muscular dystrophies. Muscle Nerve 2018;57(1):6–15.

Amyotrophic Lateral Sclerosis and the Respiratory System

Andrew T. Braun, MD, MHS[a,b],
Candelaria Caballero-Eraso, MD, PhD[a,c],
Noah Lechtzin, MD, MHS[a,*]

KEYWORDS

- Noninvasive ventilation • Diaphragm • Secretion clearance

KEY POINTS

- Amyotrophic lateral sclerosis (ALS) is an incurable disease whereby patients most commonly die of respiratory complications.
- It is important for pulmonary physicians to be aware of this and understand management options, including noninvasive and invasive ventilation and assisted cough techniques.
- Because ALS affects both upper and lower motor neurons, it causes hyperreflexia, spasticity, muscle fasciculations, muscle atrophy, and weakness.

INTRODUCTION

Amyotrophic lateral sclerosis (ALS) is a progressive neurodegenerative disorder that always affects the respiratory muscles. It is characterized by degeneration of motor neurons in the brain and spinal cord.[1] Respiratory complications, including pneumonia and progressive respiratory failure, are the most common causes of death in ALS and typically occur within 3 to 5 years of diagnosis.[2,3] Because ALS affects both upper and lower motor neurons, it causes hyperreflexia, spasticity, muscle fasciculations, muscle atrophy, and weakness. It ultimately progresses to functional quadriplegia. ALS most commonly begins in the limbs, but in about one-third of cases it begins in the bulbar muscles responsible for speech and swallowing.[4] A small proportion of cases begin with respiratory muscle weakness and can present as unexplained hypercarbic respiratory failure.[5]

Most cases of ALS are idiopathic, but approximately 10% of cases are due to identifiable genetic mutations and are inherited in an autosomal dominant manner.[6] The incidence of ALS in the United States is 1 to 2 cases per 100,000 people, and the average age of onset is in the mid-fifties. There is a male predominance of sporadic cases with a male to female ratio of almost 2:1.[7] There are now 2 medications approved by the US Food and Drug Administration for the treatment of ALS, riluzole and edaravone[8]; but in spite of therapeutic developments, the disease is uniformly fatal and the treatment is largely

Disclosures: Dr N. Lechtzin has served as a consultant with Hill-Rom, Inc, Dr A. Braun and Dr C. Caballero-Eraso have no relevant conflicts of interest or financial disclosures.
[a] Division of Pulmonary and Critical Care and Sleep Medicine, Department of Medicine, Johns Hopkins University School of Medicine, 1830 East Monument Street, Baltimore, MD 21205, USA; [b] Division of Allergy, Pulmonary, and Critical Care, Department of Medicine, University of Wisconsin School of Medicine and Public Health, 600 Highland Avenue, Madison, WI 53792, USA; [c] Medical-Surgical Unit of Respiratory Diseases, Institute of Biomedicine of Seville (IBiS), Centre for Biomedical Research in Respiratory Diseases Network (CIBERES), University Hospital Virgen del Rocío, University of Seville, Avenida Dr. Fedriani, 41009 Sevilla, Spain
* Corresponding author.
E-mail address: nlechtz@jhmi.edu

Clin Chest Med 39 (2018) 391–400
https://doi.org/10.1016/j.ccm.2018.01.003
0272-5231/18/© 2018 Elsevier Inc. All rights reserved.

supportive. Much of the therapy for ALS is directed at improving respiratory symptoms and minimizing pulmonary complications.[9] This therapy includes interventions directed at secretion clearance and ventilator support. This article describes the respiratory evaluation and treatment of individuals with ALS.

RESPIRATORY MANIFESTATIONS

ALS causes multiple problems that impact the respiratory system. **Fig. 1** provides an overview of the most relevant complications. ALS causes diffuse muscle weakness that ultimately leads to functional quadriplegia and anarthria.

Inspiratory Muscle Weakness

The major muscles of inspiration are the diaphragm, the sternocleidomastoids, the scalenes, and the external intercostals. Weakness of these muscles leads to a decrease in tidal volume, resulting in alveolar hypoventilation and subsequent respiratory insufficiency.

Expiratory Muscle Weakness

The major muscles of expiration are the abdominal muscles, including the rectus abdominis, the internal and external obliques, the transversus abdominis, and the internal intercostal muscles.[10] Decreased strength in expiratory muscles, often coincident with impaired glottic function, can lead to an ineffective cough, retention of upper airway secretions, and subsequent lower respiratory tract infections. Both the inspiratory and expiratory muscle groups become weak in ALS, but this may happen at any time in the disease course; inspiratory muscles can become weak at a different time than the expiratory muscles.

Bulbar-Innervated Muscles Dysfunction

Approximately 30% of patients with ALS present with bulbar dysfunction at the time of diagnosis, which has been linked to poor outcomes.[11] Sialorrhea, dysphagia, and dysarthria are the most important symptoms related to pharyngeal and laryngeal muscle weakness and lead to altered secretion management, decreased calorie intake, and resultant malnutrition. The direct impairment in bulbar-innervated muscles can also lead to an increased risk of aspiration during swallowing, provoking respiratory infections. The recognition of bulbar dysfunction in patients with ALS is crucial for the management of the respiratory complications and will be a key factor in assessing the indication for noninvasive ventilation (NIV) and its subsequent tolerance.

As respiratory muscles become weaker, patients will often develop dyspnea and orthopnea.[12] Additionally, progressive limb weakness can make simple tasks effortful, which can further worsen dyspnea and fatigue. Clinicians need to be aware of the need to elicit more subtle symptoms of respiratory muscle insufficiency, such as disturbed sleep, morning headache, excessive daytime somnolence, orthopnea, and fatigue. As respiratory muscle weakness progresses, patients develop a restrictive ventilatory pattern, which can lead to hypoventilation with hypoxic and hypercarbic respiratory failure. Patients frequently develop atelectasis as the disease progresses, which worsens pulmonary shunt and hypoxia. The combination of inspiratory muscle weakness, expiratory muscle weakness, and poor glottic function makes coughing ineffective; patients have difficulty clearing respiratory secretions and can develop mucous plugging and pneumonia. Bulbar weakness makes swallowing difficult, and patients frequently develop aspiration pneumonia.

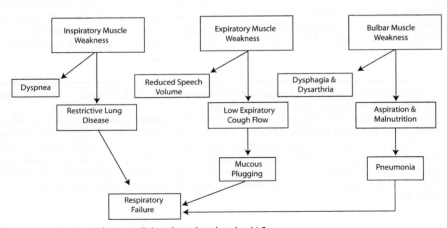

Fig. 1. The major respiratory abnormalities that develop in ALS.

Another problem faced by patients with ALS, but often overlooked by clinicians, is laryngospasm.[13] Laryngospasm can occur when bulbar involvement is relatively mild. Patients will report a sudden inability to breathe. This inability is quite distressing and can prompt emergency medical calls. It is the experience of the authors that these episodes are extremely unpleasant for patients but end spontaneously within a few minutes. Patients may find that efforts to relieve dyspnea, such as blowing a fan on one's face, may cause laryngospasm to end. Some clinicians have used medications, such as sublingual benzodiazepines, with success.

Atelectasis, hypoventilation, and microaspiration all worsen when supine and when sleeping; sleep disordered breathing can be a problem in ALS and is discussed in more detail later.

RESPIRATORY ASSESSMENT IN AMYOTROPHIC LATERAL SCLEROSIS

As respiratory complications are the most common causes of death in patients with ALS, the early and periodic evaluation of respiratory function is mandatory (**Fig. 2**). Once a diagnosis of ALS is established, signs and symptoms of respiratory failure in patients with ALS should be monitored closely (**Box 1**).[14] Although some patients with ALS do not present with overt respiratory symptoms, clinicians should be vigilant to recognize subtle symptoms, such as orthopnea, to consider initiating NIV.[15]

Pulmonary Function Testing

Respiratory function should be assessed in patients with ALS at the time of diagnosis and thereafter, every 3 to 6 months.[9]

The most frequently used test to evaluate respiratory function is upright *forced vital capacity* (FVC).[16] Additionally, although supine FVC is a more difficult spirometric measure to perform, it has higher specificity for diagnosing diaphragmatic weakness than an upright FVC. A study performed in 2002 showed that supine FVC correlates very well with diaphragm strength, as measured by transdiaphragmatic pressure (r2 = 0.76, $P<.001$).[17] Most centers consider a decrease in FVC to less than 50% of predicted, or a decrease of 20% to 25% from upright to supine FVC, as evidence of diaphragmatic weakness, at which time a consideration of NIV should be considered. However, although the timing to initiate NIV is controversial, in the last decade, many ALS centers have moved toward initiating NIV before the FVC decreases to less than 50% of predicted.[18] Although FVC correlates with survival in ALS, if hypoventilation symptoms are present, a normal FVC does not exclude significant respiratory

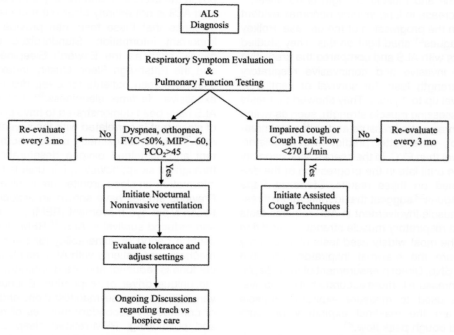

Fig. 2. Respiratory management algorithm. FVC, force vital capacity; MIP, maximal inspiratory pressure; trach, tracheostomy.

> **Box 1**
> **Symptoms and signs of respiratory issues in patients with amyotrophic lateral sclerosis**
>
> *Symptoms*
> Dyspnea
> Dyspnea with exertion[a]
> Orthopnea
> Morning headache
> Poor sleep
> Daytime somnolence
> Weak cough
> Softer speech
>
> *Signs*
> Use of accessory muscles of respiration
> Paradoxic abdominal movement
> Tachypnea
> Decreased chest movement
>
> [a] Exertion can be minimal, such as assisted transfer, speaking, eating, and so forth.

are encouraged to inhale maximally or exhale against an occluded valve and the resultant pressure generated is measured. MIP has been correlated with survival, and normal values almost always exclude inspiratory muscles weakness. However, although low MIP values have been correlated with respiratory complications, such as sleep disordered breathing, values less than the normal threshold can be difficult to interpret. In addition, when bulbar weakness is present, patients are often unable to perform this procedure correctly because of the inability to form a tight seal around the mouthpiece.[18,23] These tests can underestimate inspiratory and expiratory muscle strength. In these cases, other tests, such as SNp, should be performed.

SNp is a noninvasive test measured by inserting a nose plug connected to a pressure transducer into the nostril and having patients perform maximal sniff maneuvers. SNp has been shown to accurately reflect intrathoracic pressures.[24] This test can be performed in most patients with ALS and is sensitive to change over time. In a study evaluating the predictive accuracy of respiratory functions tests, SNp was the parameter that showed the greatest decline leading to the need for NIV initiation.[25]

Nocturnal Oximetry and Polysomnography

The role of overnight oximetry and polysomnography in the evaluation and management of patients with ALS is not entirely clear but there is growing evidence that these tests can provide clinically important information. Standardized questionnaires, such as the Epworth Sleepiness Scale and the Pittsburgh Sleep Quality Index, can be used to screen patients for sleep disruption and excessive daytime sleepiness.[26] Patients with ALS have been demonstrated to have poor quality of sleep that is correlated with the severity of their ALS.[26] Nocturnal oximetry detects both intermittent and sustained oxygen desaturation events throughout sleep; however, it is unable to provide information on sleep architecture or sleep quality. Previous studies have shown an association between rapid eye movement (REM) sleep duration and reduced survival in ALS.[27] REM sleep represents a period of vulnerability for the respiratory mechanics of patients with ALS, as skeletal muscle tone is reduced, and the diaphragm becomes the unique driver of respiration. Because of the variability in disease manifestation, and the loss of contributory secondary muscles of respiration and positioning, REM-related sleep disordered breathing and oxygen desaturation are more likely to develop. Notably, it has been shown that

muscle weakness. Although the current international guidelines recommend spirometry as the primary respiratory test in ALS,[19] it has some limitations. On one hand, the relationship between lung volume and muscle strength is nonlinear,[20] so the decrease in lung volume becomes evident only late in the progression of the disease. Polkey and colleagues[21] shed light on this. They studied 78 patients with ALS and compared the predictive power of invasive and noninvasive respiratory muscle strength tests for survival or ventilator-free survival up to 3 years. They showed that tests directly assessing muscle strength, such as twitch transdiaphragmatic pressure and sniff nasal pressure (SNp), were better predictors of ventilator-free survival than FVC. In their series, vital capacity was stable until late in the progression of the disease. Based on these results, Sferrazza Papa and colleagues[22] suggest that identification of respiratory muscle involvement in ALS requires tests specific to respiratory muscle strength in addition to FVC. The most widely used tests of inspiratory strength are the maximal inspiratory pressure (MIP) and SNp. Direct measurement of transdiaphragmatic pressure is more accurate but is invasive. The tests used to measure expiratory muscle strength are the maximal expiratory pressure (MEP) and cough peak flow.[23]

MIP and MEP are measured by a noninvasive mask or mouthpiece. For these tests, patients

patients who start using noninvasive positive pressure ventilation (NPPV) based on nocturnal desaturation rather than daytime hypoxemia have improved survival.[28] Additionally, obstructive apneas occur more frequently in patients with bulbar involvement and more advanced respiratory involvement.[29,30] It has been reported that between 17% and 76% of patients with ALS have sleep disordered breathing.[31] Nocturnal desaturation correlates with inspiratory muscle weakness and can be used as a guide for initiating NPPV. Patients with ALS can have relatively normal FVC but have nocturnal desaturation.[32] These recent studies suggest that nocturnal oximetry and possibly polysomnography should be used more frequently in the evaluation of respiratory status in ALS. The use of NPPV has been shown to improve nocturnal desaturation; but the net impact on other sleep outcomes, such as sleep efficiency, sleep arousals, and sleep architecture, are unclear.[33] A recent single-center prospective study of targeted in-hospital NPPV titration revealed improved amounts of deep sleep and gas exchange in patients with nonbulbar ALS after 1 month.[34] However, the investigators admit that the resource-heavy in-hospital titration may be a barrier for widespread application of these findings. Additionally, other sleep disorders, such as restless leg syndrome (RLS), periodic leg movements during sleep, and REM behavior disorder, can be concomitant causes of sleep disruption; targeted treatment, such as evaluation and treatment of iron deficiency in RLS, has been shown to improve sleep quality in patients with ALS.[35]

Although nocturnal gas exchange abnormalities may be relatively common in ALS, daytime hypoxia and hypercapnia are uncommon and occur late in the course of the disease.[36] Therefore, the authors do not recommend measuring arterial blood gas routinely in patients with ALS. Arterial blood gas analysis should be obtained only if patients have respiratory symptoms, disturbed sleep, morning headaches, or hypersomnolence.

TREATMENT OF RESPIRATORY COMPLICATIONS IN AMYOTROPHIC LATERAL SCLEROSIS
Improving Ventilation

Even if patients with ALS are fortunate enough to avoid a fatal aspiration event, progressive ventilatory insufficiency remains inevitable.[37,38] This progression can be forestalled with the initiation of positive pressure ventilatory support (see **Fig. 2**). NPPV has been shown to reduce the rate of FVC decline, increase cognitive function, and improve overall patient survival in ALS.[39,40] Fears

of prolonging death by initiating NPPV have been allayed by studies demonstrating an improvement in the overall quality of life in patients with ALS who use NPPV.[15,41,42]

Although protocols vary by center, bilevel ventilatory support is typically initiated with the development of respiratory symptoms, a decrease in FVC to less than 50% of predicted, elevated carbon dioxide, low MIP, or an accelerated rate of FVC decline.[28,38,40] Support is typically initiated at night (ie, in the supine position) with a nasal bilevel positive airway pressure device. Inspiratory and expiratory pressures are titrated to maintain a tidal volume of 12 to 15 mL/kg; this goal becomes increasingly more difficult to achieve with advancing weakness.[43] The setting for the initiation of NIV initiation varies by center; however, a recent study has suggested that early outpatient initiation of NIV in ALS is as effective as inpatient initiation.[44] As the disease progresses, patients will typically begin extending the use of NPPV into the daytime and often progress to continuous use. Inspiratory pressure support should be titrated higher as inspiratory muscle weakness progresses. Because of the need to gradually adjust pressure support, some have advocated using auto-titrating volume-targeted modes of NIV or the use of volume cycled ventilator modes. Although these approaches are sensible and effective, there is no high-level evidence to suggest they are superior to more standard bilevel NIV.

The use of diaphragmatic pacemakers has been investigated as a means of slowing lung function decline. These devices may decrease apneas and hypopneas during REM sleep, but randomized studies suggest they shorten survival.[45]

Ultimately, patients will require continuous ventilatory assistance. With aggressive secretion management, however, even this continuous support can be well tolerated. Once progressive bulbar weakness precludes the patients' ability to clear their secretions (even with mechanical assistance), NIV is no longer a viable treatment option. The decision must then be made whether to proceed with tracheostomy or focus on palliation.

SECRETION MANAGEMENT

The combination of immobility, weakened cough, hypersialorrhea, and dysphagia place individuals with ALS at high risk for respiratory infections. The management of oral and respiratory secretions can be one of the most difficult aspects of ALS care, and the ability to clear secretions is the main factor that determines if patients can successfully use NIV.

There are several common-sense approaches to reduce the risk for pneumonia. These approaches include vaccination against influenza and pneumococcus. Patients should be taught techniques to minimize aspiration. These techniques may include a chin tuck while swallowing or the use of a straw, but specific techniques should be taught by an experienced speech therapist. Sialorrhea can be managed with oral suctioning or with pharmacologic measures. The latter includes oral glycopyrrolate, amitriptyline, transdermal scopolamine, and sublingual hyoscyamine. Botulinum toxin injections to the salivary glands can be used in refractory cases.[13] Patients are often challenged to find the correct balance between excessively dry oral mucosa and thickened secretions versus sialorrhea.

The essential mechanism of airway protection is the ability to cough. Coughing requires a synchronization of 3 main actions: an inspiratory phase, in which lung insufflation occurs to 85% to 90% of the total lung capacity; a compressive phase, in which expiratory muscles contract the inspired volume against a closed glottis; and a forceful expiration phase, in which the glottis is rapidly opened, with a resultant escape of the pressurized air (and up to a 300 mm Hg intrathoracic pressure change).[46] This expulsion usually produces peak cough flow rates (measured via a peak flow meter during the act of coughing) of 6 L per second or greater.

In neuromuscular disease, the ability to cough is threatened by both bulbar dysfunction and respiratory muscle weakness. Without the ability to maintain a closed glottis, no amount of respiratory muscle tone or mechanical assistance will allow the production of intrathoracic pressures of sufficient magnitude to produce a viable cough. In this situation, techniques to augment cough or tracheostomy are indicated to provide airway protection. Even if sufficient glottic tone exists, the ability to cough can be hampered by the presence of either inspiratory or expiratory muscle weakness. With inspiratory weakness, cough is limited by an inability to achieve insufflation of sufficient magnitude to produce adequate expiratory flow. With expiratory muscle weakness, adequate intrathoracic pressures cannot be obtained to produce acceptable peak cough flows.[47] Inspiratory and expiratory muscle weakness can be treated with a variety of noninvasive modalities. Once patients' peak cough flow drops to less than a certain threshold (eg, 270–300 L/min), investigators have recommended patient training in assisted coughing.[47,48]

One approach to mobilizing secretions is the use of high-frequency chest wall oscillation.

Clinical trials that have assessed chest wall vests in ALS have had negative results, though there is a recent time series study using administrative data suggesting improved outcomes for patients with neuromuscular disease.[49] Other techniques, such as positive expiratory pressure devices or postural drainage, are not practical or effective in ALS, whereas mechanical insufflation-exsufflation (MIE) is a highly effective technique to expel respiratory secretions in ALS.[50]

Assisted cough can be accomplished by an abdominal thrust during a cough (either by a caregiver or a specialized belt apparatus), MIE (a device that stacks several positive pressure face-mask breaths before suddenly changing to a negative pressure), or the combination of both. The use of MIE has been shown to produce greater cough velocities than assisted cough techniques alone.[51] These processes may allow the creation and maintenance of peak cough flows greater than 160 L/min, a threshold deemed sufficient to allow airway clearance and can reduce pulmonary complications. Patients with an impaired cough should be instructed to use in-exsufflators at least twice a day and as needed.

Tracheostomy/Mechanical Ventilation and End-of-Life Care

Appropriate ventilatory support is critical for providing symptom relief, decreasing hospitalizations,[52] and improving the quality of life and survival in ALS. Invasive mechanical ventilation (via a tracheostomy: tracheostomy positive pressure ventilation [TPPV]) is an option in specific circumstances: when NIV is not able to maintain adequate ventilation because of the progression of the disease, when the presence of bulbar-innervated muscle impairment does not permit tolerance of NIV, and when poor control and clearance of secretions are not mitigated by mechanical cough techniques. It is important to note that many individuals with ALS do not choose to pursue tracheostomy, even if these conditions are present.

Invasive mechanical ventilation is strongly associated with prolonged survival in ALS. However, an improvement in the quality of life is less clear.[19] Patients with TPPV continue to experience disease progression. For this reason, some patients eventually progress to a locked-in state in which they are unable to communicate or move. Fortunately, improved communication devices, such as eye-gaze controlled speech synthesizers, can usually maintain patients' ability to communicate. It is important for patients and family members to recognize that the care patients using invasive ventilation require is complex. TPPV patients will require special care of the stoma, cannula hygiene, and techniques of secretions aspiration. Clinicians must ensure that patients and caregivers are well instructed in order to be able to manage the tracheostomy at home. Previous studies have analyzed both the prevalence of depression in patients with ALS with TPPV and their caregivers. A retrospective study, which analyzed the quality of life in patients with ALS after tracheostomy after an acute respiratory failure, showed that 15% of the patients with ALS were severely depressed and 85% regret the decision to proceed with the tracheostomy.[53] In a prospective study performed in 71 individuals with ALS, the patients who decided to receive invasive ventilation support were younger and received more supportive care. Both the patients and their caregivers displayed a high burden of depression symptoms at baseline, but this declined overtime.[54] Other studies have described that invasive ventilation in patients with ALS causes an increase in the caregivers' burden and reduces their quality of life.[55,56]

TPPV is a costly treatment and has significant emotional and social impacts on patients and caregivers. There is high variability of the acceptance of this invasive treatment, owing to cultural and demographic issues.[57] A recent study that analyzed the similarities and differences in ALS management between Europe, the United States, and Japan showed that despite similar guidelines for NIV and tracheostomy-invasive ventilation in these countries, the prevalence of TPPV in Japan was clearly higher than that reported for the United States or Europe. Moreover, the rate of TPPV also varied between European countries, with Italy having the highest prevalence of tracheostomy and England the lowest.[58]

As ALS has a somewhat predictable course, it is important to discuss with patients and caregivers the potential invasive and noninvasive management options as soon as possible, aiming to avoid these decisions in the context of abrupt clinical deterioration and to give patients and families time to reflect.[59] Making a decision in a rushed and acute context can impact patients' health and quality of life. More recently, the recognition that some patients with ALS develop frontotemporal dementia poses additional challenges for clinicians and families when a decision, such as invasive treatment, is entertained.[60] Once a goals-of-care discussion is held and end-of-life decisions have been settled, written documents should be completed.

PALLIATIVE CARE

Because ALS is a progressive disease affecting different organ systems, and to date a curative treatment is unknown, an ALS diagnosis has a profound impact on patients and families. It has been shown that a multidisciplinary team (MDT) improves the quality of life and survival in patients with ALS. An MDT should include a specialist in palliative care from the time of diagnosis in order to improve the quality of life of patients by providing emotional and psychological support and relief of symptoms.[61] Although palliative care support varies between countries, there are some international guidelines that try to standardize the palliative care approach in different countries.[62]

WITHDRAWAL OF LIFE SUPPORT

An important issue to discuss with patients and family members is that decisions can change over the disease course. Legal and ethical precedents generally support the right of patients to discontinue any treatment, including mechanical ventilation. However, there is no current consensus regarding how palliative medications should be administered and how to transition patients with ALS off of mechanical ventilation. Nevertheless, most authorities agree that clinicians should ensure that symptoms, such as anxiety and dyspnea, are well controlled and that medications, such as sedatives and analgesics, should be administered to avoid and relieve pain and discomfort.

SUMMARY

ALS is a rapidly progressive neuromuscular disease. Our understanding of the pathophysiology of ALS has improved, and a new drug was approved to treat ALS in 2017. But the prognosis still remains grim, and survival from disease diagnosis is only a few years on average. Most patients die of pulmonary complications; therefore, it is critical that pulmonary physicians understand the disease and how to properly manage respiratory complications. Patients with ALS should have close pulmonary follow-up with regular measurement of pulmonary function. Spirometry is the single most frequently used parameter to gauge respiratory status; but other measures, such as SNp and sleep studies, can be useful. Management of respiratory insufficiency should address both ventilator support and secretion clearance. NPPV is a mainstay of therapy for ALS and has been shown to improve survival in both observational and experimental studies. Few patients with ALS in the United States choose to use long-term ventilation via tracheostomy, but it can sustain survival and, in the right setting, maintain an acceptable quality of life.

Pulmonologists have therapies that can improve survival and quality of life for individuals with ALS more than any other treatment. It is important for pulmonologists to be familiar with ALS and be actively involved in the care of these patients.

REFERENCES

1. Rowland LP, Shneider NA. Amyotrophic lateral sclerosis. N Engl J Med 2001;344(22):1688–700.
2. Lechtzin N, Wiener CM, Clawson L, et al. Hospitalization in amyotrophic lateral sclerosis: causes, costs, and outcomes. Neurology 2001;56(6):753–7.
3. Brown RH, Al-Chalabi A. Amyotrophic lateral sclerosis. N Engl J Med 2017;377(2):162–72.
4. Tandan R, Bradley WG. Amyotrophic lateral sclerosis: part 1. Clinical features, pathology, and ethical issues in management. Ann Neurol 1985; 18(3):271–80.
5. de CM, Matias T, Coelho F, et al. Motor neuron disease presenting with respiratory failure. J Neurol Sci 1996;139(Suppl):117–22.
6. Mulder DW, Kurland LT, Offord KP, et al. Familial adult motor neuron disease: amyotrophic lateral sclerosis. Neurology 1986;36(4):511–7.
7. Robberecht W, Philips T. The changing scene of amyotrophic lateral sclerosis. Nat Rev Neurosci 2013;14(4):248–64.
8. Voelker R. Antioxidant drug approved for ALS. JAMA 2017;317(23):2363.
9. Miller RG, Jackson CE, Kasarskis EJ, et al. Practice parameter update: the care of the patient with amyotrophic lateral sclerosis: drug, nutritional, and respiratory therapies (an evidence-based review): report of the Quality Standards Subcommittee of the American Academy of Neurology. Neurology 2009;73(15): 1218–26.
10. Wijdicks EFM. The neurology of acutely failing respiratory mechanics. Ann Neurol 2017;81(4):485–94.
11. Louwerse ES, Visser CE, Bossuyt PM, et al. Amyotrophic lateral sclerosis: mortality risk during the course of the disease and prognostic factors. The Netherlands ALS Consortium. J Neurol Sci 1997; 152(Suppl 1):S10–7.
12. Just N, Bautin N, Danel-Brunaud V, et al. The Borg dyspnoea score: a relevant clinical marker of inspiratory muscle weakness in amyotrophic lateral sclerosis. Eur Respir J 2010;35(2):353–60.
13. Kuhnlein P, Gdynia HJ, Sperfeld AD, et al. Diagnosis and treatment of bulbar symptoms in amyotrophic lateral sclerosis. Nat Clin Pract Neurol 2008;4(7): 366–74.
14. Farrero E, Prats E, Povedano M, et al. Survival in amyotrophic lateral sclerosis with home mechanical ventilation: the impact of systematic respiratory assessment and bulbar involvement. Chest 2005; 127(6):2132–8.
15. Bourke SC, Bullock RE, Williams TL, et al. Noninvasive ventilation in ALS: indications and effect on quality of life. Neurology 2003;61(2):171–7.
16. Czaplinski A, Yen AA, Appel SH. Forced vital capacity (FVC) as an indicator of survival and disease progression in an ALS clinic population. J Neurol Neurosurg Psychiatry 2006;77(3):390–2.
17. Lechtzin N, Wiener CM, Shade DM, et al. Spirometry in the supine position improves the detection of diaphragmatic weakness in patients with amyotrophic lateral sclerosis. Chest 2002;121(2):436–42.
18. Lechtzin N, Scott Y, Busse AM, et al. Early use of non-invasive ventilation prolongs survival in subjects with ALS. Amyotroph Lateral Scler 2007;8(3):185–8.
19. EFNS Task Force on Diagnosis and Management of Amyotrophic Lateral Sclerosis, Andersen PM, Abrahams S, Borasio GD, et al. EFNS guidelines on the clinical management of amyotrophic lateral sclerosis (MALS)–revised report of an EFNS task force. Eur J Neurol 2012;19(3):360–75.
20. De Troyer A, Borenstein S, Cordier R. Analysis of lung volume restriction in patients with respiratory muscle weakness. Thorax 1980;35(8):603–10.
21. Polkey MI, Lyall RA, Yang K, et al. Respiratory muscle strength as a predictive biomarker for survival in amyotrophic lateral sclerosis. Am J Respir Crit Care Med 2017;195(1):86–95.
22. Sferrazza Papa GF, Pellegrino GM, Di Marco F, et al. Predicting survival in amyotrophic lateral sclerosis: should we move forward from vital capacity? Am J Respir Crit Care Med 2017;195(1):144–5.
23. Lechtzin N. Respiratory effects of amyotrophic lateral sclerosis: problems and solutions. Respir Care 2006;51(8):871–81 [discussion: 881–4].
24. Fitting JW, Paillex R, Hirt L, et al. Sniff nasal pressure: a sensitive respiratory test to assess progression of amyotrophic lateral sclerosis. Ann Neurol 1999;46(6):887–93.
25. Tilanus TBM, Groothuis JT, TenBroek-Pastoor JMC, et al. The predictive value of respiratory function tests for non-invasive ventilation in amyotrophic lateral sclerosis. Respir Res 2017;18(1):144.
26. Lo Coco D, Mattaliano P, Spataro R, et al. Sleep-wake disturbances in patients with amyotrophic lateral sclerosis. J Neurol Neurosurg Psychiatry 2011;82(8):839–42.
27. Arnulf I, Similowski T, Salachas F, et al. Sleep disorders and diaphragmatic function in patients with amyotrophic lateral sclerosis. Am J Respir Crit Care Med 2000;161(3 Pt 1):849–56.
28. Pinto A, de Carvalho M, Evangelista T, et al. Nocturnal pulse oximetry: a new approach to

establish the appropriate time for non-invasive ventilation in ALS patients. Amyotroph Lateral Scler Other Motor Neuron Disord 2003;4(1):31–5.

29. Ahmed RM, Newcombe RE, Piper AJ, et al. Sleep disorders and respiratory function in amyotrophic lateral sclerosis. Sleep Med Rev 2016;26: 33–42.

30. Quaranta VN, Carratu P, Damiani MF, et al. The prognostic role of obstructive sleep apnea at the onset of amyotrophic lateral sclerosis. Neurodegener Dis 2017;17(1):14–21.

31. Bourke SC, Gibson GJ. Sleep and breathing in neuromuscular disease. Eur Respir J 2002;19(6): 1194–201.

32. Elman LB, Siderowf AD, McCluskey LF. Nocturnal oximetry: utility in the respiratory management of amyotrophic lateral sclerosis. Am J Phys Med Rehabil 2003;82(11):866–70.

33. Katzberg HD, Selegiman A, Guion L, et al. Effects of noninvasive ventilation on sleep outcomes in amyotrophic lateral sclerosis. J Clin Sleep Med 2013;9(4): 345–51.

34. Vrijsen B, Buyse B, Belge C, et al. Noninvasive ventilation improves sleep in amyotrophic lateral sclerosis: a prospective polysomnographic study. J Clin Sleep Med 2015;11(5):559–66.

35. Lo Coco D, Piccoli F, La Bella V. Restless legs syndrome in patients with amyotrophic lateral sclerosis. Mov Disord 2010;25(15):2658–61.

36. Vitacca M, Clini E, Facchetti D, et al. Breathing pattern and respiratory mechanics in patients with amyotrophic lateral sclerosis. Eur Respir J 1997; 10(7):1614–21.

37. Borasio GD, Gelinas DF, Yanagisawa N. Mechanical ventilation in amyotrophic lateral sclerosis: a cross-cultural perspective. J Neurol 1998;245(Suppl 2): S7–12.

38. Hopkins LC, Tatarian GT, Pianta TF. Management of ALS: respiratory care. Neurology 1996;47(4 Suppl 2):S123–5.

39. Pinto AC, Evangelista T, Carvalho M, et al. Respiratory assistance with a noninvasive ventilator (Bipap) in MND/ALS patients - survival rates in a controlled trial. J Neurol Sci 1995;129:19–26.

40. Aboussouan LS, Khan SU, Meeker DP, et al. Effect of noninvasive positive-pressure ventilation on survival in amyotrophic lateral sclerosis. Ann Intern Med 1997;127(6):450–3.

41. Lyall RA, Donaldson N, Fleming T, et al. A prospective study of quality of life in ALS patients treated with noninvasive ventilation. Neurology 2001; 57(1):153–6.

42. Bourke SC, Tomlinson M, Williams TL, et al. Effects of non-invasive ventilation on survival and quality of life in patients with amyotrophic lateral sclerosis: a randomised controlled trial. Lancet Neurol 2006; 5(2):140–7.

43. Bach JR, Goncalves MR, Hon A, et al. Changing trends in the management of end-stage neuromuscular respiratory muscle failure: recommendations of an international consensus. Am J Phys Med Rehabil 2013;92(3):267–77.

44. Bertella E, Banfi P, Paneroni M, et al. Early initiation of nighttime NIV in an outpatient setting. A randomized non inferiority study in ALS patients. Eur J Phys Rehabil Med 2017;53(6):892–9.

45. Gonzalez-Bermejo J, Morelot-Panzini C, Tanguy ML, et al. Early diaphragm pacing in patients with amyotrophic lateral sclerosis (RespiStimALS): a randomised controlled triple-blind trial. Lancet Neurol 2016;15(12):1217–27.

46. Chernick V. Physiology of cough. In: Haddad G, editor. Basic mechanisms of pediatric respiratory disease. St. Louis (MO): BC Decker; 2002. p. 179–83.

47. Filart RA, Bach JR. Pulmonary physical medicine interventions for elderly patients with muscular dysfunction. Clin Geriatr Med 2003;19(1):189–204, viii–ix.

48. Hanayama K, Ishikawa Y, Bach JR. Amyotrophic lateral sclerosis. Successful treatment of mucous plugging by mechanical insufflation-exsufflation. Am J Phys Med Rehabil 1997;76(4):338–9.

49. Lechtzin N, Wolfe LF, Frick KD. The impact of high-frequency chest wall oscillation on healthcare use in patients with neuromuscular diseases. Ann Am Thorac Soc 2016;13(6):904–9.

50. Bach JR. Amyotrophic lateral sclerosis: prolongation of life by noninvasive respiratory AIDS. Chest 2002; 122(1):92–8.

51. Mustfa N, Aiello M, Lyall RA, et al. Cough augmentation in amyotrophic lateral sclerosis. Neurology 2003;61(9):1285–7.

52. Bach JR, Bianchi C, Aufiero E. Oximetry and indications for tracheotomy for amyotrophic lateral sclerosis. Chest 2004;126(5):1502–7.

53. Vianello A, Arcaro G, Palmieri A, et al. Survival and quality of life after tracheostomy for acute respiratory failure in patients with amyotrophic lateral sclerosis. J Crit Care 2011;26(3):329.e7-14.

54. Albert SM, Whitaker A, Rabkin JG, et al. Medical and supportive care among people with ALS in the months before death or tracheostomy. J Pain Symptom Manage 2009;38(4):546–53.

55. Gelinas DF, O'Connor P, Miller RG. Quality of life for ventilator-dependent ALS patients and their caregivers. J Neurol Sci 1998;160(Suppl 1):S134–6.

56. Kaub-Wittemer D, Steinbuchel N, Wasner M, et al. Quality of life and psychosocial issues in ventilated patients with amyotrophic lateral sclerosis and their caregivers. J Pain Symptom Manage 2003;26(4): 890–6.

57. Rabkin J, Ogino M, Goetz R, et al. Japanese and American ALS patient preferences regarding TIV (tracheostomy with invasive ventilation): a

cross-national survey. Amyotroph Lateral Scler Frontotemporal Degener 2014;15(3–4):185–91.

58. Takei K, Tsuda K, Takahashi F, et al. An assessment of treatment guidelines, clinical practices, demographics, and progression of disease among patients with amyotrophic lateral sclerosis in Japan, the United States, and Europe. Amyotroph Lateral Scler Frontotemporal Degener 2017;18(sup1):88–97.

59. Heritier Barras AC, Adler D, Iancu Ferfoglia R, et al. Is tracheostomy still an option in amyotrophic lateral sclerosis? Reflections of a multidisciplinary work group. Swiss Med Wkly 2013;143:w13830.

60. Goldstein LH, Abrahams S. Changes in cognition and behaviour in amyotrophic lateral sclerosis: nature of impairment and implications for assessment. Lancet Neurol 2013;12(4):368–80.

61. Mitsumoto H, Bromberg M, Johnston W, et al. Promoting excellence in end-of-life care in ALS. Amyotroph Lateral Scler Other Motor Neuron Disord 2005; 6(3):145–54.

62. Oliver DJ, Borasio GD, Caraceni A, et al. A consensus review on the development of palliative care for patients with chronic and progressive neurological disease. Eur J Neurol 2016;23(1):30–8.

Metabolic Myopathies and the Respiratory System

Patrick Koo, MD, ScM*, Jigme M. Sethi, MD

KEYWORDS

- Metabolic myopathies • Glycogen storage disease • Mitochondrial disease • Lipid • Purine
- Metabolism • Myopathy

KEY POINTS

- Primary care providers and pulmonologists are inexperienced in diagnosing and treating metabolic myopathies, and there is a paucity of literature to guide management decisions.
- A defect in lipid metabolism can cause exercise intolerance usually later in exercise when glycogen stores are exhausted and the energy source is switched to fatty acid oxidation.
- Mitochondrial dysfunction can present in adulthood and may constitute a substantial proportion of patients seen in a tertiary care dyspnea clinic.
- Cardiopulmonary exercise testing is useful in differentiating among glycogen storage disease, disease of lipid metabolism, and mitochondrial disease being the cause of myopathy.
- Management of metabolic myopathies using nonpharmacologic therapy, such as noninvasive ventilation, pulmonary toileting, special diets, and judicious exercise prescription, has been the mainstay of treatment.

INTRODUCTION: NATURE OF THE PROBLEM

Most of the inherited metabolic myopathic diseases are caused by a deficiency of an enzyme responsible for glycogen, lipid, or purine metabolism or by a defective transporter or mitochondrial electron transport chain protein. Although several metabolic diseases have been associated with respiratory disorders, they are uncommon, usually present in the younger population, have variable symptoms, and mimic other neuromuscular disorders. For the most part, respiratory physicians are inexperienced in diagnosing and treating these diseases, and there is a paucity of literature to guide management decisions.

With the inherited metabolic diseases, multiple organs are usually affected. Although several anatomic components of the respiratory system such as the airways, pulmonary interstitium and the pulmonary arterial tree may be affected by metabolic disorders, this review focuses on myopathies affecting the respiratory system and causing dyspnea, impaired exercise tolerance, or respiratory failure. The mechanism of exercise intolerance for each of the diseases is discussed in detail elsewhere in this article.

OVERVIEW OF THE METABOLIC MYOPATHIES

Contracting muscles use multiple substrates to supply energy for contraction. For high-intensity, short-duration contractions, the substrate of choice is glucose, which is derived from the breakdown of muscle glycogen. Thus, disorders of glycolysis or glycogenolysis present with muscle cramps, weakness, and rhabdomyoglobinuria during high-intensity muscle contraction. Glycogen

The authors have no conflict of interest to disclose.
Department of Respiratory, Critical Care, and Sleep Medicine, University of Tennessee College of Medicine Chattanooga, Erlanger Health System, 975 East 3rd Street, C-735, Chattanooga, TN 37403, USA
* Corresponding author.
E-mail address: drpkoo@gmail.com

Clin Chest Med 39 (2018) 401–410
https://doi.org/10.1016/j.ccm.2018.02.001
0272-5231/18/© 2018 Elsevier Inc. All rights reserved.

accumulates in the muscle cell in these glycogen storage diseases (GSD).

For sustained, endurance-type muscle activity or during fasting, free fatty acids in the fatty acid acetyl-coenzyme A form are used for energy. The fatty acid acetyl-coenzyme A substrates are bound to carnitine by carnitine palmitoyl transferase I, translocated across the mitochondrial membrane by carnitine translocases and released into the mitochondrial matrix by carnitine palmitoyl transferase II, for oxidation. Defects in this pathway cause myopathy during sustained activity and in fasting states.

The purine nucleotide cycle in muscle allows the synthesis of adenosine triphosphate (ATP) from the high energy bond of adenosine diphosphate or adenosine diphosphate during anaerobic exercise when oxygen supplies are limited. The resulting adenosine monophosphate (AMP) is converted to inosine monophosphate and ammonia by adenylate deaminase. Adenylsuccinate diffuses out of the cell preventing accumulation of AMP and allowing anaerobic synthesis of ATP to continue. Deficiency of myoadenylate deaminase ultimately interferes with the synthesis of ATP during anaerobic conditions causing a myopathy.

Impairment of oxidative phosphorylation localized to the mitochondria is due to defects in either maternally inherited mitochondrial DNA (mtDNA) or defects in the autosomally inherited nuclear genome that also encode mitochondrial proteins. The various protein subunits of the components of the oxidative phosphorylation cascade are encoded by genes from both genomes and each mitochondrion may have 2 to 10 copies of mtDNA, some normal and some mutant. This is the basis for the phenomenon of genetic heteroplasmy, with varying relative proportions of wild-type and mutant DNA in each affected individual and cell and tissue. In some cases, complementation may allow defects of mtDNA to be compensated for by other copies of normal mtDNA in the same mitochondrion. Further, even in normal cells, mtDNA mutations accumulate with aging, rendering the cell more susceptible to impairments of ATP synthesis. This genetic complexity underpins the variable age of presentation, severity of illness, and distribution of tissue involvement in patients with these disorders and prevents ready genotype–phenotype correlations. Clinical disease is expressed primarily in tissues with the highest oxygen requirements and, hence, myopathy is a constant feature, but multiple organ systems are affected, especially the central nervous system, retina and optic nerve, and cardiac and endocrine systems. A characteristic feature of all mitochondrial myopathies is the abnormal proliferation and accumulation of mitochondria in a subsarcolemmal location. With the Gomori trichrome stain, muscles fibers have a characteristic ragged red fiber appearance.[1,2]

METABOLIC MYOPATHIES AFFECTING THE RESPIRATORY SYSTEM
Glycogen Storage Diseases

Deficiency in glycogen metabolism is the mechanism for GSD. It is inherited genetically as an autosomal-recessive disorder. The incidence of GSD is approximately 1 case per 20,000 to 43,000 live births.[3] In GSD, the absence of a particular enzyme blocks glycogen processing to produce ATP. As a result of impaired metabolism, glycogen accumulates in skeletal and cardiac muscle. There are 12 types of GSD.[4] Types II and V GSD are known to affect the respiratory system.

Type II GSD is caused by a deficiency in α-glucosidase deficiency, which impairs the degradation of glycogen to glucose. This disease is also known as acid maltase deficiency or Pompe disease.[5] There are 3 known subtypes of Pompe disease: classical (complete enzyme deficiency), a nonclassical infantile form, and a late-onset form. The classical form is associated with early mortality in the first year of life.[6] The late-onset subtype occurs later in life starting during childhood or even during adulthood. It is a milder form that affects the skeletal muscles and not the cardiac muscle.[7,8] It may cause severe diaphragm weakness, which eventually could lead to alveolar hypoventilation and chronic hypercapnic respiratory failure. Additionally, the reduced inspiratory pressure generated by a weakened diaphragm may result in an ineffective cough owing to reduced inspired volumes, leading to recurrent pneumonias and atelectasis.[6]

Type V GSD, also known as McArdle disease, affects only the skeletal muscles. It is caused by a deficiency of myophosphorylase, which is an isoform of glycogen phosphorylase.[9,10] The deficiency of this enzyme prevents breakdown of glycogen into glucose-1-phosphate. Interestingly, patients with this disease complain of exercise intolerance, but they do not produce lactic acid during anaerobic exercise owing to the glycolysis pathway being proximally blocked and preventing pyruvate synthesis, which is required for lactate production. Additionally, owing to the pathway being hindered proximally, the amount of substrate for oxidative phosphorylation is also limited leading to exercise intolerance.[11] The lack of lactate production during initial exercise is pathognomonic for McArdle disease, and the disease is tested by measuring lactate concentrations during the forearm exercise test.[12,13] The symptoms of McArdle disease are muscle fatigue, weakness, and myalgias during exercise. Although these patients are limited early on during exercise, with prolonged exercise, they may encounter a "second wind" phenomenon in which the tolerance to exercise improves owing to extramuscular substrates being used for energy production.[14,15]

Diseases of Lipid and Purine Metabolism

Alternatives to glucose metabolism for energy production are the use of mitochondrial fatty acid oxidation and purine metabolism. Fatty acids are processed through the beta-oxidation pathway in the mitochondria. Clinical myopathy caused by CPT I deficiency in muscle has not been reported.[16] Our discussion focuses on CPT II deficiency, which causes adult-onset myopathy. Patients with CPT II deficiency have myalgias, muscle stiffness, fatigue, and rhabdomyolysis during periods when fatty acids are used to produce energy. These states include fasting and prolonged exercise.[17] In relation to the respiratory system, there is 1 case report of respiratory insufficiency in a patient with CPT II deficiency.[18]

Myoadenylate (AMP) deaminase deficiency is localized to skeletal muscle. This enzyme helps with the repletion of ATP in anaerobic conditions as described elsewhere in this article.[19] Deficiency of AMP deaminase causes myalgias and cramps during exercise and, thus, exercise intolerance. Rhabdomyolysis and myoglobinuria could also be present.

Mitochondrial Diseases

As discussed, the clinical presentation of mitochondrial diseases is variable, because symptoms and severity may be different depending on the patient, the organs involved, and the rate of disease progression. The prevalence of mitochondrial disorders is approximately 1 per 10,000.[20] In 1 study, mitochondrial myopathy was the final diagnosis in 8.5% of adult patients referred to a tertiary care dyspnea clinic.[21] The primary symptoms of mitochondrial myopathies are muscle weakness and exercise intolerance. In the cohort mentioned, respiratory muscle weakness was absent. Additionally, mitochondrial myopathies are associated with dysfunction of other organ systems that require high energy demand, and these organ systems include the central nervous, cardiac, and endocrine systems. Mitochondrial myopathies should be considered in patients who present with muscle weakness, exercise intolerance, and multiorgan dysfunction.[22] Rare cases of

respiratory muscle weakness presenting with acute hypercapnic respiratory failure requiring intubation and mechanical ventilation, caused by cytochrome oxidase deficiency and an isolated defect of succinate-cytochrome C reductase activity, have been described.[23]

There are several phenotypes of mitochondrial myopathies, and they affect different age ranges and have different organ involvement and severity. We only discuss those phenotypes that affect the ability to exercise and are associated with respiratory failure in adults. In rare cases, isolated myopathy can be present in which only skeletal muscles are affected. These patients present with exercise intolerance, muscle weakness, elevated creatine kinase, myalgia, and myoglobinuria.[24–26]

The following mitochondrial myopathies that affect multiple organ systems have been associated with respiratory failure owing to pathology in the brain stem or respiratory muscle weakness. Chronic progressive external ophthalmoplegia (CPEO) is a mild form of mitochondrial myopathy that can present during childhood or adulthood. It causes ophthalmoplegia, bilateral ptosis, and proximal myopathy. CPEO with pigmentary retinopathy is known as Kearns-Sayre syndrome, which is a more severe form compared with CPEO. Although Kearns-Sayre syndrome mainly affects the retina, cardiac conduction system, and cerebellum, patients with this disease can also develop diabetes mellitus, sensorineural hearing loss, proximal myopathy, and respiratory muscle weakness. Although there are no large studies examining the development of respiratory failure in Kearns-Sayre syndrome, cases of Kearns-Sayre syndrome associated with respiratory failure have been described.[27,28] Objectively, a reduction in vital capacity, forced expiratory volume in 1 second, and peak expiratory flow has been noted in CPEO.[29]

Patients with mitochondrial encephalomyopathy with lactic acidosis and stroke-like episodes and myoclonic epilepsy with ragged red fibers may develop significant myopathy leading to respiratory failure from alveolar hypoventilation.

PATIENT HISTORY

A patient may present with 1 or more of the following[30,31]:

- Exercise intolerance;
- "Second wind" phenomenon (pain and ability to exercise improves after a certain duration of activity);
- Generalized or localized progressive muscle weakness;

- Muscle cramps or myalgia;
- Pigmenturia;
- Positional dyspnea;
- Unexplained dyspnea in the setting of muscle weakness; or
- Family history of myopathy.

PHYSICAL EXAMINATION

Abnormal findings on physical examination[30,31]
- Low oxygen saturation.
- Short stature.
- Extraocular muscle weakness.
- Muscle atrophy.
- Diffuse proximal or distal decrease in muscle power.
- Abnormal chest wall expansion.

DIAGNOSTIC TESTING

Metabolic myopathies negatively affect muscles owing to defects in metabolism that cause a decreased availability of a substrate for energy production. Patients with these disorders present with exercise intolerance and fatigue. Mitochondrial disorders are the best characterized in the literature in relation to abnormalities found on pulmonary function and exercise testing.

Arterial Blood Gas Sampling and Pulmonary Function Testing

When a patient first presents with respiratory complaints and the presence of a metabolic myopathy is being considered, an arterial blood gas would be helpful in characterizing the type of respiratory failure. Some of the aforementioned metabolic myopathies may cause alveolar hypoventilation, which could lead to chronic hypercapnia. Depending on these findings, pulmonary function and respiratory muscle strength testing may be obtained to better describe the abnormality.

The various pulmonary function abnormalities depend on the area of the respiratory system that is affected. Some of the metabolic myopathies affect the skeletal muscles and, therefore, accessory skeletal muscles used for expiration may be impaired, resulting in a higher expiratory reserve and reserve volumes at the end of expiration.[32] The diaphragm, which is the primary muscle of inspiration, is involved in Pompe disease.[33] With diaphragm dysfunction, a reduction in the forced vital capacity and forced expiratory volume in 1 second may be seen in conjunction with a decrease in total lung capacity, indicating a restrictive ventilatory defect. The diffusing capacity in these cases is normal. Diaphragm dysfunction is assessed with measuring the maximal inspiratory

pressure, maximal expiratory pressure, and seated and supine vital capacities. An increase in the maximal expiratory pressure to maximal inspiratory pressure ratio or a decrease in the vital capacity from the seated to supine position suggests diaphragm dysfunction.[34] The sniff test (which uses fluoroscopy to visualize diaphragm excursion) or ultrasound confirmation of diaphragmatic thickening can be used to confirm the diagnosis of diaphragm dysfunction[35] (see Taro Minami and colleagues' article, "Assessing Diaphragm Function in Chest Wall and Neuromuscular Diseases," in this issue for further details.)

Cardiopulmonary Exercise Testing

Cardiopulmonary exercise testing is routinely used in evaluating exercise intolerance when other commonly ordered diagnostic examinations, such as pulmonary function tests, are unrevealing. It provides additional information about the cardiovascular, respiratory, and muscular system functioning as a unit. During exercise, respiration and blood flow increases to help supply oxygen to muscles and to remove carbon dioxide from them. Use of the skeletal muscles also produces lactic acid, a byproduct of anaerobic metabolism. Measurements of oxygen consumption, carbon dioxide elimination, and lactic acid generation can help to identify the disease process.[36]

Cardiopulmonary exercise testing can be completed on a cycle ergometer or treadmill. Hemodynamic measurements, including heart rate, blood pressure, and respiratory rate are obtained at rest and during exercise. Sampling of venous and/or arterial blood for lactate and blood gas before, during, and after exercise is performed to obtain measurements of other parameters involved in respiration. A detailed description, protocol, and recommendations of cardiopulmonary exercise testing are presented elsewhere.[37]

Glycogen storage disorders negatively affect the muscle by preventing influx of carbohydrates into the ATP cycle. McArdle disease physiology has been extensively studied, and the changes during exercise have been well reported in literature (**Table 1**). As mentioned, lactic acid is not produced during exercise and, therefore, an absent anaerobic threshold is expected. Exercise capacity is reduced, which leads to a lower oxygen consumption. The heart rate and cardiac output are high, but the overall tissue extraction of oxygen is low owing to the inability of the muscle to fully use oxygen for oxidative phosphorylation (low oxygen pulse). Because lactic acid is not produced and equilibration of acidemia is not required, the ratio of minute volume to carbon dioxide

Table 1
Comparison of relative physiologic responses between defects of glycogenolysis and glycolysis and defects of mitochondria

	Defects of Glycogenolysis and Glycolysis	Mitochondrial Myopathies
Peak exercise $\dot{V}_{O2}$	Reduced; often <50% predicted. "Second-wind" phenomenon in McArdle disease.	Reduced; variable, but often <50% predicted.
Anaerobic threshold	Absent.	Occurs early; usually well below 40% of predicted peak V_{O2}.
$\dot{V}_E/\dot{V}_{CO2}$	May be normal or mildly elevated throughout exercise. Normal (25–40) or high (>40) at peak exercise.	Probably normal (25–30) or somewhat increased (30–35) before respiratory compensation point. May be normal (25–40) or high (>40) at peak exercise.
$\dot{V}_E/\dot{V}_{O2}$	May be slightly elevated during exercise. Usually low (<25) at peak exercise.	Probably normal before lactic acidosis threshold (20–30). Very high at peak exercise (>50). Large increment (>25) from nadir to peak values.
Peak exercise heart rate	Close to normal predicted value.	Close to normal predicted value.
Peak exercise oxygen-pulse	Low, usually <60% predicted.	Low, usually <60% predicted.
Chronotropic index	High (male, >45 L^{-1}; female, >70 L^{-1}).	High (male, >45 L^{-1}; female, >70 L^{-1}).
Respiratory exchange ratio	Low throughout exercise and at peak exercise (<0.9). Low during recovery (<1.1).	Very high at peak exercise (>1.5).
End-tidal partial pressure of carbon dioxide	May be normal or slightly low throughout exercise. Usually normal at peak exercise (35–40 mm Hg), but low values (<35 mm Hg) possible if hyperventilation present.	Uncertain. May be normal or mildly reduced below respiratory compensation point. May be normal (35–45 mm Hg) or low (<35 mm Hg) at peak exercise.
End-tidal partial pressure of oxygen	Low (<100 mm Hg) at peak exercise.	Likely to be very high (>120 mm Hg) at peak exercise.
Peripheral capillary hemoglobin oxygen concentration	Normal (>95%).	Normal (>95%).
$\dot{V}_{O2}$-work rate slope	High (>12 mL min^{-1} W^{-1}).	Uncertain.
Blood lactate	No increase.	Early and persistent increase. Peak level may be excessive (eg, 12–15 mmol/L).
Blood ammonia	Very high, often >200 µmol/L at peak exercise and during the first few minutes of recovery.	Uncertain. Any increase likely to occur early.
Creatine kinase	Increased at rest and throughout exercise (>300 U/L^{-1}).	Often normal or only slightly elevated. Significant elevations (>300 U/L^{-1}) in a minority.

Adapted from Riley MS, Nicholls DP, Cooper CB. Cardiopulmonary exercise testing and metabolic myopathies. Ann Am Thorac Soc 2017;14(Supplemental_1):S133; with permission.

production is normal and hyperventilation is absent. The buffering of lactic acid to produce carbon dioxide is absent, which leads to low minute ventilation to oxygen consumption. Because glycolysis and oxidative phosphorylation are impaired, the source of energy production is shifted to lipid metabolism, which decreases the respiratory exchange ratio.[38]

Table 2
Metabolic myopathies and disease-specific treatments

Disease	Pharmacologic Treatments	Reference
Pompe disease	Enzyme replacement therapy (α-glucosidase)	Raben et al,[39] 2005; Kuperus et al,[40] 2017
	Chaperone therapy	Porto et al,[41] 2009; Parenti & Andria,[42] 2011
McArdle disease	No disease-specific therapy available	
CPT II deficiency	No disease-specific therapy available	
Myoadenylate deaminase deficiency	No disease-specific therapy available	
Mitochondrial disease	No disease-specific therapy available	

Mitochondrial dysfunction affects the generation of ATP from oxidative phosphorylation in the electron transport chain. Glycolysis is intact and, therefore, lactic acid is produced in mitochondrial myopathies. Lactic acid levels increase earlier on owing to the muscle's dependence on glycolysis for energy. The work rate is impaired, leading to a decrease in oxygen consumption. The heart rate and cardiac output are increased. Given that there is absence of oxidative phosphorylation during exercise, oxygen extraction in the tissue is reduced and, therefore, oxygen-pulse is reduced. With elevation in lactic acid, compensation for acidemia and increased bicarbonate buffering are expected. Elevation of $\dot{V}_E/\dot{V}_{CO2}$, $\dot{V}_E/\dot{V}_{O2}$, and $\dot{V}_{CO2}/\dot{V}_{O2}$ may be observed. Hyperventilation is appropriate given the lactic acid production during exercise and reflected as normal to low end-tidal carbon dioxide levels.[38]

Table 3
Metabolic myopathies and nonpharmacologic treatments

Disease	Nonpharmacologic Treatments	Reference
Pompe disease	Noninvasive mechanical ventilation	Mellies et al,[43] 2005; Ambrosino et al,[44] 2013
	Inhaled bronchodilators	Kishnani et al,[45] 2006; Cupler et al,[46] 2012
	Airway clearance techniques, cough assist	Kishnani et al,[45] 2006; Cupler et al,[46] 2012; Finder et al,[47] 2004; Chatwin et al,[48] 2003
	Inspiratory muscle training	Finder et al,[47] 2004
McArdle disease	Glucose infusion	Ørngreen & Vissing,[49,50] 2017; Haller & Vissing,[51] 2002
	Oral sucrose	Ørngreen & Vissing,[49] 2017; Anderson et al,[52] 2008
	High-carbohydrate diet	Ørngreen & Vissing,[49] 2017; Anderson & Vissing,[53] 2008
	Oral creatine	Ørngreen & Vissing,[49] 2017; Vorgerd et al,[54] 2000
CPT II deficiency	Glucose infusion	Ørngreen & Vissing,[49] 2017; Ørngreen et al,[55] 2002
	High-carbohydrate diet	Ørngreen & Vissing,[49] 2017; Ørngreen et al,[56] 2003
Myoadenylate deaminase deficiency	Ribose	Wagner et al,[57] 1991; Gross et al,[58] 1991
Mitochondrial disease	Noninvasive mechanical ventilation	Pfeffer & Chinnery,[2] 2013; Howard & Davidson,[59] 2003
	Creatine	Tarnopolsky et al,[60] 1997
	Carnitine	Gimenes et al,[61] 2015
	Coenzyme Q10	Bresolin et al,[62] 1990

Table 4
Evaluation of outcome

Disease	Prognosis	Reference
Pompe disease	The median age at the time of diagnosis: 38 y 5-y survival after diagnosis: 95% 10-y survival after diagnosis: 83% 20-y survival after diagnosis: 65% 30-y survival after diagnosis: 40%	Güngör et al,[63] 2011
McArdle disease	Symptoms of the disease are usually present during childhood, but the diagnosis is not made until after 30 y of age. It is not associated with a decrease in survival.	Quinlivan et al,[10] 2010
CPT II deficiency	Age of onset is variable. The myopathic form is associated with good prognosis.	Wieser,[64] 2004
Myoadenylate deaminase deficiency	Age of onset is variable. It is not associated with a decrease in survival.	Mercelis et al,[65] 1987
Mitochondrial disease	Age of onset and prognosis vary depending on type of mitochondrial myopathy. However, the age of onset is usually before the age of 20 y. It is associated with premature mortality. Age of mortality is about 40 y.	DiMauro & Hirano,[66] 2003; Barends et al,[67] 2016

PHARMACOLOGIC TREATMENT OPTIONS

Metabolic myopathies occur through genetic mutations, which cause a deficiency in certain enzymes of metabolism, and they have been difficult to treat owing to limited available therapy. Research for disease-specific treatments is ongoing. These treatments include enzyme replacement therapy and chaperone therapy. Although these treatments are available, experience using these therapies is limited, and they are expensive. The diseases under discussion with disease-specific treatments are presented in **Table 2**.

NON-PHARMACOLOGIC TREATMENT OPTIONS

There are no definitive treatments for many of the metabolic myopathies that have been discussed. For those with disease-specific treatments, therapeutic options are still in their infancy, and evidence for these treatments are sparse; further research is ongoing. Therefore, the management of most of the metabolic myopathies involves supportive and maintenance care to minimize symptoms, such as myalgia and exercise intolerance. Additionally, these treatments can help with the clearance of secretions, and the prevention of aspiration and alveolar hypoventilation (**Tables 3** and **4**).

SUMMARY

- Primary care providers and pulmonologist are inexperienced in diagnosing and treating these disorders, and there is a paucity of literature to guide management decisions.
- Pompe disease (type II GSD) and McArdle disease (type V GSD) are commonly associated with exercise intolerance. Pompe disease also causes diaphragm dysfunction, which may lead to chronic hypercapnic respiratory failure form alveolar hypoventilation. McArdle disease has been well-studied physiologically. It is known for the absence of lactic acid during exercise.
- A defect in lipid metabolism can cause exercise intolerance, usually later in exercise when glycogen stores are exhausted and the energy source is switched to fatty acid oxidation.
- Mitochondrial dysfunction can present in adulthood and may constitute a substantial proportion of patients seen in a tertiary care dyspnea clinic.
- Cardiopulmonary exercise testing is useful in differentiating among GSD, disease of lipid metabolism, and mitochondrial disease being the cause of myopathy.
- Although the available disease-specific treatments are promising, experience is lacking, and they are expensive.

- Management of metabolic myopathies using nonpharmacologic therapy, such as noninvasive ventilation, pulmonary toileting, special diets, and judicious exercise prescription has been mainstay in treating symptoms of metabolic myopathies.

REFERENCES

1. Rose MR. Mitochondrial myopathies: genetic mechanisms. Arch Neurol 1998;55(1):17–24.

2. Pfeffer G, Chinnery PF. Diagnosis and treatment of mitochondrial myopathies. Ann Med 2013;45(1): 4–16.

3. Ozen H. Glycogen storage diseases: new perspectives. World J Gastroenterol 2007;13(18):2541–53.

4. Hicks J, Wartchow E, Mierau G. Glycogen storage diseases: a brief review and update on clinical features, genetic abnormalities, pathologic features, and treatment. Ultrastruct Pathol 2011;35(5): 183–96.

5. Mellies U, Lofaso F. Pompe disease: a neuromuscular disease with respiratory muscle involvement. Respir Med 2009;103(4):477–84.

6. Fukuda T, Roberts A, Plotz PH, et al. Acid alpha-glucosidase deficiency (Pompe disease). Curr Neurol Neurosci Rep 2007;7(1):71–7.

7. Bembi B, Cerini E, Danesino C, et al. Diagnosis of glycogenosis type II. Neurology 2008;71(23 Suppl 2):S4–11.

8. Winkel LP, Hagemans ML, van Doorn PA, et al. The natural course of non-classic Pompe's disease; a review of 225 published cases. J Neurol 2005;252(8): 875–84.

9. McArdle B. Myopathy due to a defect in muscle glycogen breakdown. Clin Sci 1951;10(1):13–35.

10. Quinlivan R, Buckley J, James M, et al. McArdle disease: a clinical review. J Neurol Neurosurg Psychiatry 2010;81(11):1182–8.

11. Kitaoka Y. McArdle disease and exercise physiology. Biology (Basel) 2014;3(1):157–66.

12. Hogrel JY, Laforêt P, Ben Yaou R, et al. A non-ischemic forearm exercise test for the screening of patients with exercise intolerance. Neurolog 2001; 56(12):1733–8.

13. Kazemi-Esfarjani P, Skomorowska E, Jensen TD, et al. A nonischemic forearm exercise test for McArdle disease. Ann Neurol 2002;52(2):153–9.

14. Vissing J, Lewis SF, Galbo H, et al. Effect of deficient muscular glycogenolysis on extramuscular fuel production in exercise. J Appl Physiol (1985) 1992; 72(5):1773–9.

15. Robertshaw HA, Raha S, Kaczor JJ, et al. Increased PFK activity and GLUT4 protein content in McArdle's disease. Muscle Nerve 2008;37(4):431–7.

16. Bonnefont JP, Djouadi F, Prip-Buus C, et al. Carnitine palmitoyltransferases 1 and 2: biochemical, molecular and medical aspects. Mol Aspects Med 2004;25(5–6):495–520.

17. Liang WC, Nishino I. State of the art in muscle lipid diseases. Acta Myol 2010;29:351–6.

18. DiMauro S, DiMauro PM. Muscle carnitine palmitoyl-transferase deficiency and myoglobinuria. Science 1973;182(4115):929–31.

19. Sabina RL, Swain JL, Olanow CW, et al. Myoadenylate deaminase deficiency. Functional and metabolic abnormalities associated with disruption of the purine nucleotide cycle. J Clin Invest 1984;73(2): 720–30.

20. Tonin P, Lewis P, Servidei S, et al. Metabolic causes of myoglobinuria. Ann Neurol 1990;27(2): 181–5.

21. Flaherty KR, Wald J, Weisman IM, et al. Unexplained exertional limitation: characterization of patients with a mitochondrial myopathy. Am J Respir Crit Care Med 2001;164(3):425–32.

22. Schaefer AM, McFarland R, Blakely EL, et al. Prevalence of mitochondrial DNA disease in adults. Ann Neurol 2008;63(1):35–9.

23. Cros D, Palliyath S, DiMauro S, et al. Respiratory failure revealing mitochondrial myopathy in adults. Chest 1992;101(3):824–8.

24. Andreu AL, Bruno C, Dunne TC, et al. A nonsense mutation (G15059A) in the cytochrome b gene in a patient with exercise intolerance and myoglobinuria. Ann Neurol 1999;45(1):127–30.

25. McFarland R, Taylor RW, Chinnery PF, et al. A novel sporadic mutation in cytochrome c oxidase subunit II as a cause of rhabdomyolysis. Neuromuscul Disord 2004;14(2):162–6.

26. Massie R, Wong LJ, Milone M. Exercise intolerance due to cytochrome b mutation. Muscle Nerve 2010;42(1):136–40.

27. Barohn RJ, Clanton T, Sahenk Z, et al. Recurrent respiratory insufficiency and depressed ventilatory drive complicating mitochondrial myopathies. Neurology 1990;40(1):103–6.

28. Sanaker PS, Husebye ES, Fondenes O, et al. Clinical evolution of Kearns-Sayre syndrome with polyendocrinopathy and respiratory failure. Acta Neurol Scand Suppl 2007;187:64–7.

29. Smits BW, Heijdra YF, Cuppen FW, et al. Nature and frequent of respiratory involvement in chronic progressive external ophthalmoplegia. J Neurol 2011; 258(11):2020–5.

30. Barohn RJ, Dimachkie MM, Jackson CE. A pattern recognition approach to patients with a suspected myopathy. Neurol Clin 2014;32(3):569–93.

31. Lilleker JB, Keh YS, Roncaroli F, et al. Metabolic myopathies: a practical approach. Pract Neurol 2018; 18(1):14–26.

32. Shahrizalia N, Kinnear WJ, Wills AJ. Respiratory involvement in inherited primary muscle conditions. J Neurol Neurosurg Psychiatry 2006;77(10):1108–15.

33. Johnson EM, Roberts M, Mozaffar T, et al. Pulmonary function tests (maximum inspiratory pressure, maximum expiratory pressure, vital capacity, forced vital capacity) predict ventilator use in late-onset Pompe disease. Neuromuscul Disord 2016;26(2): 136–45.

34. Koo P, Oyeng'o DO, Gartman EJ, et al. The maximal expiratory-to-inspiratory ratio and supine vital capacity as screening tests for diaphragm dysfunction. Lung 2017;195(1):29–35.

35. McCool FD, Tzelepis GE. Dysfunction of the diaphragm. N Engl J Med 2012;366(10):932–42.

36. Wasserman K, Hansen JE, Sue DY, et al. Principles of exercise testing and interpretation. 5th edition. Philadelphia: Lippincott, Williams, and Wilkins; 2012.

37. American Thoracic Society; American College of Chest Physicians. ATS/ACCP statement on cardiopulmonary exercise testing. Am J Respir Crit Care Med 2003;167(2):211–77.

38. Riley MS, Nicholls DP, Cooper CB. Cardiopulmonary exercise testing and metabolic myopathies. Ann Am Thorac Soc 2017;14(Supplemental_1): S129–39.

39. Raben N, Fukuda T, Gilbert AL, et al. Replacing acid alpha-glucosidase in Pompe disease: recombinant and transgenic enzymes are equipotent, but neither completely clears glycogen from type II muscle fibers. Mol Ther 2005;11(1):48–56.

40. Kuperus E, Kruijshaar ME, Wens SCA, et al. Long-term benefit of enzyme replacement therapy in Pompe disease: a 5-year prospective study. Neurology 2017;89(23):2365–73.

41. Porto C, Cardone M, Fontana F, et al. The pharmacological chaperone N-butyldeoxynojirimycin enhances enzyme replacement therapy in Pompe disease fibroblasts. Mol Ther 2009;17(6):964–71.

42. Parenti G, Andria G. Pompe disease: from new views on pathophysiology to innovative therapeutic strategies. Curr Pharm Biotechnol 2011;12(6):902–15.

43. Mellies U, Stehling F, Dohna-Schwake C, et al. Respiratory failure in Pompe disease: treatment with noninvasive ventilation. Neurology 2005;64(8): 1465–7.

44. Ambrosino N, Confalonieri M, Crescimanno G, et al. The role of respiratory management of Pompe disease. Respir Med 2013;107(8):1124–32.

45. Kishnani PS, Steiner RD, Bali D, et al. Pompe disease diagnosis and management guideline. Genet Med 2006;8(5):267–88.

46. Cupler EJ, Berger KI, Leshner RT, et al. AANEM consensus committee on late-onset Pompe disease. Muscle Nerve 2012;45(3):319–33.

47. Finder JD, Birnkrant D, Carl J, et al, American Thoracic Society. Respiratory care of the patient with Duchenne muscular dystrophy: ATS consensus statement. Am J Respir Crit Care Med 2004;170:456–65.

48. Chatwin M, Ross E, Hart N, et al. Cough augmentation with mechanical insufflation/exsufflation in patients with neuromuscular weakness. Eur Respir J 2003;21:502–8.

49. Ørngreen MC, Vissing J. Treatment opportunities in patients with metabolic myopathies. Curr Treat Options Neurol 2017;19(11):37.

50. Vissing J, Haller RG. The effect of oral sucrose on exercise tolerance in patients with McArdle's disease. N Engl J Med 2003;349(26):2503–9.

51. Haller RG, Vissing K. Spontaneous "second wind" and glucose-induced second "second wind" in McArdle disease: oxidative mechanisms. Arch Neurol 2002;59:1395–402.

52. Anderson ST, Haller RG, Vissing J. Effect of oral sucrose shortly before exercise on work capacity in McArdle disease. Arch Neurol 2008;65(6): 786–9.

53. Anderson ST, Vissing J. Carbohydrate- and protein-rich diets in McArdle disease: effects on exercise capacity. J Neurol Neurosurg Psychiatry 2008; 79(12):1359–63.

54. Vorgerd M, Grehl T, Jager M, et al. Creatine therapy in myophosphorylase deficiency (McArdle disease): a placebo-controlled crossover trial. Arch Neurol 2000;57(7):956–63.

55. Ørngreen MC, Olsen DB, Vissing J. Exercise intolerance in carnitine palmitoyltransferase II deficiency with IV and oral glucose. Neurology 2002;59(7): 1046–51.

56. Ørngreen MC, Ejstrup R, Vissing J. Effect of diet on exercise tolerance in carnitine palmitoyltransferase II deficiency. Neurology 2003;61(4): 559–61.

57. Wagner DR, Gresser U, Zöllner N. Effects of oral ribose on muscle metabolism during bicycle ergometer in AMPD-deficient patients. Ann Nutr Metab 1991;35(5):297–302.

58. Gross M, Kormann B, Zöllner N. Ribose administration during exercise: effects on substrates and products of energy metabolism in healthy subjects and a patient with myoadenylate deaminase deficiency. Klin Wochenschr 1991;69(4): 151–5.

59. Howard RS, Davidson C. Long term ventilation in neurogenic respiratory failure. J Neurol Neurosurg Psychiatry 2003;74(Suppl 3):iii24–30.

60. Tarnopolsky MA, Roy BD, MacDonald JR. A randomized, controlled trial of creatine monohydrate in patients with mitochondrial cytopathies. Muscle Nerve 1997;20:1502–9.

61. Gimenes AC, Bravo DM, Nápolis M, et al. Effect of L-carnitine on exercise performance in patients with mitochondrial myopathy. Braz J Med Biol Res 2015;48(4):354–62.

62. Bresolin N, Doriguzzi C, Ponzetto C, et al. Ubidecarenone in the treatment of mitochondrial myopathies:

a multi-center double-blind trial. J Neurol Sci 1990;
100(1–2):70–8.

63. Güngör D, de Vries JM, Hop WC, et al. Survival and
associated factors in 268 adults with Pompe disease
prior to treatment with enzyme replacement therapy.
Orphanet J Rare Dis 2011;6:34.

64. Wieser T. Carnitine palmitoyltransferase II
deficiency. In: Adam MP, Ardinger HH,
Pagon RA, et al, editors. GeneReviews®. Seattle
(WA): University of Washington, Seattle; 2004. p.
1993–2018. Available at: https://www.ncbi.nlm.
nih.gov/books/NBK1253/. Accessed Mar 16,
2017.

65. Mercelis R, Martin JJ, de Barsy T, et al. Myoadenylate deaminase deficiency: absence of correlation
with exercise intolerance in 452 muscle biopsies.
J Neurol 1987;234(6):385–9.

66. DiMauro S, Hirano M. Mitochondrial DNA deletion
syndromes. In: Adam MP, Ardinger HH, Pagon RA,
et al, editors. GeneReviews®. Seattle (WA): University of Washington, Seattle; 2003. p. 1993–2018.
Available at: https://www.ncbi.nlm.nih.gov/books/
NBK1203/. Accessed May 3, 2011.

67. Barends M, Verschuren L, Morava E, et al. Causes of
death in adults with mitochondrial disease. JIMD
Rep 2016;26:103–13.

Traumatic Spinal Cord Injury
Pulmonary Physiologic Principles and Management

Gregory J. Schilero, MD[a,b,*], William A. Bauman, MD[a,b,c], Miroslav Radulovic, MD[a,b]

KEYWORDS

- Pulmonary function • Spinal cord injury • Respiratory muscle strength
- Restrictive airway dysfunction • Airway dynamics • Respiratory symptoms • Sleep apnea

KEY POINTS

- Respiratory complications, principally pneumonia, are the primary cause for premature mortality among individuals who have suffered traumatic spinal cord injury, both during the early acute post-injury period and thereafter.
- Due to paralysis of respiratory muscles, traumatic injury to the cervical and upper thoracic spinal cord is associated with restrictive pulmonary dysfunction and respiratory muscle weakness, with greater compromise of expiratory as compared with inspiratory muscle function.
- A significant number of persons with cervical spinal cord injury manifest obstructive physiology characterized by reduction in baseline airway caliber, bronchodilator responsiveness, and nonspecific airway hyperreactivity, although the clinical significance of these findings are unclear.
- Chest physiotherapeutic techniques appear to be effective early adjuncts to prevent atelectasis and promote respiratory clearance during weaning attempts and to help prevent respiratory complications, such as pneumonia, among subjects with high cervical spinal cord injury.
- The prevalence of sleep-disordered breathing among subjects with tetraplegia far exceeds that witnessed in the general population, and implies a unique underlying physiology among these individuals.

INTRODUCTION

Traumatic injury to the cervical and upper thoracic spinal cord is associated with variable degrees of pulmonary dysfunction and disability dependent on the level and completeness of injury. The purpose of this article was to detail the pulmonary function and mechanisms of pulmonary physiologic impairment associated with traumatic spinal cord injury (SCI), and interventions to prevent pulmonary complications associated with attendant decreases in respiratory muscle strength and impaired cough. We

Disclosure: None of the authors have any financial interests in subject matter or materials discussed in this article.
[a] Department of Medicine, The Icahn School of Medicine at Mount Sinai, 1 Gustave L. Levy Place, New York, NY 10029, USA; [b] Rehabilitation Research & Development Center of Excellence for the Medical Consequences of Spinal Cord Injury, The James J. Peters VAMC, 130 West Kingsbridge Road, Bronx, NY 10468, USA; [c] Department of Rehabilitation Medicine, The Icahn School of Medicine at Mount Sinai, 1 Gustave L. Levy Place, New York, NY 10029, USA
* Corresponding author. Department of Medicine, The Icahn School of Medicine at Mount Sinai, 1 Gustave L. Levy Place, New York, NY 10029.
E-mail address: Gregory.Schilero@va.gov

Clin Chest Med 39 (2018) 411–425
https://doi.org/10.1016/j.ccm.2018.02.002
0272-5231/18/Published by Elsevier Inc.

examine temporal changes in pulmonary function following traumatic SCI and focus on the physiologic principles that govern and affect the ability to breathe spontaneously without ventilatory support. Various interventions discussed include chest physiotherapy, pharmacologic and nonpharmacologic techniques to improve respiratory muscle strength, and electrical pacing techniques. Sleep-disordered breathing also is discussed because of its high prevalence in this population, including current thoughts regarding pathophysiology and management. This review does not address spinal shock, the acute care of the spinal cord–injured patient (including ventilator or tracheostomy management), pulmonary embolism, or management of respiratory complications. With regard to diaphragmatic pacing, the reader is directed to Anthony F. DiMarcos' article, "Diaphragm Pacing," in this issue.

EPIDEMIOLOGY

Significant and lifelong neurologic deficits are all too often the dramatic consequence of traumatic SCI. According to 2017 estimates compiled by the National Spinal Cord Injury Data Center, the annual incidence of traumatic SCI in the United States is approximately 54 cases per 1 million people, or 17,500 new cases per year, and affects approximately 285,000 persons (range 245,000–345,000).[1] Compared with the 1970s, men still comprise approximately 80% of victims of SCI, although the average age at injury has increased from 28.7 years to 42.2 years, a consequence of our aging population and an increase in injuries resulting from falls among older individuals.[2] There has been a corresponding decrease in the percentage of SCIs resulting from vehicular crashes (47% to 38%), although this remains the most common etiology, followed by falls (31%), acts of violence (14%), sports-related injuries (9%), medical/surgical complications (5%), and others (4%).[1,2] Notwithstanding the attendant emotional and physical challenges of SCI, the socioeconomic impact across a lifetime is substantial; according to the National SCI Statistical Center, the estimated lifetime medical cost for an individual injured at age 25 with low tetraplegia is approximately $3.5 million.[1]

The past 40 years have witnessed a substantial improvement in the acute management and short-term 2-year survival in persons with SCI, although the mortality risk remains high during this period, ranging from 3.1% to 21.0%.[3–10] Pulmonary complications pose the greatest risk during the first 2 years postinjury, and include pneumonia, pulmonary edema, respiratory failure, and thromboembolism.[11,12] Despite improved early survival and shorter initial hospital lengths of stay, according to a recent study of data from the National Spinal Cord Injury Model System, the life expectancy for those surviving beyond 2 years postinjury compared with an age-matched noninjured population has declined slightly over the past 30 years, and overall long-term survival for persons with SCI remains significantly less than that of the general population regardless of injury level.[1,13] Historical data also identify a shift in the principal cause of mortality during the chronic phase of SCI; mortality related to urosepsis and renal failure has now been supplanted by sepsis and pulmonary complications, particularly pneumonia.[1,14,15] Thus, pulmonary complications are now a primary cause for morbidity and mortality in the SCI population, regardless of time postinjury.

OVERVIEW OF RESPIRATORY MUSCLE FUNCTION

The principal muscle of inspiration is the diaphragm innervated by the phrenic nerve arising from cervical nerve roots C3 to C5. Dome-shaped, the diaphragm consists of a central tendon and skeletal muscle fibers that insert laterally along the inner surface of the lower 6 ribs and anteromedially along the costal cartilages. The region of diaphragm that closely abuts the lower ribs at functional residual capacity defines the zone of apposition which normally constitutes 30% of total rib cage surface area.[16] With inspiration and muscle shortening, the diaphragm descends and the zone of apposition decreases, thereby increasing the thoracic cavity, displacing abdominal contents caudally, and elevating the lower rib cage.[17] The external intercostal muscles and parasternal portion of the internal intercostals supplied by corresponding thoracic spinal nerves have a synergistic action with the diaphragm during inspiration, serving to elevate the 2nd through 12th ribs.[18,19] Accessory muscles of inspiration, including the sternocleidomastoid (cranial nerve [CN] XI), scalene (C2–C7), and upper trapezius (CN XI) muscles, function to elevate the upper ribs and sternum.[16]

Generally, during quiet breathing, expiration is a passive process, although recruitment of expiratory muscles is essential for force generation during active processes, such a cough or exercise. The principal muscles of expiration are the internal intercostals and the abdominal muscles. The interosseous internal intercostals are innervated by corresponding thoracic nerves, and their major function is to lower the rib cage (from the 2nd to the 12th ribs). The abdominal muscles involved in active expiration include the rectus abdominis (T5 to L1), and the external and internal oblique muscles (lower 6 intercostal nerves, subcostal nerve), which compress both rib cage and abdomen. Accessory muscles include the clavicular portion of the pectoralis major (C5–C7) and latissimus dorsi (C6–C8).[16]

Optimal function of the diagram is contingent on intact intercostal and abdominal muscle function. In patients with cervical or thoracic SCI, paralysis of intercostal and abdominal musculature impairs diaphragm performance. The tethering effect of the inspiratory intercostal muscles is no longer present in SCI. Therefore, when the diaphragm contracts and lowers pleural pressure, the intercostals can no longer counterbalance the deflationary effects of negative intrapleural pressure on the upper rib cage. Consequently, there is paradoxic inward motion of the upper rib cage during inspiration. In addition, abdominal muscle paralysis increases abdominal compliance, resulting in greater diaphragm shortening for a given tidal volume. The combination of reduced abdominal compliance and paradoxic

inward motion of the upper rib cage results in a decrease in diaphragmatic efficiency (less volume inhaled for a given amount of diaphragmatic work), and an increased oxygen cost of breathing.[20-23]

A schematic showing levels of innervation of the inspiratory and expiratory muscles is shown in **Fig. 1**.

ASSESSMENT OF MOTOR AND SENSORY IMPAIRMENT FOLLOWING SPINAL CORD INJURY

The American Spinal Injury Impairment Scale (AIS) is used to classify the extent of motor and sensory impairment following SCI.[24] Tetraplegia refers to impairment or loss of motor and/or sensory function in the cervical segments (C1–C8), whereas paraplegia refers to impairment or loss of motor and/or sensory function involving the thoracic (T1–T12), lumbar (L1–L5), or sacral segments (S1–S5) of the spinal cord. Motor complete injuries are characterized by complete absence of motor functional preservation below the neurologic level and either a corresponding absence (AIS A) or preservation of sensory function (AIS B). Motor incomplete lesions have variable degrees of residual motor function (AIS C and AIS D) (**Table 1**). The degree of ventilatory muscle impairment is

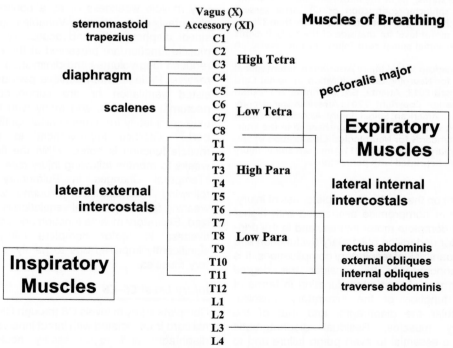

Fig. 1. Respiratory muscles and SCI. (*From* Schilero GJ, Spungen AM, Bauman WA, et al. Pulmonary function and spinal cord injury. Respir Physiol Neurobiol 2009;166(3):130; with permission.)

Table 1
American Spinal Injury Association impairment scale (AIS)
A   Complete cord injury. No motor or sensory function is preserved in the sacral segments S4–5.
B   Sensory incomplete. Sensory but not motor function is preserved below the neurologic level and includes the sacral segments (light touch or pin prick at S4–5 or deep anal pressure) AND no motor function is preserved more than 3 levels below the motor level on either side of the body.
C   Motor incomplete. Motor function is preserved below the neurologic level and more than half of key muscle functions below the neurologic level of injury have a muscle grade <3 (Grades 0–2).
D   Motor incomplete. Motor function is preserved below the neurologic level and at least half (half or more) of key muscle functions below the neurologic level of injury have a muscle grade ≥3.
E   Normal. Sensation and motor function are graded as normal in all segments and the patient had prior deficits.

Muscle function is graded using the International Standards for Neurologic Classification of Spinal Cord Injury. For an individual to receive a grade of C or D (ie, motor incomplete status), he or she must have either (1) voluntary anal sphincter contraction or (2) sacral sensory sparing with sparing of motor function more than 3 levels below the motor level for that side of the body. Patients without an initial spinal cord injury do not receive an AIS grade.

From American Spinal Injury Association: International Standards for Neurological Classification of Spinal Cord Injury, revised 2013; Atlanta, GA. Reprinted 2013. Used with permission. Copyright © 2013 American Spinal Injury Association. American Spinal Injury Association (ASIA) impairment scale (AIS) remained unchanged in the International Standards for Neurological Classification of Spinal Cord Injury (ISNCSCI). © 2011 American Spinal Injury Association. Reprinted with permission.

contingent on the level and completeness of injury, with greater compromise associated with higher cord and complete motor injuries, and is the principal factor underlying pulmonary dysfunction and the attendant risk of respiratory complications. It is useful conceptually to consider the degree of impairment of respiratory function in terms of residual function of the inspiratory muscles, in particular the diaphragm, and that of the expiratory muscles. Residual diaphragmatic function is essential to avert pump failure and to spontaneously breathe without ventilatory support, whereas expiratory muscle function is essential for maintenance of cough strength and effectiveness to reduce the propensity for atelectasis and pneumonia.

Key injury levels as they pertain to the degree of physiologic impairment and recovery are as follows.

Injury Level C1–C3

Complete injury is associated with near-complete absence of function of the muscles of inspiration, principally the diaphragm (C3–C5) and external intercostals (T1–T12), resulting in respiratory pump failure. The muscles of expiration, including the internal intercostals and abdominal muscles, are also nonfunctional. Survival is therefore contingent on the immediate institution of ventilatory support. These patients will most likely be full-time ventilator-dependent, although techniques such as glossopharyngeal or "frog" breathing might facilitate brief ventilator-free periods, and certain individuals might be candidates for diaphragmatic pacing.[25] The indications for diaphragmatic pacing are discussed separately (see section on "Methods to Improve Respiratory Muscle Strength and Pulmonary Function").

Injury Level C3–C5

Mechanical ventilation is frequently required in the first few days to weeks after injury due to respiratory muscle weakness or as a consequence of atelectasis or pneumonia.[3] Variable degrees of residual diaphragmatic and accessory inspiratory muscle function are preserved at the expense of reduced lung volumes and diminished pulmonary reserve. Patients often achieve periods of unassisted ventilation or are supported through nocturnal ventilation, and many with time graduate completely from mechanical ventilatory support.[25] Gradual improvement in respiratory muscle function is noted within the first several weeks to months following injury (see section on "Temporal Changes in Pulmonary Function following Traumatic SCI"), during which time weaning from mechanical ventilation is often realized. Expiratory muscle function and cough effectiveness in motor complete injury will be significantly impaired due to paralysis of expiratory muscles.

Injury Level C6–C8

Complete injury at levels C6 through C8 of the spinal cord is associated with intact innervation to the diaphragm and to accessory neck muscles compatible with independent breathing, although the facilitative effects of intact intercostal and abdominal muscles on diaphragmatic function are not present. Expiratory muscle function, due to paralysis primarily of the internal intercostals and abdominal muscles, remains significantly impaired. Forced expiration and the ability to generate effective cough in these individuals lies with residual innervation of accessory muscles, principally the clavicular portion of the pectoralis major (C5–C7) and possibly to the latissimus dorsi (C6–C8).[26–28] Thus, these individuals remain vulnerable to respiratory failure as a consequence of increased ventilatory loads as might occur in association with pneumonia or retained secretions.[22]

Failure of individuals with cervical SCI to wean off mechanical ventilatory support may be a consequence of accompanying bulbar weakness stemming from injury to lower cranial nerves. The resultant weakness in pharyngeal and palatal muscles leads to recurrent aspiration and impaired airway protection dictating the need for long-term tracheostomy to facilitate airway clearance. Those persons with intact bulbar function but still requiring ventilatory support alternatively have a better chance of graduating to partial or complete noninvasive ventilation by using techniques such as glossopharyngeal breathing coupled with manually assisted cough ("quad cough") and other forms of chest physiotherapy, and be potentially good candidates for diaphragmatic pacing.[29,30]

Injury Level T1–T12

Thoracic-level SCI is associated with preserved diaphragmatic function notwithstanding some loss of intercostal muscle strength and the stabilizing effects of intact abdominal musculature. The major concern of thoracic-level SCI is the impact on residual expiratory muscle function and cough strength. Cough effectiveness improves as the level of thoracic injury decreases. This is a consequence of progressively greater preservation of expiratory intercostal and abdominal muscle function.

CHEST PHYSIOTHERAPY

Chest physiotherapeutic techniques may prove especially beneficial following acute injury and during the weaning process to promote lung expansion and augment secretion clearance, and also may play a role among those with chronic SCI in association with acute chest infection or as clinically indicated.[3,31] These techniques include manually assisted cough ("quad cough"), mechanical insufflation-exsufflation, suction catheters, therapeutic bronchoscopy, and conventional deep breathing exercises accompanied by

frequent changes in body position and postural drainage.[32–35]

The manually assisted or "quad cough" is performed by situating the subject in a supine or slightly upright posture while being straddled by a therapist whose hands are placed under the left and right costal margins. The subject then inhales to total lung capacity, and the therapist applies vigorous pressure to the abdomen timed to coincide with cough efforts. Contraindications include the presence of an abdominal aortic aneurysm or prosthesis, or an inferior vena cava filter.

The mechanical insufflation-exsufflation device consists of insufflation of the lungs with positive pressure, followed by application of negative-pressure that creates a peak and sustained high flow enough to provide adequate shear and velocity to loosen and remove secretions toward the mouth for suctioning or expectoration.[34] The device can deliver in-exsufflation via a mask or a tracheostomy tube, and peak expiratory flows of 6 to 11 L/s can be achieved. Potential, albeit rare, complications include abdominal distention, aggravation of gastroesophageal reflux, hemoptysis, chest and abdominal discomfort, acute cardiovascular effects, and pneumothorax. The device can be used as frequently as every 5 minutes.[33]

Bronchoscopy, as compared with use of suction catheters, allows for direct visualization of the airway and is perhaps the most effective method of secretion clearance. Performance of quad coughs during the bronchoscopic procedure might enhance secretion clearance by mobilizing secretions not otherwise bronchoscopically visible.[33]

TEMPORAL CHANGES IN PULMONARY FUNCTION FOLLOWING TRAUMATIC SPINAL CORD INJURY

The period immediately following traumatic SCI, referred to as spinal shock, is characterized by flaccid paralysis and areflexia below the level of injury.[36] Following cervical SCI, vital capacity and expiratory flows are generally at their lowest, and values of forced vital capacity less than 25% of predicted identify those individuals likely to develop respiratory failure requiring ventilatory support. Significant increases in vital capacity occur within 5 weeks of injury, with approximate doubling of vital capacity within 3 months.[37] Continued improvement in pulmonary function is noted during the remainder of the first year following cervical SCI, during which time pulmonary function parameters, including vital capacity (VC), inspiratory capacity (IC), total lung capacity (TLC), and inspiratory and expiratory flow rates increase, whereas functional residual capacity (FRC) decreases.[33,38–40] Early improvements in pulmonary function have been attributed to functional decline in the level of SCI coincident with resolution of inflammation and edema above the injury level,[38] and subsequently to improvement in diaphragm function,[33,41–44] in the performance of accessory neck muscles,[45] to the change from flaccid to spastic paralysis,[46] and to increased rib cage stability.[38,43]

ASSESSMENT OF PULMONARY FUNCTION AMONG SUBJECTS WITH CHRONIC SPINAL CORD INJURY
Testing Considerations

Precise measurement of height used to calculate predicted pulmonary function values is problematic among persons with SCI, most of whom cannot stand. Because recalled height may not be accurate, and arm span measurements appear even less reliable, it is recommended that supine length be measured for use in calculating predicted values for pulmonary function.[47] The use of modified ATS/ERS standards for the performance of spirometry also might be necessary for the subset of patients with SCI who are unable to meet acceptable standards due to excessive back-extrapolated volume and/or expiratory efforts lasting less than 6 seconds. Although most subjects with SCI are able to perform spirometry in accordance with acceptable standards for the able-bodied,[48–50] the minority who cannot are generally those with neurologically complete cervical cord injury and lower baseline levels of forced vital capacity (FVC) and forced expiratory volume in 1 second (FEV1). Modification of ATS/ERS standards to permit excessive back-extrapolated volume and expiratory efforts of less than 6 seconds duration allows for 88% of subjects with chronic SCI to provide acceptable and reproducible spirometric efforts.[49]

For measurement of maximal inspiratory and expiratory pressures (MIP and MEP, respectively), a flange-style mouthpiece is generally used. However, in a study of 50 subjects with tetraplegia, MEP values obtained using a tube-style mouthpiece were significantly greater than those obtained by use of an intraoral flange-style mouthpiece due to perioral air leaks around the latter device.[51]

Restrictive Dysfunction

Neuromuscular weakness in persons with chronic tetraplegia and high paraplegia is classically associated with spirometric and lung volume measurements demonstrating restrictive ventilatory defects highlighted by reduction in VC, peak expiratory flow, TLC, expiratory reserve volume (ERV) and IC, as well as an increase in residual volume (RV) and little change in FRC.[40,52–61] Following acute injury, VC was shown to correlate well with other spirometric and lung volume parameters, indicating that during the acute period, VC is a good surrogate of overall ventilatory function.[60] The higher the level of injury, the greater the reduction in pulmonary function parameters (**Fig. 2**),[58] with incomplete injury mitigating FVC loss in tetraplegia.[57,58] Three large cross-sectional studies have assessed spirometry in patients with chronic SCI.[52,62,63] Adjusting for neurologic level and completeness of SCI, Jain and colleagues[62] noted that lower FEV1 values were significantly related to older age, more years since injury, greater lifetime cigarette smoking in pack-years, previous chest injury or operation, a history of clinician-diagnosed asthma, self-report of wheeze, and a lower MIP. A lower FEV1/FVC ratio was associated with older age, greater lifetime cigarette smoking in pack-years, previous chest injury or operation, self-report of wheeze, and greater body mass index (BMI).[62] Similarly, in the study by Almenoff and colleagues,[52] smoking was associated with reduction in FEV1/FVC in patients with tetraplegia and paraplegia, whereas in the study by Linn and colleagues,[63] a consistent effect of smoking was not observed, although reduction in FEV1 was associated with a greater number of years since injury. In addition to level and completeness of injury, determinants of full lung volumes (TLC, FRC, RV, and ERV) included decrease in these parameters with increasing BMI and longer time since injury, increase in FRC and RV with total pack-years of smoking, and increase in RV associated with physician-diagnosed chronic obstructive pulmonary disease.[64]

In a cross-sectional analysis including 455 subjects from 2 large outpatient populations, regression analysis was used to determine % predicted FVC in motor complete SCI; the FVC fell below 80% of predicted, indicating a threshold level for restrictive dysfunction at the T4 injury level and above[58] (see **Fig. 2**). For individuals with C4-C5 motor complete SCI, this model predicts an FVC of 45% to 52% of predicted, very similar to the adjusted FVC value of 55% reported by Jain and colleagues,[62] thus identifying moderate to severe restrictive dysfunction associated with high cervical cord injury.

Airway Dynamics (Obstructive Physiology and Airway Hyperreactivity)

The weight of evidence from numerous studies assessing changes in spirometric indices and

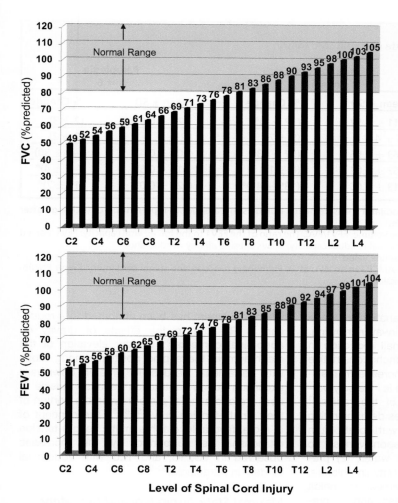

Fig. 2. Level of injury and pulmonary function abnormality. (*Adapted from* Linn WS, Spungen AM, Gong H Jr, et al. Forced vital capacity in two large outpatient populations with chronic spinal cord injury. Spinal Cord 2001;39(5):263–8; with permission.)

specific airway conductance is that subjects with chronic stable tetraplegia have reduced baseline airway caliber and that many exhibit bronchodilator responsiveness following inhalation of either an inhaled beta-2 adrenergic agonist or anticholinergic agent (ipratropium bromide) (**Table 2**), and that these findings are unique to cervical SCI and not evident in lower-level paraplegia (T7 and below).[52,65–70] A recent comparison study demonstrated that the bronchodilator effect of ipratropium bromide was greater than that of the beta-2 agonist albuterol, thereby suggesting by the specific action of anticholinergic agents that heightened cholinergic airway tone exists in tetraplegia.[65] The cumulative findings support the hypothesis that reduced airway caliber and bronchodilator responsiveness in tetraplegia is due to interruption of sympathetic innervation to the lung arising from the upper 6 thoracic nerve roots, thereby resulting in unopposed parasympathetic innervation to airways carried by vagal nerve

fibers. Although controversial, and in contrast to earlier studies, the presence of functional sympathetic innervation of human airways is supported by histochemical and ultrastructural studies demonstrating sympathetic fibers reaching the level of secondary bronchi and terminal bronchioles,[71,72] and from studies of dorsal sympathectomy for essential hyperhydrosis that revealed reduction in expiratory flows 6 months following surgery compared with values before surgery.[73–75] Despite these observations, the clinical role of bronchodilators in the management of patients with SCI is unclear, although they are often used empirically in a variety of settings.

Individuals with tetraplegia, but not those with low paraplegia, demonstrate airway hyperreactivity (AHR) in response to methacholine, histamine, and ultrasonically nebulized distilled water.[76–79] Responders to histamine demonstrated reduction in surrogate spirometric indices of airway size and airway size relative to lung size.[80] Similar to the

Table 2
Response to ipratropium bromide in spinal cord injury

Pulmonary Function Parameter	Tetraplegia n = 6		Paraplegia n = 6	
	Mean ± SD	% Change	Mean ± SD	% Change
FEV1, L	2.11 ± 0.57	(12 ± 6)[a]	3.24 ± 0.64	(2 ± 3)
FEV1/FVC ratio	75 ± 4	(5 ± 7)	82 ± 7	(0 ± 2)
ERV, L	0.63 ± 0.56	(57 ± 63)[a]	1.09 ± 0.45	(−7 ± 30)
FRC, L	2.67 ± 1.02	(0 ± 10)	3.16 ± 0.58	(−5 ± 4)[a]
sGaw, $cmH_2O^{-1}s^{-1}$	0.13 ± 0.05	(135 ± 47)[a]	0.26 ± 0.02	(19 ± 7)[a]

Values are mean ± SD for prebronchodilator measurements. Numbers in parentheses represent percent change after administration of ipratropium bromide.

Abbreviations: ERV, Expiratory reserve volume; FEV1/FVC, The ratio of the FEV1 to the forced vital capacity; FEV1, Forced expired volume in 1 second; FRC, functional residual capacity; sGaw, specific airway conductance.

[a] $P<.05$ for percent change from baseline value.

Adapted from Schilero GJ, Spungen AM, Bauman WA, et al. Pulmonary function and spinal cord injury. Respir Physiol Neurobiol 2009;166(3):133; with permission.

bronchodilator studies, one explanation for these findings would be preexisting airway narrowing, in that findings of a further small reduction in airway caliber induced by a bronchoconstrictive agent would produce a large increase in resistance, because airway resistance is inversely proportional to the fourth power of the radius.[81] Support came from further studies demonstrating the ability of: (1) pretreatment with ipratropium bromide to attenuate hyperresponsiveness to ultrasonically nebulized distilled water; (2) pretreatment with baclofen and oxybutynin chloride, both with anticholinergic properties, to inhibit methacholine hyperresponsiveness; and (3) pretreatment with metaproterenol to attenuate methacholine and histamine-induced hyperresonsiveness.[76,79,82,83] Other factors in addition to reduced baseline airway caliber, however, might be needed to explain histamine-induced AHR in subjects with tetraplegia, because neither pretreatment with ipratropium bromide nor administration of baclofen or oxybutynin chloride attenuated responsiveness to histamine.[77,83,84]

Like bronchodilator responsiveness, the clinical implications of AHR among subjects with chronic tetraplegia is unknown, although a recent Canada-wide survey of chronic respiratory disease found that after adjusting for age, sex, and smoking status, SCI was associated with significantly increased odds of asthma and chronic obstructive pulmonary disease.[85]

Effects of Body Position

In contrast to able-bodied individuals, FVC and FEV1 are significantly higher supine as compared with a sitting position.[86–89] The increase in VC when recumbent has been attributed to a reduction in RV due to the effects of gravity on abdominal contents.[89] Greater elevation of the diaphragm in the supine position among those with tetraplegia results in greater downward excursion during contraction because muscle fibers are operating at a more favorable portion of their length-tension curve.[54,87,89] The concept of a more favorable diaphragmatic length-tension relationship is supported by the increases observed in VC, IC, and TLC with abdominal binders in tetraplegia.[90–93]

Maximal Static Inspiratory and Expiratory Mouth Pressures

Maximal mouth static respiratory pressures (MIP, MEP), considered surrogate measures of global inspiratory and expiratory muscle strength and more sensitive than spirometry for detection of early muscle weakness, are reduced among persons with tetraplegia, and in contrast to healthy subjects, MIP is higher than MEP due to greater compromise of expiratory muscle function.[54,94,95] Gounden[95] found a mean MEP in the sitting position of 48 cmH2O and mean MIP of −64 cmH2O among 30 subjects with C5–C8 complete motor lesions of more than 6 months' duration. Static mouth pressures correlated with level of injury among subjects with complete motor lesions, but not among those with incomplete lesions.[67]

Lung and Rib Cage Compliance

Synchronous contraction of neck muscles among subjects with high tetraplegia acts to pull the sternum cranially and to expand the upper rib cage, but paradoxically results in inward displacement of the lateral walls of the lower rib cage.[20,96] Conversely, isolated diaphragmatic contraction is generally associated with expansion of the lower rib cage and collapse of the upper rib cage.[21,23,93,94,97–99] This abnormal coupling between the diaphragm and the upper rib cage is felt due to loss of intercostal muscle activity and increased compliance of the abdominal wall.[21,98,100,101] With time, this rib cage paradox decreases,[23] possibly because of the development of bony rib cage stiffness, increased strength of cervical accessory muscles, and improved coupling of various rib cage elements.[46] The increase in rib cage stiffness is thought to stem from ankylosis of joints due to chronic inability of subjects to inhale deeply and to increased spasticity of intercostal muscles.[46] In addition to reduction in rib cage compliance, there is a decrease in lung compliance that occurs within 1 month after injury that is felt more likely due to microatelectasis than to altered surfactant properties of the lungs.[23,46,53,54,100,102] Overall, decreases in chest wall and lung compliance coupled with increased abdominal wall compliance contribute to increased work of breathing in tetraplegia,[102–105] and possibly to respiratory muscle fatigue.[33]

RESPIRATORY SYMPTOMS

The symptom of breathlessness appears to be more prevalent among subjects with neurologically complete cervical SCI compared with those with lower-level injury. Using a modified respiratory symptom questionnaire developed for use in general epidemiologic studies among 180 subjects with SCI, breathlessness, the most prevalent symptom, was associated with level of injury: 73% in high tetraplegia (C5 and above not requiring chemical ventilation), 58% in low tetraplegia (C6 to C8), 43% in high paraplegia (T1–T7), and 29% in low paraplegia (T8–L3).[106] The prevalence of other symptoms, including chronic cough, phlegm, or wheeze, ranged from 18% to 30%, and did not differ significantly among the 4 groups. Of interest, in a subsequent analysis of the data, independent predictors of breathlessness were associated with level of injury and lung volume parameters (reduced TLC and ERV), whereas independent predictors of a combined symptom of cough + phlegm and/or wheeze were linked to smoking and FEV1 <60% predicted.[107] In other studies, breathlessness was more prevalent among those with neurologically complete cervical injury, those requiring a motorized wheelchair for daily activities, and those persons with SCI considered nonathletes.[108–110]

METHODS TO IMPROVE RESPIRATORY MUSCLE STRENGTH AND PULMONARY FUNCTION

Several interventional studies in persons with SCI have investigated whether inspiratory and expiratory resistive or threshold training, involving relatively inexpensive portable devices, are effective for improving respiratory muscle strength. Most studies have been uncontrolled and not comparable because of diverse protocols, heterogeneity of subject characteristics, or differences in training techniques. Since 2006, there have been 3 systematic reviews of respiratory muscle training in persons with SCI, and similar conclusions have been drawn; respiratory muscle training may realize increases in VC and static mouth pressures (MIP, MEP), although the effect size is small, and in many cases the data inconclusive.[111–113] Further, there is no evidence of carryover beyond the training. Insufficient data exist to make conclusions regarding the effects of respiratory muscle training on endurance, quality of life, exercise performance, or pulmonary complications.[111,113] In one well-designed trial, based on knowledge of residual function of expiratory muscles following cervical SCI, repetitive training of the clavicular portion of the pectoralis major via isometric exercise for 6 weeks among subjects with tetraplegia resulted in marked improvement in maximal isometric muscle strength and ERV, and a decrease in RV.[114] Also of interest, normocapnic hyperpnea, a technique that involves both inspiratory and expiratory muscle training via breathing at high minute ventilation, when compared with sham training for 8 weeks among 14 individuals with acute SCI, was associated with significant improvement in maximal voluntary ventilation and improved MIP and MEP.[115] The limitation of these techniques, however, lies in the difficulty in their implementation on a wider scale due to the substantive nature of the training and the methodologies involved. With regard to use of an abdominal binder to improve respiratory function, a systematic review and meta-analysis found a lack of sufficient evidence to either support or discourage use in persons with SCI.[116]

In highly motivated ventilator-dependent patients with SCI who have been shown to have intact phrenic nerve function, diaphragmatic pacing either by conventional thoracotomy and electrode placement directly upon the phrenic nerves, or via a newer and less invasive laparoscopic approach entailing insertion of electrodes directly into the diaphragm in proximity to the phrenic nerves, holds promise for achieving ventilator independence.[117,118] Preoperative testing by fluoroscopic evaluation of diaphragm excursion during simultaneous phrenic nerve stimulation is generally required, as phrenic nerve damage is quite common in association with SCI, and precludes diaphragmatic pacing if present. After implantation, a period of diaphragm reconditioning is required. Although there are no randomized studies, significant improvement in quality of life has been reported, and success defined by either partial or complete freedom from ventilatory support is achieved in many subjects.[117,118] Surgical implantation of electrodes at T9, T11, and L1 levels also has been described to improve expiratory muscle function and cough effectiveness in highly selected patients.[119] Stimulated efforts achieve maximal airway pressures approaching that seen in the able-bodied, and with greater efficacy when compared with magnetic stimulation situated at T10 posteriorly or by placement of surface electrodes along the anterolateral abdominal wall. Implantation, however, is invasive and requires hemi-laminectomy along with attendant surgical risks.[119]

Preliminary investigations have been performed involving beta-2 adrenergic agonists to improve respiratory muscle strength in persons with SCI. Precedent comes from studies of oral beta-2 adrenergic agonist administration in young men eliciting anabolic effects on skeletal muscle,[120] and augmentation in muscle strength among patients with facioscapulohumeral muscular dystrophy.[121] In subjects with tetraplegia, oral beta-2 agonists were shown to amplify total work output during functional electrical stimulation of leg muscles,[122] and to improve forearm muscle size and strength.[123] On the basis of these reports, salmeterol, a long-acting beta-2 adrenergic agonist known to exhibit systemic absorption following inhalation,[124] was administered via inhalation (50 mcg twice daily) to 11 subjects with chronic stable tetraplegia in a randomized, double-blind, placebo-controlled, crossover trial. Significant improvements compared with matching placebo were seen in lung volumes (FVC, FEV1, ERV) and static mouth pressures (MIP and MEP) after 4 weeks of twice-daily administration, suggesting improvement in lung function and respiratory muscle strength (**Table 3**).[125] The medication was well tolerated, and no adverse events were reported.

SLEEP-DISORDERED BREATHING

The prevalence of sleep-disordered breathing among subjects with tetraplegia has been reported to be as high as 83% in the first year following injury,[126] and among those with chronic injury in the range of 27% to 77%.[127–133] Reports of obstructive sleep apnea (OSA) predominate in the

Table 3
Effect of salmeterol on respiratory parameters among subjects with tetraplegia (n = 11)

Parameter	Baseline	Placebo	Salmeterol
FVC, L	3.11 ± 0.38	3.22 ± 0.41	3.36 ± 0.41[a,b]
FEV1, L	2.40 ± 0.51	2.52 ± 0.49	2.74 ± 0.52[a,b]
PEF, L/s	4.63 ± 1.13	5.01 ± 1.06	5.78 ± 1.20[a,b]
MIP, cmH$_2$O	−72.5 ± 18.6	−73.9 ± 21.5	−81.6 ± 20.8[a,b]
MEP, cmH$_2$O	40.9 ± 16.1	45.9 ± 19.2	51.3 ± 20.0[a,b]

The data are mean ± SD.
Abbreviations: FVC, forced vital capacity; FEV1, forced expired volume in 1 second; MEP, maximal expiratory pressure; MIP, maximal inspiratory pressure; PEF, peak expiratory flow.
[a] $P<.001$ compared with baseline.
[b] $P<.05$ compared with placebo.
Adapted from Grimm DR, Schilero GJ, Spungen AM, et al. Salmeterol improves pulmonary function in persons with tetraplegia. Lung 2006;184(6):338; with permission.

literature, although a recent investigation suggested a high prevalence of central apnea.[131] Symptom assessment as a tool to screen for OSA in this population appears to be relatively nondiscriminatory given the high prevalence of sleep disturbances reported regardless of cause.[131,134] The incidence of OSA among subjects with paraplegia does not appear different from that encountered in the general population, although the numbers of these subjects included in most studies are small. Possible etiologies for the high prevalence of sleep-disordered breathing among those with tetraplegia in addition to respiratory muscle weakness include sleep-related hypoventilation,[131] decreased pharyngeal cross-sectional area,[135] unopposed parasympathetic stimulation of mucosal and vessel walls of the upper airway,[136] preferential adoption of a supine sleeping position, loss of lean tissue mass and fat redistribution in the neck,[137] or compensatory neck muscle hypertrophy.[138] The long-term consequences of OSA in this population are not known, although treatment adherence with continuous positive airway pressure is low (20%–50%).[131,133,138,139]

REFERENCES

1. National Spinal Cord Injury Statistical Center, facts and figures at a glance. Birmingham (AL): University of Alabama at Birmingham; 2017. Available at: nscisc.uab.edu.

2. Chen Y, He Y, DeVivo MJ. Changing demographics and injury profile of new traumatic spinal cord injuries in the United States, 1972-2014. Arch Phys Med Rehabil 2016;97(10):1610–9.
3. Claxton AR, Wong DT, Chung F, et al. Predictors of hospital mortality and mechanical ventilation in patients with cervical spinal cord injury. Can J Anaesth 1998;45(2):144–9.
4. DeVivo MJ. Sir Ludwig Guttmann Lecture: trends in spinal cord injury rehabilitation outcomes from model systems in the United States: 1973-2006. Spinal Cord 2007;45(11):713–21.
5. DeVivo MJ, Jackson AB, Dijkers MP, et al. Current research outcomes from the model spinal cord injury care systems. Arch Phys Med Rehabil 1999;80(11):1363–4.
6. Lenehan B, Street J, Kwon BK, et al. The epidemiology of spinal cord injury in British Columbia, Canada. Spine (Phila Pa 1976) 2012;37(4):321–9.
7. Schoenfeld AJ, Sielski B, Rivera KP, et al. Epidemiology of cervical spine fractures in the US military. Spine J 2012;12(9):777–83.
8. Sekhon LH, Fehlings MG. Epidemiology, demographics, and pathophysiology of acute spinal cord injury. Spine (Phila Pa 1976) 2001;26(24 Suppl):S2–12.
9. Strauss DJ, Devivo MJ, Paculdo DR, et al. Trends in life expectancy after spinal cord injury. Arch Phys Med Rehabil 2006;87(8):1079–85.
10. Varma A, Hill EG, Nicholas J, et al. Predictors of early mortality after traumatic spinal cord injury; a population-based study. Spine 2010;35(7):778–83.
11. DeVivo MJ, Kartus PL, Stover SL, et al. Cause of death for patients with spinal cord injuries. Arch Intern Med 1989;149(8):1761–6.
12. Wuermser LA, Ho CH, Chiodo AE, et al. Spinal cord injury medicine. 2. Acute care management of traumatic and nontraumatic injury. Arch Phys Med Rehabil 2007;88(3 Suppl 1):S55–61.
13. Shavelle RM, DeVivo MJ, Brooks JC, et al. Improvements in long-term survival after spinal cord injury? Arch Phys Med Rehabil 2015;96(4):645–51.
14. Krause JS, Cao Y, DeVivo MJ, et al. Risk and protective factors for cause-specific mortality after spinal cord injury. Arch Phys Med Rehabil 2016;97(10):1669–78.
15. van den Berg ME, Castellote JM, de Pedro-Cuesta J, et al. Survival after spinal cord injury: a systematic review. J Neurotrauma 2010;27(8):1517–28.
16. Terson de Paleville DG, McKay WB, Folz RJ, et al. Respiratory motor control disrupted by spinal cord injury: mechanisms, evaluation, and restoration. Transl Stroke Res 2011;2(4):463–73.
17. Derenne JP, Macklem PT, Roussos C. The respiratory muscles: mechanics, control, and pathophysiology. Am Rev Respir Dis 1978;118(1):119–33.
18. Han JN, Gayan-Ramirez G, Dekhuijzen R, et al. Respiratory function of the rib cage muscles. Eur Respir J 1993;6(5):722–8.
19. Maarsingh EJ, van Eykern LA, Sprikkelman AB, et al. Respiratory muscle activity measured with a noninvasive EMG technique: technical aspects and reproducibility. J Appl Physiol (1985) 2000;88(6):1955–61.
20. De Troyer A, Estenne M, Vincken W. Rib cage motion and muscle use in high tetraplegics. Am Rev Respir Dis 1986;133(6):1115–9.
21. Estenne M, De Troyer A. Relationship between respiratory muscle electromyogram and rib cage motion in tetraplegia. Am Rev Respir Dis 1985;132(1):53–9.
22. Manning H, McCool FD, Scharf SM, et al. Oxygen cost of resistive-loaded breathing in quadriplegia. J Appl Physiol (1985) 1992;73(3):825–31.
23. Scanlon PD, Loring SH, Pichurko BM, et al. Respiratory mechanics in acute quadriplegia. Lung and chest wall compliance and dimensional changes during respiratory maneuvers. Am Rev Respir Dis 1989;139(3):615–20.
24. Kirshblum SC, Burns SP, Biering-Sorensen F, et al. International standards for neurological classification of spinal cord injury (revised 2011). J Spinal Cord Med 2011;34(6):535–46.
25. Berlowitz DJ, Wadsworth B, Ross J. Respiratory problems and management in people with spinal cord injury. Breathe (Sheff) 2016;12(4):328–40.
26. De Troyer A, Estenne M. The expiratory muscles in tetraplegia. Paraplegia 1991;29(6):359–63.
27. De Troyer A, Estenne M, Heilporn A. Mechanism of active expiration in tetraplegic subjects. N Engl J Med 1986;314(12):740–4.
28. Fujiwara T, Hara Y, Chino N. Expiratory function in complete tetraplegics: study of spirometry, maximal expiratory pressure, and muscle activity of pectoralis major and latissimus dorsi muscles. Am J Phys Med Rehabil 1999;78(5):464–9.
29. Bach JR. Noninvasive respiratory management of high level spinal cord injury. J Spinal Cord Med 2012;35(2):72–80.
30. Bach JR. Continuous noninvasive ventilation for patients with neuromuscular disease and spinal cord injury. Semin Respir Crit Care Med 2002;23(3):283–92.
31. Slack RS, Shucart W. Respiratory dysfunction associated with traumatic injury to the central nervous system. Clin Chest Med 1994;15(4):739–49.
32. Bach JR. Noninvasive respiratory management and diaphragm and electrophrenic pacing in neuromuscular disease and spinal cord injury. Muscle Nerve 2013;47(2):297–305.
33. Brown R, DiMarco AF, Hoit JD, et al. Respiratory dysfunction and management in spinal cord

injury. Respir Care 2006;51(8):853–68 [discussion: 869–70].

34. Homnick DN. Mechanical insufflation-exsufflation for airway mucus clearance. Respir Care 2007; 52(10):1296–305 [discussion: 1306–7].

35. Reid WD, Brown JA, Konnyu KJ, et al. Physiotherapy secretion removal techniques in people with spinal cord injury: a systematic review. J Spinal Cord Med 2010;33(4):353–70.

36. Ditunno JF, Little JW, Tessler A, et al. Spinal shock revisited: a four-phase model. Spinal Cord 2004; 42(7):383–95.

37. Ledsome JR, Sharp JM. Pulmonary function in acute cervical cord injury. Am Rev Respir Dis 1981;124(1):41–4.

38. Haas F, Axen K, Pineda H, et al. Temporal pulmonary function changes in cervical cord injury. Arch Phys Med Rehabil 1985;66(3):139–44.

39. Mueller G, de Groot S, van der Woude L, et al. Time-courses of lung function and respiratory muscle pressure generating capacity after spinal cord injury: a prospective cohort study. J Rehabil Med 2008;40(4):269–76.

40. Bluechardt MH, Wiens M, Thomas SG, et al. Repeated measurements of pulmonary function following spinal cord injury. Paraplegia 1992; 30(11):768–74.

41. Axen K, Pineda H, Shunfenthal I, et al. Diaphragmatic function following cervical cord injury: neurally mediated improvement. Arch Phys Med Rehabil 1985;66(4):219–22.

42. McKinley W, McNamee S, Meade M, et al. Incidence, etiology, and risk factors for fever following acute spinal cord injury. J Spinal Cord Med 2006; 29(5):501–6.

43. McMichan JC, Michel L, Westbrook PR. Pulmonary dysfunction following traumatic quadriplegia. Recognition, prevention, and treatment. JAMA 1980;243(6):528–31.

44. Oo T, Watt JW, Soni BM, et al. Delayed diaphragm recovery in 12 patients after high cervical spinal cord injury. A retrospective review of the diaphragm status of 107 patients ventilated after acute spinal cord injury. Spinal Cord 1999;37(2):117–22.

45. Frisbie JH, Binard J. Low prevalence of prostatic cancer among myelopathy patients. J Am Paraplegia Soc 1994;17(3):148–9.

46. Estenne M, De Troyer A. The effects of tetraplegia on chest wall statics. Am Rev Respir Dis 1986; 134(1):121–4.

47. Garshick E, Ashba J, Tun CG, et al. Assessment of stature in spinal cord injury. J Spinal Cord Med 1997;20(1):36–42.

48. Ashba J, Garshick E, Tun CG, et al. Spirometry–acceptability and reproducibility in spinal cord injured subjects. J Am Paraplegia Soc 1993; 16(4):197–203.

49. Kelley A, Garshick E, Gross ER, et al. Spirometry testing standards in spinal cord injury. Chest 2003;123(3):725–30.

50. Miller MR, Hankinson J, Brusasco V, et al. Standardisation of spirometry. Eur Respir J 2005;26(2): 319–38.

51. Tully K, Koke K, Garshick E, et al. Maximal expiratory pressures in spinal cord injury using two mouthpieces. Chest 1997;112(1):113–6.

52. Almenoff PL, Spungen AM, Lesser M, et al. Pulmonary function survey in spinal cord injury: influences of smoking and level and completeness of injury. Lung 1995;173(5):297–306.

53. Forner JV. Lung volumes and mechanics of breathing in tetraplegics. Paraplegia 1980;18(4):258–66.

54. Fugl-Meyer AR, Grimby G. Ventilatory function in tetraplegic patients. Scand J Rehabil Med 1971; 3(4):151–60.

55. Hemingway A, Bors E, Hobby RP. An investigation of the pulmonary function of paraplegics. J Clin Invest 1958;37(5):773–82.

56. Kokkola K, Moller K, Lehtonen T. Pulmonary function in tetraplegic and paraplegic patients. Ann Clin Res 1975;7(2):76–9.

57. Linn WS, Adkins RH, Gong H Jr, et al. Pulmonary function in chronic spinal cord injury: a cross-sectional survey of 222 southern California adult outpatients. Arch Phys Med Rehabil 2000;81(6): 757–63.

58. Linn WS, Spungen AM, Gong H Jr, et al. Forced vital capacity in two large outpatient populations with chronic spinal cord injury. Spinal Cord 2001;39(5): 263–8.

59. Ohry A, Molho M, Rozin R. Alterations of pulmonary function in spinal cord injured patients. Paraplegia 1975;13(2):101–8.

60. Roth EJ, Nussbaum SB, Berkowitz M, et al. Pulmonary function testing in spinal cord injury: correlation with vital capacity. Paraplegia 1995;33(8): 454–7.

61. Fugl-Meyer AR. Effects of respiratory muscle paralysis in tetraplegic and paraplegic patients. Scand J Rehabil Med 1971;3(4):141–50.

62. Jain NB, Brown R, Tun CG, et al. Determinants of forced expiratory volume in 1 second (FEV1), forced vital capacity (FVC), and FEV1/FVC in chronic spinal cord injury. Arch Phys Med Rehabil 2006;87(10):1327–33.

63. Linn WS, Spungen AM, Gong H Jr, et al. Smoking and obstructive lung dysfunction in persons with chronic spinal cord injury. J Spinal Cord Med 2003;26(1):28–35.

64. Stepp EL, Brown R, Tun CG, et al. Determinants of lung volumes in chronic spinal cord injury. Arch Phys Med Rehabil 2008;89(8):1499–506.

65. Schilero GJ, Hobson JC, Singh K, et al. Bronchodilator effects of ipratropium bromide and albuterol

sulfate among subjects with tetraplegia. J Spinal Cord Med 2018;41(1):42–7.

66. Radulovic M, Schilero GJ, Wecht JM, et al. Airflow obstruction and reversibility in spinal cord injury: evidence for functional sympathetic innervation. Arch Phys Med Rehabil 2008;89(12):2349–53.

67. Mateus SR, Beraldo PS, Horan TA. Cholinergic bronchomotor tone and airway caliber in tetraplegic patients. Spinal Cord 2006;44(5):269–74.

68. Schilero GJ, Grimm DR, Bauman WA, et al. Assessment of airway caliber and bronchodilator responsiveness in subjects with spinal cord injury. Chest 2005;127(1):149–55.

69. Schilero GJ, Grimm D, Spungen AM, et al. Bronchodilator responses to metaproterenol sulfate among subjects with spinal cord injury. J Rehabil Res Dev 2004;41(1):59–64.

70. Spungen AM, Dicpinigaitis PV, Almenoff PL, et al. Pulmonary obstruction in individuals with cervical spinal cord lesions unmasked by bronchodilator administration. Paraplegia 1993;31(6):404–7.

71. Laitinen A, Partanen M, Hervonen A, et al. Electron microscopic study on the innervation of the human lower respiratory tract: evidence of adrenergic nerves. Eur J Respir Dis 1985;67(3):209–15.

72. Partanen M, Laitinen A, Hervonen A, et al. Catecholamine- and acetylcholinesterase-containing nerves in human lower respiratory tract. Histochemistry 1982;76(2):175–88.

73. Vigil L, Calaf N, Codina E, et al. Video-assisted sympathectomy for essential hyperhidrosis: effects on cardiopulmonary function. Chest 2005;128(4):2702–5.

74. Tseng MY, Tseng JH. Thoracoscopic sympathectomy for palmar hyperhidrosis: effects on pulmonary function. J Clin Neurosci 2001;8(6):539–41.

75. Noppen M, Vincken W. Thoracoscopic sympathicolysis for essential hyperhidrosis: effects on pulmonary function. Eur Respir J 1996;9(8):1660–4.

76. Grimm DR, Arias E, Lesser M, et al. Airway hyperresponsiveness to ultrasonically nebulized distilled water in subjects with tetraplegia. J Appl Physiol (1985) 1999;86(4):1165–9.

77. Fein ED, Grimm DR, Lesser M, et al. The effects of ipratropium bromide on histamine-induced bronchoconstriction in subjects with cervical spinal cord injury. J Asthma 1998;35(1):49–55.

78. Singas E, Lesser M, Spungen AM, et al. Airway hyperresponsiveness to methacholine in subjects with spinal cord injury. Chest 1996;110(4):911–5.

79. Dicpinigaitis PV, Spungen AM, Bauman WA, et al. Bronchial hyperresponsiveness after cervical spinal cord injury. Chest 1994;105(4):1073–6.

80. Grimm DR, Chandy D, Almenoff PL, et al. Airway hyperreactivity in subjects with tetraplegia is associated with reduced baseline airway caliber. Chest 2000;118(5):1397–404.

81. Cockcroft DW, Davis BE. The bronchoprotective effect of inhaling methacholine by using total lung capacity inspirations has a marked influence on the interpretation of the test result. J Allergy Clin Immunol 2006;117(6):1244–8.

82. DeLuca RV, Grimm DR, Lesser M, et al. Effects of a beta2-agonist on airway hyperreactivity in subjects with cervical spinal cord injury. Chest 1999;115(6):1533–8.

83. Singas E, Grimm DR, Almenoff PL, et al. Inhibition of airway hyperreactivity by oxybutynin chloride in subjects with cervical spinal cord injury. Spinal Cord 1999;37(4):279–83.

84. Grimm DR, DeLuca RV, Lesser M, et al. Effects of GABA-B agonist baclofen on bronchial hyperreactivity to inhaled histamine in subjects with cervical spinal cord injury. Lung 1997;175(5):333–41.

85. Cragg JJ, Warner FM, Kramer JK, et al. A Canada-wide survey of chronic respiratory disease and spinal cord injury. Neurology 2015;84(13):1341–5.

86. Ali J, Qi W. Pulmonary function and posture in traumatic quadriplegia. J Trauma 1995;39(2):334–7.

87. Baydur A, Adkins RH, Milic-Emili J. Lung mechanics in individuals with spinal cord injury: effects of injury level and posture. J Appl Physiol (1985) 2001;90(2):405–11.

88. Chen CF, Lien IN, Wu MC. Respiratory function in patients with spinal cord injuries: effects of posture. Paraplegia 1990;28(2):81–6.

89. Estenne M, De Troyer A. Mechanism of the postural dependence of vital capacity in tetraplegic subjects. Am Rev Respir Dis 1987;135(2):367–71.

90. Goldman JM, Rose LS, Williams SJ, et al. Effect of abdominal binders on breathing in tetraplegic patients. Thorax 1986;41(12):940–5.

91. Hart N, Laffont I, de la Sota AP, et al. Respiratory effects of combined truncal and abdominal support in patients with spinal cord injury. Arch Phys Med Rehabil 2005;86(7):1447–51.

92. Maloney FP. Pulmonary function in quadriplegia: effects of a corset. Arch Phys Med Rehabil 1979;60(6):261–5.

93. McCool FD, Pichurko BM, Slutsky AS, et al. Changes in lung volume and rib cage configuration with abdominal binding in quadriplegia. J Appl Physiol (1985) 1986;60(4):1198–202.

94. Fugl-Meyer AR, Grimby G. Rib-cage and abdominal volume ventilation partitioning in tetraplegic patients. Scand J Rehabil Med 1971;3(4):161–7.

95. Gounden P. Static respiratory pressures in patients with post-traumatic tetraplegia. Spinal Cord 1997;35(1):43–7.

96. Danon J, Druz WS, Goldberg NB, et al. Function of the isolated paced diaphragm and the cervical accessory muscles in C1 quadriplegics. Am Rev Respir Dis 1979;119(6):909–19.

97. Mead J, Banzett RB, Lehr J, et al. Effect of posture on upper and lower rib cage motion and tidal volume during diaphragm pacing. Am Rev Respir Dis 1984;130(2):320–1.

98. Moulton A, Silver JR. Chest movements in patients with traumatic injuries of the cervical cord. Clin Sci 1970;39(3):407–22.

99. Urmey W, Loring S, Mead J, et al. Upper and lower rib cage deformation during breathing in quadriplegics. J Appl Physiol (1985) 1986;60(2):618–22.

100. De Troyer A, Heilporn A. Respiratory mechanics in quadriplegia. The respiratory function of the intercostal muscles. Am Rev Respir Dis 1980;122(4):591–600.

101. Goldman MD, Mead J. Mechanical interaction between the diaphragm and rib cage. J Appl Physiol 1973;35(2):197–204.

102. Stone DJ, Keltz H. The effect of respiratory muscle dysfunction on pulmonary function. Studies in patients with spinal cord injuries. Am Rev Respir Dis 1963;88:621–9.

103. Bergofsky EH. Quantiation of the function of respiratory muscles in normal individuals and quadriplegic patients. Arch Phys Med Rehabil 1964;45:575–80.

104. Bergofsky EH. Mechanism for respiratory insufficiency after cervical cord injury; a source of alveolar hypoventilation. Ann Intern Med 1964;61:435–47.

105. Silver JR. The oxygen cost of breathing in tetraplegic patients. Paraplegia 1963;1:204–14.

106. Spungen AM, Grimm DR, Lesser M, et al. Self-reported prevalence of pulmonary symptoms in subjects with spinal cord injury. Spinal Cord 1997;35(10):652–7.

107. Spungen AM, Grimm DR, Schilero G, et al. Relationship of respiratory symptoms with smoking status and pulmonary function in chronic spinal cord injury. J Spinal Cord Med 2002;25(1):23–7.

108. Ayas NT, DiMarco AF, Hoit JD, et al. Breathlessness in spinal cord injury depends on injury level. J Spinal Cord Med 1999;22(2):97–101.

109. Grandas NF, Jain NB, Denckla JB, et al. Dyspnea during daily activities in chronic spinal cord injury. Arch Phys Med Rehabil 2005;86(8):1631–5.

110. Wien MF, Garshick E, Tun CG, et al. Breathlessness and exercise in spinal cord injury. J Spinal Cord Med 1999;22(4):297–302.

111. Berlowitz DJ, Tamplin J. Respiratory muscle training for cervical spinal cord injury. Cochrane Database Syst Rev 2013;(7):CD008507.

112. Sheel AW, Reid WD, Townson AF, et al. Effects of exercise training and inspiratory muscle training in spinal cord injury: a systematic review. J Spinal Cord Med 2008;31(5):500–8.

113. Van Houtte S, Vanlandewijck Y, Gosselink R. Respiratory muscle training in persons with spinal cord injury: a systematic review. Respir Med 2006;100(11):1886–95.

114. Estenne M, Knoop C, Vanvaerenbergh J, et al. The effect of pectoralis muscle training in tetraplegic subjects. Am Rev Respir Dis 1989;139(5):1218–22.

115. Van Houtte S, Vanlandewijck Y, Kiekens C, et al. Patients with acute spinal cord injury benefit from normocapnic hyperpnoea training. J Rehabil Med 2008;40(2):119–25.

116. Wadsworth BM, Haines TP, Cornwell PL, et al. Abdominal binder use in people with spinal cord injuries: a systematic review and meta-analysis. Spinal Cord 2009;47(4):274–85.

117. DiMarco AF, Onders RP, Ignagni A, et al. Inspiratory muscle pacing in spinal cord injury: case report and clinical commentary. J Spinal Cord Med 2006;29(2):95–108.

118. Le Pimpec-Barthes F, Legras A, Arame A, et al. Diaphragm pacing: the state of the art. J Thorac Dis 2016;8(Suppl 4):S376–86.

119. DiMarco AF, Kowalski KE, Geertman RT, et al. Lower thoracic spinal cord stimulation to restore cough in patients with spinal cord injury: results of a National Institutes of Health-sponsored clinical trial. Part I: methodology and effectiveness of expiratory muscle activation. Arch Phys Med Rehabil 2009;90(5):717–25.

120. Martineau L, Horan MA, Rothwell NJ, et al. Salbutamol, a beta 2-adrenoceptor agonist, increases skeletal muscle strength in young men. Clin Sci (Lond) 1992;83(5):615–21.

121. Kissel JT, McDermott MP, Natarajan R, et al. Pilot trial of albuterol in facioscapulohumeral muscular dystrophy. FSH-DY Group. Neurology 1998;50(5):1402–6.

122. Murphy RJ, Hartkopp A, Gardiner PF, et al. Salbutamol effect in spinal cord injured individuals undergoing functional electrical stimulation training. Arch Phys Med Rehabil 1999;80(10):1264–7.

123. Signorile JF, Banovac K, Gomez M, et al. Increased muscle strength in paralyzed patients after spinal cord injury: effect of beta-2 adrenergic agonist. Arch Phys Med Rehabil 1995;76(1):55–8.

124. Bennett JA, Harrison TW, Tattersfield AE. The contribution of the swallowed fraction of an inhaled dose of salmeterol to it systemic effects. Eur Respir J 1999;13(2):445–8.

125. Grimm DR, Schilero GJ, Spungen AM, et al. Salmeterol improves pulmonary function in persons with tetraplegia. Lung 2006;184(6):335–9.

126. Berlowitz DJ, Brown DJ, Campbell DA, et al. A longitudinal evaluation of sleep and breathing in the first year after cervical spinal cord injury. Arch Phys Med Rehabil 2005;86(6):1193–9.

127. Berlowitz DJ, Spong J, Gordon I, et al. Relationships between objective sleep indices and symptoms in a community sample of people with

tetraplegia. Arch Phys Med Rehabil 2012;93(7): 1246–52.

128. Burns SP, Little JW, Hussey JD, et al. Sleep apnea syndrome in chronic spinal cord injury: associated factors and treatment. Arch Phys Med Rehabil 2000;81(10):1334–9.

129. Leduc BE, Dagher JH, Mayer P, et al. Estimated prevalence of obstructive sleep apnea-hypopnea syndrome after cervical cord injury. Arch Phys Med Rehabil 2007;88(3):333–7.

130. McEvoy RD, Mykytyn I, Sajkov D, et al. Sleep apnoea in patients with quadriplegia. Thorax 1995;50(6):613–9.

131. Sankari A, Bascom A, Sowmini O, et al. Sleep disordered breathing in chronic spinal cord injury. J Clin Sleep Med 2014;10(1):65–72.

132. Short DJ, Stradling JR, Williams SJ. Prevalence of sleep apnoea in patients over 40 years of age with spinal cord lesions. J Neurol Neurosurg Psychiatry 1992;55(11):1032–6.

133. Stockhammer E, Tobon A, Michel F, et al. Characteristics of sleep apnea syndrome in tetraplegic patients. Spinal Cord 2002;40(6):286–94.

134. Biering-Sorensen F, Biering-Sorensen M. Sleep disturbances in the spinal cord injured: an epidemiological questionnaire investigation, including a normal population. Spinal Cord 2001;39(10):505–13.

135. Hoffstein V, Zamel N, Phillipson EA. Lung volume dependence of pharyngeal cross-sectional area in patients with obstructive sleep apnea. Am Rev Respir Dis 1984;130(2):175–8.

136. Wasicko MJ, Hutt DA, Parisi RA, et al. The role of vascular tone in the control of upper airway collapsibility. Am Rev Respir Dis 1990;141(6):1569–77.

137. Spungen AM, Adkins RH, Stewart CA, et al. Factors influencing body composition in persons with spinal cord injury: a cross-sectional study. J Appl Physiol (1985) 2003;95(6):2398–407.

138. Burns SP, Kapur V, Yin KS, et al. Factors associated with sleep apnea in men with spinal cord injury: a population-based case-control study. Spinal Cord 2001;39(1):15–22.

139. Berlowitz DJ, Spong J, Pierce RJ, et al. The feasibility of using auto-titrating continuous positive airway pressure to treat obstructive sleep apnoea after acute tetraplegia. Spinal Cord 2009;47(12): 868–73.

Obesity Hypoventilation Syndrome

Imran H. Iftikhar, MD[a],*, Joshua Roland, MD[b,c]

KEYWORDS

- Obesity hypoventilation syndrome • Obstructive sleep apnea • CPAP • Bilevel PAP

KEY POINTS

- Obesity hypoventilation syndrome is a disorder characterized by alveolar hypoventilation during sleep and wakefulness.
- The disorder involves a complex interaction between impaired respiratory mechanics, ventilatory drive, and sleep-disordered breathing.
- Available treatment options include noninvasive positive airway pressure therapies and weight loss.

INTRODUCTION

Obesity hypoventilation syndrome (OHS) has also been referred to as Pickwickian syndrome, because those with OHS have been classically described to have similarities with the boy "*Joe*," *Mr Wardle's* servant in Charles Dickens' *The Posthumous Papers of the Pickwick Club*.[1] He is the "fat boy" who is described by Dickens as "*a fat and red-faced boy in a state of somnolency,*" and as "*Young Dropsy.*" Although the association of obesity and hypersomnolence was known for a long time, the term, "Pickwickian syndrome," as such, was popularized by Burwell and colleagues[2] in a case report in which they noted similarities between the boy "Joe" and their patient.

DEFINITION

OHS is defined as daytime hypercapnia ($Paco_2$ >45 mm Hg) in an obese patient (body mass index [BMI] $\geq$30 kg/m^2) with sleep-disordered breathing after all known causes of hypoventilation have been excluded, such as severe obstructive pulmonary disorders (chronic obstructive pulmonary disease [COPD]) or restrictive chest wall deformities, severe hypothyroidism, neuromuscular disease, or central hypoventilation syndromes.[3] The term "sleep-disordered breathing" in the definition could mean obstructive sleep apnea (OSA) or sleep-hypoventilation (a >10 mm Hg increase in $Paco_2$ during sleep compared with awake $Paco_2$ or $Paco_2$ >55 mm Hg during sleep for 10 minutes).

In addition to the above diagnostic criteria, the use of calculated serum bicarbonate levels greater than 27 mEq/L from arterial blood gas and/or calculated base excess of greater than 2 mmol/L have also been debated.[4] Proponents think that these metrics are longer-term measures of exposure to elevated levels of $Paco_2$, and unlike $Paco_2$ and Pao_2, are unlikely to change with a few breaths of hypoventilation or hyperventilation.[4] Based on a retrospective analysis of 525 patients, cutoff values of calculated bicarbonate from capillary blood gas analysis had a sensitivity of 85.7% and specificity

Disclosure Statement: None to disclose.
[a] Division of Pulmonary, Allergy, Critical Care and Sleep Medicine, Department of Medicine, The Emory Sleep Center, Emory University School of Medicine, 613 Michael Street, Northeast, Atlanta, GA 30329, USA; [b] Emory Sleep Medicine Fellowship, Emory Sleep Center, 12 Executive Park Drive NE, Atlanta, GA 30329, USA; [c] Division of Pulmonary, Allergy, Critical Care and Sleep Medicine, Emory University School of Medicine, 613 Michael Street, Northeast, Atlanta, GA 30329, USA
* Corresponding author. Division of Pulmonary, Allergy, Critical Care and Sleep Medicine, Emory University School of Medicine, 615 Michael Street, Northeast, Atlanta, GA.
E-mail address: imran.hasan.iftikhar@emory.edu

Clin Chest Med 39 (2018) 427–436
https://doi.org/10.1016/j.ccm.2018.01.006
0272-5231/18/© 2018 Elsevier Inc. All rights reserved.

chestmed.theclinics.com

of 89.5%.[5] The counterargument is that using a high bicarbonate level indicating metabolic alkalosis would not differentiate a primary from a compensatory process.[6] Because most obese patients are frequently found to be on diuretics or corticosteroids, they are prone to developing primary metabolic alkalosis with a mild compensatory hypercapnia. Differentiating that from a distinct OHS related abnormality is difficult. Although the debate continues, everyone agrees that an elevated serum bicarbonate level should alert the astute clinician to consider OHS as a diagnosis or patients at risk of developing OHS.

EPIDEMIOLOGY

The true prevalence of OHS in the general population is unknown. Littleton and Mokhlesi[3] in 2009 estimated the prevalence of OHS in the adult US population to be 0.15% to 0.3%, an estimate based on population facts known then (prevalence of severe obesity [BMI >40 kg/m^2] in United States being 3.0%, with half of them having OSA, and 10%–20% of those having OHS). However, based on a 2010 estimate,[7] the prevalence of severe obesity then was 6.55% (6.40–6.70), meaning thereby that the prevalence of OHS in the adult US population was perhaps 0.3% to 0.6% in 2010.

PATHOPHYSIOLOGY

OHS represents a more severe form of disease on a spectrum that includes conditions such as mild to moderate obesity to eucapnic morbid obesity and the hypercapnic obese state in OHS. Manuel and colleagues[8] in a prospective observational cohort study of obese patients examined ventilatory responses and polysomnographic parameters in obese patients with normal base excess, obese patients with elevated base excess but normal Paco$_2$, and patients with OHS. The group with elevated base excess demonstrated similar percentages of nocturnal hypoxemia as well as response to daytime hypoxic and hypercapnic challenge as seen in patients with OHS. The study offers compelling evidence that the obese group with elevated base excess represents a "form fruste" or a pre-OHS syndrome. The authors explain 3 possible physiologic derangements that occur in OHS patients in later discussion.

Altered Respiratory Physiology

Several respiratory physiologic derangements that occur in OHS are a function of the obesity itself (Fig. 1). Some of these are explained in later discussion.

Lung volumes and respiratory compliance

Obese individuals have decreased functional residual capacity and expiratory reserve volume. Compared with subjects who are of normal weight, respiratory system compliance has been shown to be about 20% less in eucapnic obese individuals and almost 60% less in patients with OHS.[9] Low lung volumes and the upper airway adiposity lead to reduced tracheal tug and make the upper airway prone to collapsibility.[10] Respiratory compliance is also reduced primarily because of the shift of the operating point for tidal breathing to a less compliant portion of the pressure-volume curve.[11] Although it seems obvious that low lung volumes and reduced respiratory compliance would also be causative factors not just in OHS but also in obese OSA–only patients, patients with OHS are more likely to have thicker necks, central as opposed to peripheral adiposity with similar BMIs, and more restrictive lung physiology than obese OSA–only patients.[12]

Increased work of breathing

Obesity may lead to expiratory flow limitation and consequently development of intrinsic positive end expiratory pressure, primarily during sleep in the supine position, which coupled with the gravitational forces of the chest wall during supine sleep increase the work of breathing for accessory muscles.[11] In addition, work of breathing worsens in the supine position with central adiposity causing cephalad projection of the diaphragm. The diaphragm is stressed in rapid eye movement sleep when the accessory muscles become atonic.

Metabolic Derangements

The combination of episodic apnea and hypopnea with prolonged hypoventilation and ineffective interevent hyperventilation leads to persistent CO$_2$ elevation, which then stimulates renal absorption of bicarbonate each night.[13] The ability to accomplish unloading of both elevated Paco$_2$ and bicarbonate load during wakefulness is determined not only by the magnitude of the load but also by the ventilatory response to CO$_2$ and by renal handling of bicarbonate,[14] which, is made worse by the increased CO$_2$ production by tissues. Sustained elevations in serum bicarbonate levels lead to increased CO$_2$ buffering capacity, attenuating the decrease in cerebrospinal fluid pH and consequently blunting the hypercapnia ventilatory response leading to diurnal hypercapnia.[14] In summary, persistence of elevated bicarbonate level not only reflects the state of chronic hypercapnia but also serves to perpetuate it.

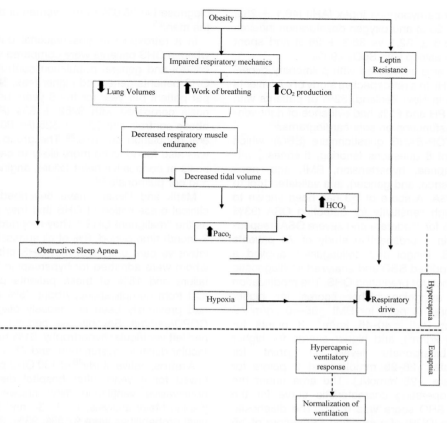

Fig. 1. Pathophysiology of OHS. Outline of interactions between factors that contribute to development of hypercapnia versus eucapnia.

Hormonal Influences

Both leptin (a protein secreted mainly by white adipose tissue) and insulin-like growth factor-1 (IGF-1) have been proposed as potential contributors to altered ventilatory control in OHS. Leptin increases in direct proportion to the degree of obesity. In the hypothalamus, its function is to inhibit appetite. It has also been shown to be a respiratory stimulant. In leptin-deficient mice with morbid obesity and hypoventilation, intraperitoneal administration of leptin over 6 weeks was shown to attenuate rapid breathing pattern, diminished lung compliance, and abnormal respiratory muscle adaptations that were seen at baseline.[15] Obesity as such is known to be associated with increased circulating levels of leptin much higher in OHS patients than in weight-matched controls, suggesting that despite sustained obesity, these individuals are likely leptin resistant.[16]

Monneret and colleagues[17] for the first time showed a significant reduction of IGF-I in OHS patients compared with the obese control group.

Serum IGF-I levels were inversely associated with $Paco_2$, and reductions in IGF-I were directly correlated with reductions in forced vital capacity and inspiratory capacity. At least in the animal model,[18] it has been shown that chronic low IGF-I levels are associated with reduced turnover of proteins in muscular fibers essential for correcting diaphragmatic strength.

CLINICAL FEATURES AND DIAGNOSIS

Symptoms of OHS overlap those of OSA; that is, patients can present with complaints of daytime hypersomnolence, witnessed apneas, loud snoring, and morning headaches. Signs of OHS most commonly seen are lower extremity edema and low resting daytime oxygen saturations. Low daytime saturation is not a typical feature of OSA; therefore, its presence should alert a clinician to consider this diagnosis in the setting of obesity and other features of OHS.

In a retrospective study by Pihtili and colleagues,[19] the incidence of OHS among OSA patients was found to be 45.1%. OHS patients had higher apnea-hypopnea index (AHI) (46.1 ± 28.2 vs 33.6 ± 25.5) and oxygen desaturation indexes (ODIs) (58.5 ± 32.1 vs 36.3 ± 26.5) and spent more time asleep with SpO_2 <90%.

OHS is also associated with pulmonary hypertension (PH). In a retrospective study of 47 patients with OHS in New Zealand, 52% of patients with OHS had PH and 63% had evidence of right ventricular dysfunction on echocardiograms.[20]

The STOP-BANG questionnaire (SBQ), which consists of 8 questions (snoring, tiredness, witnessed apnea, hypertension, BMI, age, neck circumference, and gender), is a validated tool to screen OSA. A score of ≥3 has been shown to have a high sensitivity for detecting OSA (93% and 100% for moderate and severe OSA, respectively).[21] In a prospective study of 74 patients with OHS, Bingol and colleagues[22] applied a slightly modified SBQ and analyzed its diagnostic performance for predicting OHS. The modification involved assigning higher scores for higher BMIs scores (1 point for BMI ≥35–40 kg/m², 2 points for BMI ≥40–45 kg/m², 3 points for BMI ≥45 kg/m²), and higher scores for higher serum bicarbonate levels (1 point for bicarbonate ≥26–28 mmol/L and 2 points for bicarbonate ≥28 mmol/L). The area under the receiver operating characteristic curve for the modified SBQ score was 0.755. The diagnostic odds ratio (DOR) of a modified SBQ score of ≥6 for predicting OHS was 7.5 as compared with the DOR of 3.7 for the original SBQ score of ≥6.

Cabrera Lacalzada and Dıaz-Lobato[23] have proposed grading OHS severity according to the degree of impairment of hypercapnia, hypoxemia, AHI, or BMI. Mild OHS is defined as $Paco_2$ between 46 and 60 mm Hg, Pao_2 greater than 70 mm Hg, AHI less than 5/h, and BMI 30 to 40 kg/m². Moderate is defined as $Paco_2$ between 60 and 80 mm Hg, Pao_2 60 to 70 mm Hg, AHI 5 to 15/h, and BMI 40 to 50 kg/m², and severe OHS as $Paco_2$ greater than 80 mm Hg, Pao_2 less than 60 mm Hg, AHI greater than 15/h, and BMI greater than 50 kg/m².

MORBIDITY AND MORTALITY

Because systemic inflammation, endothelial dysfunction, and insulin resistance are more pronounced in people with OHS compared with eucapnic obesity,[24] several different cardiovascular and metabolic abnormalities occur in OHS patients.

In a prospective observational study of OHS patients, approximately 71.4% of women and 61.9% of men with OHS also had PH. Severe PH (systolic pulmonary arterial pressure >70 mm Hg) was diagnosed in 28.6% of the women and 14.3% of the men.[25]

In a retrospective observational cohort study wherein OHS patients were compared with obese control and general population control subjects, OHS patients generated higher fees, $623 ± $96 per patient per year for the 5 years before diagnosis compared with $252 ± $34 (P<.001) for obese controls and $236 ± $25 (P<.001) for general population controls.[26] The group with OHS was also found to be more likely to carry a diagnosis of congestive heart failure, angina pectoris, and cor pulmonale.[26]

Marik and Desai[27] have described a unique clinical presentation of OHS that they referred to as the "malignant OHS." They reported that in an 8-month time period, 8% of all admissions to the intensive care unit (ICU) met OHS criteria, all of whom were admitted for hypercapnic respiratory failure and 18% of these patients died in the ICU from complications. About 75% of patients had previously been erroneously diagnosed for COPD/asthma. Seventy-one percent of patients had left ventricular hypertrophy, 61% had left ventricular diastolic dysfunction, and 77% had PH.

A retrospective study[28] of 130 OHS patients followed for 4 years after hospital discharge on noninvasive ventilation (NIV) showed that on Kaplan-Meier analysis, 1-, 2-, 3-, and 5-year survival probabilities were 97.5%, 93%, 88.3%, and 77.3%, respectively. A prospective study of 47 mostly untreated severely obese patients with OHS showed a much higher 18-month mortality than that for the control cohort of 103 patients with obesity alone (23% vs 9%).[29] More recently in a cross-sectional study of 302 patients, Masa and colleagues[30] examined the association between OSA severity based on tertiles of ODI and cardiovascular morbidity (defined as the presence of any of following: ischemic cardiomyopathy, chronic heart failure, stroke, PH, cardiac arrhythmia, and leg arteriopathy). The prevalence of cardiovascular morbidity decreased significantly with increasing severity of OSA based on ODI. With the exception of ischemic heart disease, the most severe ODI tertile had the lowest prevalence of PH, stroke, arrhythmia, chronic heart failure, and leg arteriopathy. Notably, chronic heart failure had the strongest inverse relationship with ODI (23.5% vs 8.1%, in the lowest and highest ODI tertiles, respectively). Although it is difficult to explain why the added burden of severe intermittent hypoxia in OHS would be associated with reduced cardiovascular morbidity, the investigators postulated that this might be due to the protective effect of "ischemic preconditioning," an adaptive mechanism in which brief repeated sublethal ischemic and reperfusion episodes confer protection from the occurrences of an acute lethal ischemia/reperfusion episode, such as in acute myocardial infarction.[31]

TREATMENT
Noninvasive Ventilation

Much debate has centered over which form of positive airway pressure (PAP) (ie, continuous PAP [CPAP] or NIV) should be the first-line or primary treatment of OHS. This is because although CPAP can effectively treat OSA, at least in theory, NIV should be more effective than CPAP (in OHS) because of its counteracting effects on the physiologic disturbances seen in OHS, such as altered ventilatory drive, increased work of breathing from chest restriction (by adiposity), and hypoventilation.[32] However, data as presented in **Table 1**, regarding the superiority of bilevel PAP, as such, over CPAP are conflicting.

In the first 2 studies[33,34] presented in **Table 1**, the type of NIV studied was pressure-preset NIV, in which inspiratory volume (V_{insp}) varies, whereas inspiratory PAP (IPAP) remains fixed. In the volume-preset NIV, conversely, V_{insp} is fixed in the ventilator, whereas the IPAP varies depending on airway resistance. In the hybrid mode, target volume based on ideal body weight is preset, and instead of a fixed IPAP, a pressure range with minimal and maximal IPAP values is set in the ventilator. With automatic calculations and adjustments made by the ventilator, IPAP smoothly transitions within a preset range to reach the set target volume. The most extensively studied hybrid mode is the average-volume assured pressure support (AVAPS). Murphy and colleagues[35] randomly allocated 50 NIV-naive patients with severe OHS (BMI: 50 ± 7 kg/m^2) either to pure pressure-preset NIV using pressure support ventilation or to AVAPS mode. Ventilator settings were individually adjusted according to a predefined protocol that included a nocturnal assessment period aimed at achieving optimal control of nocturnal ventilation. After 3 months of treatment, daytime Paco$_2$ (primary outcome) as well as health-related quality-of-life index (HRQL), lung functions, and daytime somnolence improved comparably in both groups. Both treatment strategies resulted in equivalent degrees of weight loss. Previous clinical trials[36,37] of OHS patients showing greater reductions in nocturnal transcutaneous CO$_2$ levels with this hybrid mode had a much smaller sample size and shorter follow-up period. In a more recent multicenter randomized controlled trial (RCT), Masa and colleagues[38] studied the differences in Paco$_2$, bicarbonate

levels, 6-minute walk distance, subjective daytime sleepiness, and other HRQLs in 80 patients randomized to CPAP and 71 to NIV. Although the 6-minute walk distance, forced expiratory volume in 1 second, and some aspects of HRQLs improved more in the NIV than CPAP groups, no intertreatment differences were noticed in clinical symptoms, bicarbonate levels, or Paco$_2$ after 2 months of interventions. The much-awaited Pickwick study[39] by the Spanish Sleep Network, the largest trial with the longest (36 months) follow-up, will shed further light on survival outcomes as well as comparative efficacy of NIV and CPAP.

Common Management Errors

Some common pitfalls in ambulatory management of OHS that can lead to slow and indolent worsening of daytime hypercapnia were recently described by Manthous and Mokhlesi.[40] These common errors include the following pitfalls.

Excessive oxygen administration

Hypoxemia from coexisting dependent basilar atelectasis, hypoventilation, or other coexisting pulmonary disease is not uncommon in these patients nor is the tendency to correct that with supplemental oxygen. However, administration of supplemental oxygen leads to reversal of hypoxic vasoconstriction and redistribution of blood flow to the poorly ventilated alveoli, which leads to an increase in dead space fraction, ultimately leading to hypercapnia.[41] Patients with OHS are highly sensitive to added oxygen. As much as 50%– to 100% of inspired oxygen has been shown to lead to a 3-mm Hg to as high as 10-mm Hg increase in Pco$_2$ and 3% increase in dead space fraction after 20 minutes.[41,42] Therefore, it is recommended that oxygen should be titrated to keep oxygen saturations between 89% and 92%.

Excessive administration of loop diuretics

First, treating peripheral edema with diuretics can worsen the underlying prerenal azotemia and the daytime hypercapnia. It has been postulated that acute exacerbation states of OHS that lead to worsening of hypoxemia possibly lead to a catecholamine surge, ultimately leading to increased renal vascular resistance.[43,44] Coupled with the depressed cardiac function, prerenal azotemia is only bound to worsen with early administration of diuretics, especially in acute on chronic exacerbation states of OHS. Second, contraction alkalosis associated with diuretics will only increase the existing elevated bicarbonate levels in some OHS patients, which would

Table 1
Randomized controlled trials on use of positive airway pressure devices for obesity hypoventilation syndrome

Study	Number of Participants	Follow-up Period	Comments
Pressure-preset NIV vs CPAP			
Piper et al,[34] 2008	36	12 wk	No difference in reductions in daytime $Paco_2$ and serum bicarbonate levels and in improvements in subjective daytime sleepiness. Bilevel-S group resulted in improved sleep quality and psychomotor vigilance testing
Howard et al,[33] 2017	60	12 wk	No difference in treatment failure or improvements in $Paco_2$, Pao_2, and serum bicarbonate levels. Nonsignificant between-group difference in improvement in subjective daytime sleepiness and HRQL
Volume-preset NIV hybrid mode vs CPAP			
Masa et al,[38] 2015	221	8 wk	Improved 6MWD, lung functions, HRQL with volume-preset hybrid mode NIV. No significant difference in improvements in $Paco_2$ and serum bicarbonate levels, PSG outcomes, and clinical symptoms
Volume-preset NIV hybrid mode vs pressure-preset NIV			
Storre et al,[36] 2006	10	6 wk	Comparable improvements in oxygenation, sleep quality. AVAPS led to more efficient decrease in $Paco_2$
Janssens et al,[37] 2009	12	1 night	Improved nocturnal hypoventilation but increased night time awakenings with AVAPS
Murphy et al,[35] 2012	50	12 wk	Comparable improvements in $Paco_2$, HRQL, PFTs, daytime somnolence in both groups
Bilevel-ST vs lifestyle counseling			
Borel et al,[59] 2012	35	4 wk	Improved daytime $Paco_2$ and nocturnal oxygen saturation with Bilevel-ST but no change in inflammatory, metabolic, or cardiovascular markers
Bilevel-S vs ST (low BUR) vs ST (high BUR)			
Contal et al,[60] 2013	10	1 night	Sleep quality and arousals more with high BUR. S mode was associated with more central respiratory events
Volume-preset NIV hybrid mode-automated EPAP vs fixed EPAP			
McArdle et al,[61] 2017	25 (participants included had either OHS, or COPD, or neuromuscular disease)	2 nights	No significant between-mode differences in PSG-measured sleep breathing and sleep quality outcomes, self-reported sleep quality, device comfort, and patient preference

Abbreviations: 6MWD, 6-minute walk distance; BUR, back-up rate; PFTs, pulmonary function tests; PSG, polysomnogram; S, spontaneous mode; ST, spontaneous timed mode.

lead to compensatory hypercapnia. The worsening hypoventilation and hypoxemia will potentiate greater right heart failure and pedal edema, which in turn could lead to more erroneous administration of diuretics. If treatment with a diuretic is clinically necessary, intermittent use of acetazolamide can be considered, which has been tested safely in patients with OHS.[45]

Perioperative Management

In the hospitalized setting, during NIV treatment, it is important to monitor and observe the level of consciousness, vital signs, respiratory pattern, oxygen saturation, and arterial blood gases. They require higher than usual expiratory PAP (EPAP) to prevent collapse of upper airway, and usually higher IPAP because of the high thoracic impedance. As such, EPAP should be steadily increased until witnessed apneas, snoring, and dips in oxygen saturation have disappeared, and IPAP should be increased until a steady state of oxygen saturation has been achieved. Special considerations need to be given for those requiring intubation for surgeries. During induction of anesthesia, patients with OHS should be placed in the ramp position (torso tilted with head end elevated by 25°), which improves the glottic view during intubation and reduces atelectasis. In addition, preoxygenation for more than 3 minutes can increase apnea tolerance time. One needs to be prepared and avail all specialized anesthesiology instruments and assistance, including in extreme cases use of "awake fiber-optic intubation" with concomitant use of PAP therapy.[46,47] Postoperatively, a semi-upright or lateral position is recommended for airway maintenance and better oxygenation.[48] Rapid emergence from anesthesia is recommended, and tracheal extubation should only be performed after the patient becomes fully conscious.[49] Some have even suggested that in order to accelerate emergence, use of "volatile anesthetic" should be kept to minimum and washout time from fat or muscle can be shortened by using other short-acting anesthetic adjuvants, such as remifentanil.[50] In addition, in order to avoid "opioid-induced ventilatory impairment" in patients with OHS, an opioid-sparing analgesic regimen consisting of local anesthetic–infused nerve block catheters or nonopioid adjuncts (nonsteroidal anti-inflammatory drugs) can also be considered.

Switch from Noninvasive Ventilation to Continuous Positive Airway Pressure in Ambulatory Settings

About 26% to 50% of patients suffering from OHS are diagnosed in the acute setting and often discharged on NIV on which they usually stay indefinitely until either PAP failure or nonadherence.[28,51] Whether patients can tolerate switch from NIV to CPAP has not been extensively studied. In this context, the prospective study by Orfanos and colleagues[52] conducted in France included 22 stable patients with OHS, with moderate to severe concomitant OSA and without obstructive pulmonary disease, who had been on NIV for more than 2 months. After 7 nights of washout from NIV, most patients were switched to CPAP at 2 cm above their previous EPAP on NIV. One month after the switch to CPAP, no significant differences were observed in $Paco_2$, bicarbonate levels, ODI, AHI, and adherence (NIV: 6.73 ± 2.66 hours vs CPAP: 6.8 ± 2.2 hours). Considering that NIV costs more than CPAP, the investigators calculated average savings of € 2348 per year per patient.

Bariatric Surgery

Significant weight loss can lead to improvements in lung volumes and daytime CO_2. Bariatric surgery is the most effective approach in achieving more substantial degrees of weight loss. However, a meta-analysis of studies on bariatric surgery showed that even though the BMI reduced by ~ 18 kg/m^2, and AHI reduced by 38 events per hour, the post–bariatric surgery values were still in the moderate OSA severity range (~ 16/h).[53] In a meta-analysis of RCTs comparing the effectiveness of bariatric surgery versus nonsurgical treatment of obesity, 11 RCTs with 796 participants and mean BMI of 30 to 52 kg/m^2 showed that those allocated to bariatric surgery lost more weight (mean difference: -26 kg; 95% confidence intervals [CIs]: -31 to -21 kg). These patients were also found to have greater improvement in health-related quality of life when compared with individuals who received nonsurgical weight loss therapy.[54]

De Cesare and colleagues[55] followed 102 morbidly obese patients (including 16 OHS and 22 OSA patients) after "malabsorptive surgery" (derivative biliodigestive surgery). Between 12 and 24 months postsurgery when maximum weight loss occurred, none of the 16 OHS patients fulfilled criteria for OHS as such. As such, there is relative paucity of RCTs on the effectiveness of bariatric surgery and postsurgical outcomes in OHS patients as such.

Other Management Options

Tracheostomy should only be considered when other options for treatment have failed. Although tracheostomy used to be one of the few treatment modalities available, it has since fallen out of favor, primarily because of the significant risks and complications that are associated, such as obstruction of the tube by soft tissue, displacement of the tube out of the tracheal lumen, in addition to the usual social consequences of tube placement. In 89 morbidly obese patients who were compared with a control group, morbid obesity was found to be independently associated with increased risk of tracheostomy-related complications (odds ratio: 4.4; 95% CIs: 2.1–11.7).

Acetazolamide, a carbonic anhydrase inhibitor, stimulates ventilation by decreasing the serum bicarbonate and creating metabolic acidosis. As such, acetazolamide should only be considered as an adjunct to PAP/NIV therapy.[45] Medroxyprogesterone, which acts as a respiratory stimulant at the hypothalamus through an estrogen-dependent progesterone receptor, has been shown to have mixed effects in the treatment of OHS.[56,57]

Exercise training and physical rehabilitation should be considered in OHS patients. In a recent single-center pilot RCT, 37 participants with OHS were randomized to either standard NIV or NIV and rehabilitation consisting of a program of rehabilitation physiotherapist, respiratory physician, and dietician.[58] At 3 months, there was a greater percent weight loss, increased exercise capacity, and HRQL in the rehabilitation group versus the standard of care. These effects did not persist at 12 months follow-up, probably because of attrition of participants.

SUMMARY

OHS is a frequently underdiagnosed and sometimes misdiagnosed condition. The prevalence of OHS is bound to increase given the rising epidemic of obesity in general. These patients have a poor health-related quality of life, often have prolonged hospitalizations, and face worsening comorbidities and high mortality. It is important for clinicians to keep a high index of suspicion for this condition, because early referral to sleep clinics and adequate management can help alter the course of some of the comorbidities.

REFERENCES

1. Chung F, Memtsoudis SG, Ramachandran SK, et al. Society of Anesthesia and Sleep Medicine guidelines on preoperative screening and assessment of adult patients with obstructive sleep apnea. Anesth Analg 2016;123(2):452–73.
2. Burwell CS, Robin ED, Whaley RD, et al. Extreme obesity associated with alveolar hypoventilation–a Pickwickian Syndrome. 1956. Obes Res 1994;2(4): 390–7.
3. Littleton SW, Mokhlesi B. The Pickwickian syndrome-obesity hypoventilation syndrome. Clin Chest Med 2009;30(3):467–78, vii–viii.
4. Hart N, Mandal S, Manuel A, et al. Rebuttal: 'Obesity hypoventilation syndrome (OHS): does the current definition need revisiting?'. Thorax 2014;69(10):955.
5. Macavei VM, Spurling KJ, Loft J, et al. Diagnostic predictors of obesity-hypoventilation syndrome in patients suspected of having sleep disordered breathing. J Clin Sleep Med 2013;9(9):879–84.
6. Tulaimat A, Littleton S. Defining obesity hypoventilation syndrome. Thorax 2014;69(5):491.
7. Sturm R, Hattori A. Morbid obesity rates continue to rise rapidly in the United States. Int J Obes (Lond) 2013;37(6):889–91.
8. Manuel ARG, Hart N, Stradling JR. Is a raised bicarbonate, without hypercapnia, part of the physiologic spectrum of obesity-related hypoventilation? Chest 2015;147(2):362–8.
9. Naimark A, Cherniack RM. Compliance of the respiratory system and its components in health and obesity. J Appl Physiol 1960;15:377–82.
10. Mortimore IL, Marshall I, Wraith PK, et al. Neck and total body fat deposition in nonobese and obese patients with sleep apnea compared with that in control subjects. Am J Respir Crit Care Med 1998;157(1): 280–3.
11. Lin CK, Lin CC. Work of breathing and respiratory drive in obesity. Respirology 2012;17(3):402–11.
12. Piper AJ, Yee BJ. Hypoventilation syndromes. Compr Physiol 2014;4(4):1639–76.
13. Pierce AM, Brown LK. Obesity hypoventilation syndrome: current theories of pathogenesis. Curr Opin Pulm Med 2015;21(6):557–62.
14. Norman RG, Goldring RM, Clain JM, et al. Transition from acute to chronic hypercapnia in patients with periodic breathing: predictions from a computer model. J Appl Physiol (1985) 2006;100(5):1733–41.
15. Tankersley CG, O'Donnell C, Daood MJ, et al. Leptin attenuates respiratory complications associated with the obese phenotype. J Appl Physiol (1985) 1998;85(6):2261–9.
16. Phipps PR, Starritt E, Caterson I, et al. Association of serum leptin with hypoventilation in human obesity. Thorax 2002;57(1):75–6.
17. Monneret D, Borel JC, Pepin JL, et al. Pleiotropic role of IGF-I in obesity hypoventilation syndrome. Growth Horm IGF Res 2010;20(2):127–33.
18. Lewis MI, LoRusso TJ, Fournier M. Anabolic influences of insulin-like growth factor I and/or growth hormone on the diaphragm of young rats. J Appl Physiol (1985) 1997;82(6):1972–8.
19. Pihtili A, Bingol Z, Kiyan E. The predictors of obesity hypoventilation syndrome in obstructive sleep apnea. Balkan Med J 2017;34(1):41–6.
20. Alawami M, Mustafa A, Whyte K, et al. Echocardiographic and electrocardiographic findings in patients with obesity hypoventilation syndrome. Intern Med J 2015;45(1):68–73.
21. Chung F, Yegneswaran B, Liao P, et al. STOP questionnaire: a tool to screen patients for obstructive sleep apnea. Anesthesiology 2008;108(5): 812–21.

22. Bingol Z, Pihtili A, Kiyan E. Modified STOP-BANG questionnaire to predict obesity hypoventilation syndrome in obese subjects with obstructive sleep apnea. Sleep Breath 2016;20(2):495–500.

23. Cabrera Lacalzada C, Diaz-Lobato S. Grading obesity hypoventilation syndrome severity. Eur Respir J 2008;32(3):817–8.

24. Borel JC, Roux-Lombard P, Tamisier R, et al. Endothelial dysfunction and specific inflammation in obesity hypoventilation syndrome. PLoS One 2009; 4(8):e6733.

25. Almeneessier AS, Nashwan SZ, Al-Shamiri MQ, et al. The prevalence of pulmonary hypertension in patients with obesity hypoventilation syndrome: a prospective observational study. J Thorac Dis 2017;9(3):779–88.

26. Berg G, Delaive K, Manfreda J, et al. The use of health-care resources in obesity-hypoventilation syndrome. Chest 2001;120(2):377–83.

27. Marik PE, Desai H. Characteristics of patients with the "malignant obesity hypoventilation syndrome" admitted to an ICU. J Intensive Care Med 2013; 28(2):124–30.

28. Priou P, Hamel JF, Person C, et al. Long-term outcome of noninvasive positive pressure ventilation for obesity hypoventilation syndrome. Chest 2010; 138(1):84–90.

29. Nowbar S, Burkart KM, Gonzales R, et al. Obesity-associated hypoventilation in hospitalized patients: prevalence, effects, and outcome. Am J Med 2004;116(1):1–7.

30. Masa JF, Corral J, Romero A, et al. Protective cardiovascular effect of sleep apnea severity in obesity hypoventilation syndrome. Chest 2016;150(1):68–79.

31. Lavie L, Lavie P. Ischemic preconditioning as a possible explanation for the age decline relative mortality in sleep apnea. Med Hypotheses 2006; 66(6):1069–73.

32. Noda JR, Masa JF, Mokhlesi B. CPAP or non-invasive ventilation in obesity hypoventilation syndrome: does it matter which one you start with? Thorax 2017;72(5):398–9.

33. Howard ME, Piper AJ, Stevens B, et al. A randomised controlled trial of CPAP versus non-invasive ventilation for initial treatment of obesity hypoventilation syndrome. Thorax 2017;72(5):437–44.

34. Piper AJ, Wang D, Yee BJ, et al. Randomised trial of CPAP vs bilevel support in the treatment of obesity hypoventilation syndrome without severe nocturnal desaturation. Thorax 2008;63(5):395–401.

35. Murphy PB, Davidson C, Hind MD, et al. Volume targeted versus pressure support non-invasive ventilation in patients with super obesity and chronic respiratory failure: a randomised controlled trial. Thorax 2012;67(8):727–34.

36. Storre JH, Seuthe B, Fiechter R, et al. Average volume-assured pressure support in obesity hypoventilation: a randomized crossover trial. Chest 2006;130(3):815–21.

37. Janssens JP, Metzger M, Sforza E. Impact of volume targeting on efficacy of bi-level non-invasive ventilation and sleep in obesity-hypoventilation. Respir Med 2009;103(2):165–72.

38. Masa JF, Corral J, Alonso ML, et al. Efficacy of different treatment alternatives for obesity hypoventilation syndrome. Pickwick Study. Am J Respir Crit Care Med 2015;192(1):86–95.

39. Lopez-Jimenez MJ, Masa JF, Corral J, et al. Mid- and long-term efficacy of non-invasive ventilation in obesity hypoventilation syndrome: the Pickwick's Study. Arch Bronconeumol 2016;52(3):158–65.

40. Manthous CA, Mokhlesi B. Avoiding management errors in patients with obesity hypoventilation syndrome. Ann Am Thorac Soc 2016;13(1):109–14.

41. Hollier CA, Harmer AR, Maxwell LJ, et al. Moderate concentrations of supplemental oxygen worsen hypercapnia in obesity hypoventilation syndrome: a randomised crossover study. Thorax 2014;69(4): 346–53.

42. Wijesinghe M, Williams M, Perrin K, et al. The effect of supplemental oxygen on hypercapnia in subjects with obesity-associated hypoventilation: a randomized, crossover, clinical study. Chest 2011;139(5): 1018–24.

43. Ligou JC, Nahas GG. Comparative effects of acidosis induced by acid infusion and carbon dioxide accumulation. Am J Physiol 1960;198:1201–6.

44. Sharkey RA, Mulloy EM, O'Neill SJ. Acute effects of hypoxaemia, hyperoxaemia and hypercapnia on renal blood flow in normal and renal transplant subjects. Eur Respir J 1998;12(3):653–7.

45. Raurich JM, Rialp G, Ibanez J, et al. Hypercapnic respiratory failure in obesity-hypoventilation syndrome: CO(2) response and acetazolamide treatment effects. Respir Care 2010;55(11):1442–8.

46. Cattano D, Melnikov V, Khalil Y, et al. An evaluation of the rapid airway management positioner in obese patients undergoing gastric bypass or laparoscopic gastric banding surgery. Obes Surg 2010;20(10): 1436–41.

47. Wong DT, Wang J, Venkatraghavan L. Awake bronchoscopic intubation through an air-Q(R) with the application of BIPAP. Can J Anaesth 2012;59(9): 915–6.

48. Gander S, Frascarolo P, Suter M, et al. Positive end-expiratory pressure during induction of general anesthesia increases duration of nonhypoxic apnea in morbidly obese patients. Anesth Analg 2005; 100(2):580–4.

49. Gupta A, Stierer T, Zuckerman R, et al. Comparison of recovery profile after ambulatory anesthesia with propofol, isoflurane, sevoflurane and desflurane: a systematic review. Anesth Analg 2004;98(3): 632–41. Table of contents.

50. Seet E, Chung F. Management of sleep apnea in adults - functional algorithms for the perioperative period: continuing professional development. Can J Anaesth 2010;57(9):849–64.

51. Perez de Llano LA, Golpe R, Piquer MO, et al. Clinical heterogeneity among patients with obesity hypoventilation syndrome: therapeutic implications. Respiration 2008;75(1):34–9.

52. Orfanos S, Jaffuel D, Perrin C, et al. Switch of noninvasive ventilation (NIV) to continuous positive airway pressure (CPAP) in patients with obesity hypoventilation syndrome: a pilot study. BMC Pulm Med 2017;17(1):50.

53. Greenburg DL, Lettieri CJ, Eliasson AH. Effects of surgical weight loss on measures of obstructive sleep apnea: a meta-analysis. Am J Med 2009; 122(6):535–42.

54. Gloy VL, Briel M, Bhatt DL, et al. Bariatric surgery versus non-surgical treatment for obesity: a systematic review and meta-analysis of randomised controlled trials. BMJ 2013;347:f5934.

55. De Cesare A, Cangemi B, Fiori E, et al. Early and long-term clinical outcomes of bilio-intestinal diversion in morbidly obese patients. Surg Today 2014; 44(8):1424–33.

56. Sutton FD Jr, Zwillich CW, Creagh CE, et al. Progesterone for outpatient treatment of Pickwickian syndrome. Ann Intern Med 1975;83(4):476–9.

57. Lyons HA, Huang CT. Therapeutic use of progesterone in alveolar hypoventilation associated with obesity. Am J Med 1968;44(6):881–8.

58. Mandal S, Suh ES, Harding R, et al. Nutrition and Exercise Rehabilitation in Obesity hypoventilation syndrome (NERO): a pilot randomised controlled trial. Thorax 2018;73(1):62–9.

59. Borel JC, Tamisier R, Gonzalez-Bermejo J, et al. Noninvasive ventilation in mild obesity hypoventilation syndrome: a randomized controlled trial. Chest 2012;141(3):692–702.

60. Contal O, Adler D, Borel JC, et al. Impact of different backup respiratory rates on the efficacy of noninvasive positive pressure ventilation in obesity hypoventilation syndrome: a randomized trial. Chest 2013; 143(1):37–46.

61. McArdle N, Rea C, King S, et al. Treating chronic hypoventilation with automatic adjustable versus fixed EPAP intelligent volume-assured positive airway pressure support (iVAPS): a randomized controlled trial. Sleep 2017;40(10).

Section 3: Treatment

Noninvasive Ventilation for Neuromuscular Disease

Dean R. Hess, PhD, RRT

KEYWORDS

- Face mask • Mouthpiece ventilation • Neuromuscular disease • Noninvasive ventilation

KEY POINTS

- Noninvasive ventilation (NIV) is standard practice for patients with neuromuscular respiratory failure.
- The interface distinguishes NIV from invasive ventilation.
- Selection of an appropriate interface and ventilator settings requires a close working relationship between clinicians, patients, and families.

INTRODUCTION

Noninvasive ventilation (NIV) is standard practice for patients with neuromuscular respiratory failure. Observational studies in patients with Duchenne muscular dystrophy[1] and a randomized controlled trial in patients with amyotrophic lateral sclerosis (ALS)[2] support that NIV in patients with neuromuscular disease is life prolonging. NIV with airway clearance therapy, such cough assist, are considered standard practice for patients with neuromuscular respiratory failure.[3–5] This review addresses issues related to NIV, particularly the technical aspects of NIV.

INDICATIONS

Vital capacity (VC) is commonly used to assess respiratory muscle weakness in patients with neuromuscular disease. VC less than 50% predicted is commonly used as an indication for NIV, and reimbursement is linked to this value (**Box 1**).[6] Maximum inspiratory pressure (PImax) greater than −60 cm H_2O is also used as an indication to initiate NIV. Mendoza and colleagues[7] reported that there were no cases among 161 patients whereby VC less than 50% occurred before PImax greater than −60 cm H_2O. Patients reached the PImax criterion 4.0 to 6.5 months

earlier than the VC criterion. In patients with diaphragm weakness, supine VC (orthopnea) may be a better indicator of the time to initiate NIV than an erect VC. A sniff nasal pressure can also be used, which is measured through a plug occluding one nostril during sniffs through the contralateral nostril.[8]

Overnight oximetry may be useful, as desaturation suggests nocturnal hypoventilation. Polysomnography to identify the need for NIV and titration of setting is controversial, although it was recommended in one consensus statement.[9] Recommendations from a consensus committee suggest that NIV should be initiated in patients with neuromuscular disease with symptoms (such as fatigue, dyspnea, morning headache) and one of the following physiologic criteria: $Paco_2$ 45 mm Hg or greater, nocturnal oximetry demonstrating oxygen saturation at 88% or less for 5 consecutive minutes; for progressive neuromuscular disease, maximal inspiratory pressures greater than −60 cm H_2O or forced vital capacity less than 50% predicted.[10]

NIV can be used to provide respiratory support during gastrostomy tube placement in patients with neuromuscular disease.[11] Some patients with neuromuscular disease can be successfully extubated to NIV,[12] and some patients with neuromuscular disease who have received

Respiratory Care, Massachusetts General Hospital, 55 Fruit Street, Boston, MA 02114, USA
E-mail address: dhess@mgh.harvard.edu

Clin Chest Med 39 (2018) 437–447
https://doi.org/10.1016/j.ccm.2018.01.014
0272-5231/18/© 2018 Elsevier Inc. All rights reserved.

Box 1
Medicare coverage criteria, noninvasive ventilation for restrictive thoracic disorders

Documentation in patients' medical record of a neuromuscular disease (eg, ALS) or a severe thoracic cage abnormality (eg, post-thoracoplasty for tuberculosis) and

1. An arterial blood gas $Paco_2$, done while awake and breathing the patient's fraction of inspired oxygen (Fio_2), is 45 mm Hg or greater; or sleep oximetry demonstrates oxygen saturation of 88% or less for 5 minutes or longer (minimum 2-hour recording time), done while breathing patient's prescribed Fio_2; or for a neuromuscular disease (only), maximal inspiratory pressure is greater than −60 cm H_2O or forced vital capacity is less than 50% predicted and

2. Chronic obstructive pulmonary disease does not contribute significantly to patients' pulmonary limitation.

If all of the aforementioned criteria are met, either an E0470 or E0471 (based on the judgment of the treating physician) will be covered for patients within this group of conditions for the first 3 months of therapy.

From Hess DR. The growing role of noninvasive ventilation in patients requiring prolonged mechanical ventilation. Respir Care 2012;57(6):907. [discussion: 918–20]; with permission.

tracheostomy can be successfully decannulated to NIV.[13] These patients might also be successfully transitioned to NIV with a capped tracheostomy tube and ultimately decannulated (**Fig. 1**).[14]

INTERFACE

The interface distinguishes NIV from invasive ventilation. Desirable characteristics of an interface are

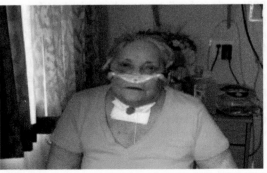

Fig. 1. NIV via nasal pillows, with a capped tracheostomy tube. (*From* O'Connor HH, White AC. Tracheostomy decannulation. Respir Care 2010;55(8):1080; with permission.)

listed in **Box 2**.[15] Interfaces are commercially available in a variety of styles and sizes (**Fig. 2**).[16,17] They can provide nasal ventilation (nasal mask or nasal pillows) and oronasal ventilation; they can fit over the entire face (total face mask); they can provide ventilation directly to the mouth (mouthpiece or oral mask); and they can be of hybrid designs (nasal pillows with oral mask). There are advantages and disadvantages of each (**Table 1**).

Types

The nasal mask fits just above the junction of the nasal bone and cartilage, directly at the sides of both nares, and just below the nose above the upper lip. Some are gel filled; others use an open cushion with an inner lip, in which pressure inside the mask pushes the cushion against the face. Nasal pillows, sometimes called nasal cushions, are available from several manufactures. This interface consists of soft plastic plugs inserted into the nares, shaped in a way that the pressure applied during inspiration helps to seal the walls of the pillows against the inner surface of the nasal vestibule.

Several interfaces fit over the nose and mouth. The oronasal mask fits just above the junction of the nasal bone and cartilage and extends below the lower lip above the jaw. The total face mask, as the name implies, fits over the entire face of patients, extending from the forehead to the jaw. A

Box 2
Desirable characteristics of an interface for noninvasive ventilation

Low dead space

Transparent

Lightweight

Easy to secure

Adequate seal with low facial pressure

Disposable or easy to clean

Nonirritating (nonallergenic)

Inexpensive

Variety of sizes: adult and pediatric

Adaptable to variations in facial anatomy

Ability to be removed quickly

Antiasphyxia mechanism

Compatible with wide range of ventilators

From Hess DR. Noninvasive ventilation in neuromuscular disease: equipment and application. Respir Care 2006;51(8):898; with permission.

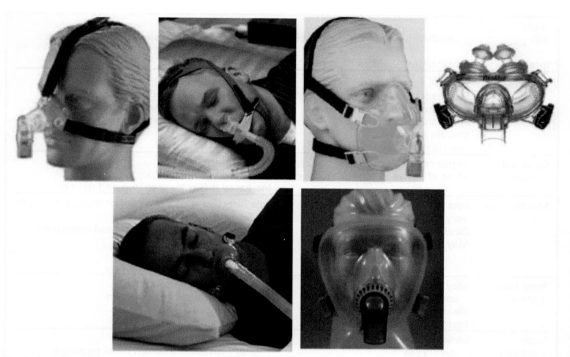

Fig. 2. Interfaces for NIV. Top (*left to right*): nasal mask, nasal pillows, oronasal mask, hybrid mask. Bottom (*left to right*): oral mask, total face. (*From* Nava S, Navalesi P, Gregoretti C. Interfaces and humidification for noninvasive mechanical ventilation. Respir Care 2009;54(1):75–78; with permission.)

hybrid mask combines an oral mask with nasal pillows.

Mouth leaks are common with a nasal interface. These leaks can affect comfort, can result in dry mouth, can result in less effective ventilation, can affect patient-ventilator interaction (trigger and cycle), and can disrupt sleep architecture.[15] One approach to a mouth leak is to coach patients to keep the mouth closed. But this is often ineffective, particularly during sleep. A chinstrap can be used, and these are variably effective. Willson and colleagues[18] found the chinstrap effective in 14 of 16 subjects, but Gonzalez and colleagues[19] reported that a chin strap was only effective in about a third of patients. If a persistent mouth leak occurs, an oronasal mask or total face mask is required. For patients receiving awake NIV, a nasal interface can be used during the daytime and an oronasal mask is used at night to minimize mouth leaks and improve sleep quality.

It has been suggested that nasal ventilation might be more efficient than oronasal ventilation. Upper airway unidirectional breathing, nose in and mouth out, reduces airway dead space[20] and might be more efficient during induction of anesthesia.[21] However, whether or not this is beneficial during NIV in patients with neuromuscular disease is not known.

Facial Skin Breakdown

A potential problem with nasal and oronasal masks is facial skin breakdown, which most commonly occurs on the bridge of the nose.[17] Perhaps the most important approach to prevent skin breakdown is to avoid strapping the mask too tightly. A mask that is too small or that is too large increases the likelihood of poor fit and facial soreness. A mask with a forehead spacer or an adjustable forehead arm can be used to reduce the pressure on the bridge of the nose. Hypoallergenic care tape can be applied to the bridge of the nose, but this is less effective after significant skin breakdown has occurred.

Trying other interfaces, sometimes on a rotational basis, may be helpful if facial skin breakdown occurs.[17] One can also consider the use of a different interface (eg, nasal pillows, mouthpiece, total face mask, or different size or manufacturer). Lemyze and colleagues[22] found that patients who switched to the total face mask (in the first 12 hours) developed fewer pressure sores despite a greater time of NIV exposure and less use of protective dressings. Schallom and colleagues[23] reported that the total face mask resulted in significantly fewer pressure ulcers and was more comfortable for patients. Yamaguti and colleagues[24] reported that the odds of facial

Table 1
Advantages and disadvantages of various types of interfaces for noninvasive ventilation

Interface	Advantages	Disadvantages
Nasal mask	Less risk for aspiration Easier secretion clearance Less claustrophobia Easier speech May be able to eat Less dead space	Mouth leak Higher resistance through nasal passages Less effective with nasal obstruction Nasal irritation and rhinorrhea Mouth dryness
Oronasal mask	Better oral leak control More effective in mouth breathers	Claustrophobia Increased aspiration risk Increased difficulty speaking and eating
Mouthpiece	Less interference with speech Very little dead space Does not require headgear May be able to eat	Less effective if patients cannot maintain mouth seal Usually requires nasal or oronasal interface at night Can result in hypersalivation Potential for orthodontic injury
Total face mask	May be more comfortable for some patients Easier to fit (one size fits all) Less facial skin breakdown	Greater risk for rebreathing Potential for drying of the eyes
Nasal pillows	Lower profile allows wearing of eyeglasses Less facial skin breakdown Simple headgear Easy to fit	Mouth leak Higher resistance through nasal passages Less effective with nasal obstruction Nasal irritation and rhinorrhea Mouth dryness
Hybrid	Better oral leak control More effective in mouth breathers Lower profile allows wearing of eyeglasses Less facial skin breakdown	Increased aspiration risk Increased difficulty speaking and eating

From Hess DR. Noninvasive ventilation in neuromuscular disease: equipment and application. Respir Care 2006;51(8):899; with permission.

skin breakdown were more than 80 times greater with an oronasal mask rather than with a total face mask. Although these studies were done in the acute care setting, there are likely implications for patients with neuromuscular disease receiving NIV.

Mouthpiece Ventilation

In some patients needing fulltime ventilation, the use of mouthpiece ventilation when awake is a reasonable option (**Fig. 3**).[25–30] An angled mouthpiece or straw-type mouthpiece, supported by a flexible arm, is placed near the mouth so that patients can access it with the lips and mouth as desired. Patients trigger the breath by creating a small negative pressure (sip and breathe) or placing their mouth on the mouthpiece (kiss and breathe). Any mode of ventilation can be used, but volume-controlled ventilation with a single-limb valveless circuit is commonly used.

An issue with mouthpiece ventilation has been alarms because traditionally ventilators were not designed to accommodate an open circuit.[31] Portable ventilators are now commercially available with a mouthpiece ventilation mode, which facilitates application of this approach.

Interface Selection

Evidence is lacking that any interface is clearly superior to others. The selection of an interface is usually determined by clinician bias, patient preference, and cost. Regardless of the device selected, it is important to optimize fit and comfort of the selected interface and ensure that straps are tight enough to minimize leaks but not so tight that comfort and tolerance are compromised. If the selected interface proves ineffective, another should be tried. Particularly for patients using NIV in the daytime as well as night, one device can be used at night and another during the day.

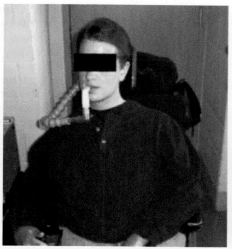
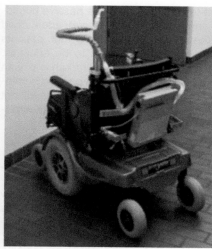

Fig. 3. Mouthpiece ventilation. Left: Patient with mouthpiece and ventilator circuit in standard position. Right: Rear view of wheelchair with ventilator and mouthpiece circuit in place. (*From* Benditt JO. Full-time noninvasive ventilation: possible and desirable. Respir Care 2006;51(9):1008. [discussion: 1012–5]; with permission.)

VENTILATOR

Years ago, the ventilator used for NIV was typically a homecare ventilator using volume-control ventilation. More recently, portable bilevel pressure-targeted ventilators were commonly used because of their superior leak compensation. There are now available portable ventilators with good leak compensation and a variety of modes.

Circuit

Critical care ventilators use a dual-limb circuit, with inspiratory and expiratory valves (**Fig. 4**).[32] In this configuration, there is separation of the inspiratory

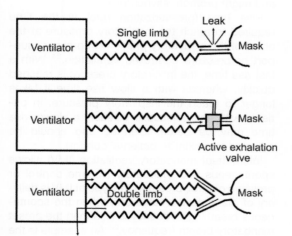

Fig. 4. Circuit configurations for NIV. (*From* Hess DR. Noninvasive Ventilation for Acute Respiratory Failure. Respir Care 2013;58(6):950–69 . [discussion: 962]; with permission.)

and expiratory gases. In the past, ventilators used for NIV in the home used a single-limb circuit with an active exhalation valve near the patient. For bilevel ventilators, a single-limb circuit is used. A leak port serves as a passive exhalation port for the patients and is incorporated into the circuit near the patient or into the interface. Some newer ventilators for NIV can use either a passive exhalation port or an active exhalation valve. The current generation of ventilators used for NIV in patients with neuromuscular disease compensate well for leaks, particularly when a passive leak port is used. Current generation ventilators used in the setting of neuromuscular disease are relatively small, portable, and with an internal battery allowing hours of ventilation.

A potential concern with the use of a single-limb circuit and a passive exhalation port is the potential for rebreathing. A major determinant of rebreathing is the flow through the circuit during exhalation. Increasing the expiratory pressure requires greater flow and, thus, decreases the amount of rebreathing. The minimum expiratory pressure setting on many ventilators with a passive leak port is 4 cm H_2O, which provides sufficient flow for carbon dioxide clearance.

Humidity

Adequate humidification during NIV is necessary for comfort. Active humidification is more effective and does not introduce additional dead space into the circuit. However, an active heated humidifier is more cumbersome and requires electrical power. A compromise is to use an active humidifier at night and a passive humidifier during the day. It is important to remember that the passive humidifier (heat and moisture exchanger) adds dead space to the circuit and requires that patients exhale through the device for it to be effective. With a significant leak, such as a mouth leak with a nasal interface, the function of a passive humidifier is compromised. A passive humidifier will not be effective if the leak port (exhalation) is incorporated into the interface.

Modes

With volume control ventilation, the ventilator delivers a fixed tidal volume and inspiratory flow pattern with each breath. The inspiratory time is usually the function of the tidal volume, inspiratory flow, and inspiratory flow pattern selected. Volume control is not commonly used for NIV, the exception being for mouthpiece ventilation. Breath-stacking maneuvers can be provided with volume control but not pressure control or pressure support ventilation. Martinez and colleagues[33] reported a high rate of NIV tolerance in subjects with ALS receiving volume control ventilation.

With pressure support, the pressure applied to the airway is fixed for each breath and there is no backup rate or fixed inspiratory time. For some ventilators, the level of pressure support is applied as the pressure above the baseline positive end-expiratory pressure (PEEP). With other ventilators, the inspiratory positive airway pressure (IPAP) and expiratory positive airway pressure (EPAP) are set. With this approach, the difference between the IPAP and EPAP is the level of pressure support. On some ventilators, pressure support is the spontaneous mode.

With pressure support, every breath is triggered by the patients. The ability of the ventilator to compensate for leaks has an important effect on triggering. If the leak is great, that can affect the ability of the patients to trigger, leading to either missed trigger or auto-trigger. Triggers have traditionally assessed a pressure or flow change to initiate inspiration. Some ventilators are volume triggered, which is a variation on flow triggering. Another approach is Auto-Trak, in which a shape signal is created by offsetting the actual patient flow by 15 L/min and delaying it for a 300-millisecond period. A change in patient flow will cross the shape signal, causing the ventilator to trigger to inspiration (or cycle to exhalation). The clinician can adjust the trigger on some ventilators but not on others. Some ventilators use redundant triggering mechanisms to improve sensitivity. The trigger should be set to minimize patient effort without auto-triggering.

Pressure support is usually flow cycled.[34,35] If the leak flow is greater than the flow cycle criteria, the inspiratory phase will continue indefinitely. However, there is usually a secondary time cycle, which is fixed on some ventilators (eg, 3 seconds) but adjustable on others. Several strategies can be used to address the issue of prolonged inspiration with pressure support.[36] Unintentional leaks should be minimized, and the use of a ventilator with good leak compensation should be used. Some ventilators allow the flow cycle criteria to be adjusted, with a higher flow cycle used in the presence of leaks.

Pressure control ventilation is similar to pressure support. The ventilator applies a fixed pressure with each breath. Trigger and rise time are similar between pressure support and pressure control. But there are 2 differences between pressure support and pressure control: there is a minimum rate set with pressure control and the inspiratory time is fixed with pressure control. The backup rate is beneficial in the setting of apnea or periodic breathing. The fixed inspiratory time with pressure control is beneficial when the inspiratory phase does not match the neural inspiratory phase of the patients (ie, the inspiratory phase on the ventilator is too long or too short with pressure support). In chronic stable patients with neuromuscular disease, Chadda and colleagues[37] reported that volume control, pressure control, and pressure support had similar effects on alveolar ventilation and respiratory muscle unloading. Some ventilators have a timed mode, which is triggered and cycled by the ventilator at the set rate and inspiratory time. This mode provides little interaction between patients and the ventilator and might promote asynchrony.

Rise time (pressurization rate) is the time required to reach the inspiratory pressure at the onset of the inspiratory phase with pressure support or pressure controlled ventilation.[34] With a fast rise time, the inspiratory pressure is reached quickly, whereas with a slow rise time it takes longer to reach the inspiratory pressure. In patients with neuromuscular disease, a slower rise time may be better tolerated and should be adjusted to maximize patients' comfort.

Intermittent mandatory ventilation (IMV) allows spontaneous and mandatory (volume control or pressure control) breaths. One type of IMV is delivery of mandatory breaths only when the spontaneous breathing frequency is less than the preset mandatory breath frequency.[38] An example is the spontaneous/times mode available on some NIV ventilators. With this mode, pressure support is delivered if patients trigger the ventilator. However, pressure control is delivered if patients becomes apneic. This mode is very commonly used in patients with neuromuscular disease receiving NIV.

Average volume-assured pressure support (AVAPS) is an adaptive pressure support mode that adjusts the pressure to maintain a target tidal volume.[39] AVAPS maintains a tidal volume equal to or greater than the target tidal volume by automatically controlling the pressure support between the minimum and maximum IPAP settings. It averages tidal volume over time and changes the IPAP gradually over several minutes. If patient effort decreases, AVAPS automatically increases IPAP to maintain the target tidal volume. On the other hand, if patient effort increases, AVAPS will reduce IPAP. A limitation of AVAPS is that support is reduced if patient effort causes tidal volume to exceeds the target.

In a bench study, Lujan and colleagues[40] found that the presence of unintentional leaks interfered with ventilator performance using adaptive pressure support modes. Inspiratory leaks resulted in a reduction in pressure support, without a guarantee of delivered tidal volume. Nicholson and colleagues[41] performed a retrospective chart review of patients with ALS using either pressure support or AVAPS. Compared with AVAPS, the tidal volume was significantly lower for pressure support. However, the difference was small: 356 mL (5.5 mL/kg ideal body weight) versus 390 mL (5.9 mL/kg ideal body weight). Hours of use per day, breathing frequency, and minute ventilation were not significantly different between groups. It remains to be determined whether this small difference in tidal volume translates into better clinical outcomes.

Oxygen and Aerosol

Oxygen[42] and inhaled bronchodilators[43] can be administered with NIV. However, patients with neuromuscular disease generally have normal lungs; thus, oxygen and bronchodilators are usually not necessary. In the setting of desaturation, airway clearance and perhaps an increase in ventilator support are necessary; the appropriate response is usually not oxygen and bronchodilators.

MONITORING
Tidal Volume and Ventilating Pressures

Normal tidal volume is 6 to 8 mL/kg predicted body weight. Because patients with neuromuscular respiratory failure have normal lungs, it would seem reasonable to target this tidal volume during NIV. Larger tidal volumes have been associated

with poorer outcomes in hospitalized patients with acute respiratory failure. The relationship between tidal volume and outcome has not been reported for patients with chronic respiratory failure. Some have recommended a pressure support of at least 10 cm H_2O (span pressure).[44] Most current-generation ventilators for NIV display tidal volume, allowing ventilating pressure to be set to achieve a target tidal volume.

Expiratory pressure (EPAP or PEEP) is often set at 4 to 5 cm H_2O. This pressure level is necessary with a passive circuit to avoid rebreathing. It also has the benefit of maintaining lung volume. However, this level of expiratory pressure produces hyperinflation in some patients, producing a sensation of not being able to exhale fully. PEEP should not be used with mouthpiece ventilation because it produces a nuisance flow through the open circuit.

Higher settings for NIV in patients with neuromuscular disease are not necessarily better. Higher PEEP results in a higher inspiratory pressure, potentially decreasing patient tolerance. The use of higher levels of PEEP (EPAP) can stimulate expiratory muscle activation. Other problems related to high inspiratory pressures include increased leak, ineffective inspiratory efforts,[45] central apnea,[46] and glottic closure.[47]

Rate

A rate or 12 of 15 breaths per minute is typically set to guard against apnea, particularly during sleep. In patients who are able to trigger the ventilator, a set rate is less important when awake. If the rate is set too high, some patients complain that the breath comes too soon. Some ventilators have a dual settings option, so that separate nighttime and daytime settings can be used, such as pressure support during the day and a mode with a rate at night. If tachypnea occurs during NIV, one should assess for auto-triggering or the need to increase the level of support.

Asynchrony

Asynchrony occurs when the timing on the ventilator does not match that of the respiratory center. During NIV, asynchrony is often the result of leaks.[36] To prevent trigger asynchrony, the sensitivity should be a compromise between trigger difficulty and auto-triggering. Cycle asynchrony can occur if the inspiratory time is set too short (double triggering) or too long (active exhalation). This asynchrony can be addressed by appropriately setting the flow cycle criteria with pressure support or the inspiratory time with pressure control or volume control.

Leak

Leaks are a reality with NIV, and devices that use a passive exhalation port require the presence of a leak. A leak during NIV can be the intentional leak through the passive exhalation port or unintentional leaks in the circuit, at the interface, or from the mouth (with a nasal interface) or the nose (with an oral interface). In the past, pressure ventilation was preferred over volume ventilation because of better leak compensation. But some current-generation ventilators compensate for leaks with either pressure ventilation or volume ventilation when a passive circuit is used. Some current-generation ventilators use redundant leak estimation algorithms. An unintentional leak less than 0.5 L/s is generally well tolerated.[48] Some ventilators track the leak rate and display this on the ventilator screen.

Pulse Oximetry

Pulse oximetry has become ubiquitous. Its role in the management of patients with neuromuscular disease receiving NIV is controversial. Because the lungs are normal, oxygen saturation measured by pulse oximetry (SpO_2) should be greater than 95% breathing room air. A decreased SpO_2 is likely the result of hypoventilation, suggesting that the level of NIV should be increased, or retained secretions, suggesting the need for airway clearance therapy.

Capnography and Transcutaneous Monitoring

The measurement of end-tidal Pco_2 is potentially beneficial in patients with neuromuscular disease. Because these patients have normal gas exchange, the end-tidal Pco_2 should be a reasonable proxy for arterial Pco_2. In spontaneously breathing patients, it can be measured with a cannula, mouthpiece, or mask. Evaluation of end-tidal Pco_2 becomes problematic with NIV.[49] Placing the sensor in the ventilator circuit biases the measurement because of continuous gas flow, which is worsened in the presence of unintentional leak or if the leak port is in the interface. Thus, caution is necessary if capnography is used during NIV. Devices are commercially available to measure transcutaneous Pco_2 and SpO_2 in a single probe, but these are not commonly used in patients with neuromuscular disease receiving NIV.

Alarms

Alarm settings are a balance between safety and nuisance. For patients receiving full ventilatory support, appropriate disconnect and decreased ventilation alarms should be set. For such patients, a second ventilator should be available; family members and care providers should be taught how to administer bag-mask ventilation.

Tele-Monitoring

In first-generation tele-monitoring systems, data from sensors are communicated via telephone to a database and relayed to the clinical team. In second generation nonimmediate systems, the clinical team recognizes important changes in patients' condition, but the response may be delayed the system is only available at certain times. Third-generation systems have analytical and decision-making support continuously staffed by clinicians. To date, these systems have had mixed results in the management of patients with NIV. But systems reported thus far have not included ventilator data.[5]

Current-generation ventilators for NIV monitor and track several parameters. These parameters are stored and can be periodically reviewed by a clinician (**Fig. 5**). This ability has the potential to allow the clinician to intervene if adjustments to settings are necessary. Some ventilators even allow the clinician to access the ventilator remotely by modem to make changes to settings and monitor the response. Whether tele-monitoring, including gas exchange (eg, pulse oximetry), ventilator data (eg, tidal volume, breathing frequency, hours of use), and patient symptoms, leads to better outcomes (eg, fewer hospital admissions) is yet to be determined.

SELECTION OF SETTINGS

Although much has been written about the technical aspects of interfaces and ventilators, the initiation of NIV is an art. Some tolerate NIV immediately, but many need time to become fully comfortable. Ideally patients are introduced to NIV before its use is urgent. This practice allows time to adjust the interface type and ventilator settings to maximize the benefit. To improve tolerance, it might be necessary to begin with subtherapeutic settings and then adjust upward as tolerance improves. Patients who are intolerant of nighttime use can apply NIV in the daytime, during naps, and with a distraction, such as television, to acclimate. Although acclimation is necessary for some patients, they should quickly advance their use to nocturnal NIV and daytime use as necessary, with the use of therapeutic settings. Encouragement of family and clinicians (physicians, respiratory therapists, nurses, physical therapists) is immensely important.

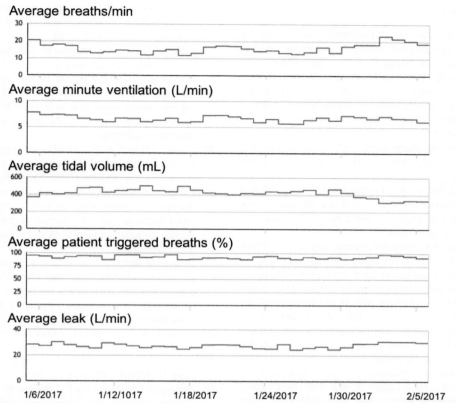

Fig. 5. Example of the output from a ventilator used for NIV in a patient with neuromuscular disease.

Once comfortable and therapeutic settings are achieved, sometimes an arterial blood gas is obtained. However, the need for blood gases is infrequent. If the SpO_2 is greater than 95% breathing room air, it is unlikely that there is significant hypercapnia. The effect of NIV is often assessed subjectively through symptoms, such as good sleep quality, no morning headache, and daytime alertness. Patients often report an improvement in these symptoms with the initiation of NIV.

NEGATIVE PRESSURE VENTILATORS

The tank ventilator, or iron lung, is the prototype negative pressure ventilator.[15] Patients lie supine with their head protruding though a porthole at the end. The chest cuirass is a rigid shell fitting over the anterior portion of the chest or over the chest and abdomen. The pneumowrap (raincoat, poncho, or wrap) consists of a parka suspended over a rigid plastic or metal chest piece. The cuirass and the pneumowrap are powered with a negative pressure ventilator. An issue of concern with negative pressure ventilators is the risk of upper airway obstruction.

Several devices provide ventilation by displacing the abdominal contents. The pneumobelt is a cloth corset containing an inflatable rubber bladder fitted over the abdomen and inflated intermittently by a positive pressure ventilator. It is effective only when patients are sitting at greater than 30°. Inflation of the bladder displaces the diaphragm upward and assists with exhalation, and deflation of the bladder allows passive downward motion of the diaphragm and an associated inhaled tidal volume. The rocking bed functions by rocking patients in a vertical axis over an arc of 40° to 45°. The force of gravity on the abdomen affects the diaphragm motion and tidal volume.

Negative pressure ventilators and devices that displace the abdominal contents are virtually obsolete, and few current-generation clinicians have experience with their use. Moreover, these devices are no longer commercially available; thus, they are primarily of historical interest.

SUMMARY

NIV is the standard practice for patients with neuromuscular respiratory failure. Selection of an appropriate interface and ventilator settings requires a close working relationship between clinicians, patients, and families.

REFERENCES

1. Bach JR, Martinez D. Duchenne muscular dystrophy: continuous noninvasive ventilatory support prolongs survival. Respir Care 2011;56(6):744–50.

2. Bourke SC, Tomlinson M, Williams TL, et al. Effects of non-invasive ventilation on survival and quality of life in patients with amyotrophic lateral sclerosis: a randomised controlled trial. Lancet Neurol 2006; 5(2):140–7.

3. Panitch HB. Respiratory implications of pediatric neuromuscular disease. Respir Care 2017;62(6): 826–48.

4. Hind M, Polkey MI, Simonds AK. AJRCCM: 100-year anniversary. homeward bound: a centenary of home mechanical ventilation. Am J Respir Crit Care Med 2017;195(9):1140–9.

5. Simonds AK. Home mechanical ventilation: an overview. Ann Am Thorac Soc 2016;13(11):2035–44.

6. Hess DR. The growing role of noninvasive ventilation in patients requiring prolonged mechanical ventilation. Respir Care 2012;57(6):900–18 [discussion: 918–20].

7. Mendoza M, Gelinas DF, Moore DH, et al. A comparison of maximal inspiratory pressure and forced vital capacity as potential criteria for initiating non-invasive ventilation in amyotrophic lateral sclerosis. Amyotroph Lateral Scler 2007;8(2):106–11.

8. Lofaso F, Nicot F, Lejaille M, et al. Sniff nasal inspiratory pressure: what is the optimal number of sniffs? Eur Respir J 2006;27(5):980–2.

9. Finder JD, Birnkrant D, Carl J, et al. Respiratory care of the patient with Duchenne muscular dystrophy: ATS consensus statement. Am J Respir Crit Care Med 2004;170(4):456–65.

10. Clinical indications for noninvasive positive pressure ventilation in chronic respiratory failure due to restrictive lung disease, COPD, and nocturnal hypoventilation–a consensus conference report. Chest 1999;116(2):521–34.

11. Banfi P, Volpato E, Valota C, et al. Use of noninvasive ventilation during feeding tube placement. Respir Care 2017;62(11):1474–84.

12. Bach JR, Goncalves MR, Hamdani I, et al. Extubation of patients with neuromuscular weakness: a new management paradigm. Chest 2010;137(5):1033–9.

13. Bach JR, Saporito LR, Shah HR, et al. Decanulation of patients with severe respiratory muscle insufficiency: efficacy of mechanical insufflation-exsufflation. J Rehabil Med 2014;46(10):1037–41.

14. O'Connor HH, White AC. Tracheostomy decannulation. Respir Care 2010;55(8):1076–81.

15. Hess DR. Noninvasive ventilation in neuromuscular disease: equipment and application. Respir Care 2006;51(8):896–911 [discussion: 911–2].

16. Nava S. Behind a mask: tricks, pitfalls, and prejudices for noninvasive ventilation. Respir Care 2013; 58(8):1367–76.

17. Nava S, Navalesi P, Gregoretti C. Interfaces and humidification for noninvasive mechanical ventilation. Respir Care 2009;54(1):71–84.

18. Willson GN, Piper AJ, Norman M, et al. Nasal versus full face mask for noninvasive ventilation in chronic respiratory failure. Eur Respir J 2004;23(4):605–9.

19. Gonzalez J, Sharshar T, Hart N, et al. Air leaks during mechanical ventilation as a cause of persistent hypercapnia in neuromuscular disorders. Intensive Care Med 2003;29(4):596–602.

20. Jiang Y, Liang Y, Kacmarek RM. The principle of upper airway unidirectional flow facilitates breathing in humans. J Appl Physiol (1985) 2008;105(3):854–8.

21. Liang Y, Kimball WR, Kacmarek RM, et al. Nasal ventilation is more effective than combined oral-nasal ventilation during induction of general anesthesia in adult subjects. Anesthesiology 2008; 108(6):998–1003.

22. Lemyze M, Mallat J, Nigeon O, et al. Rescue therapy by switching to total face mask after failure of face mask-delivered noninvasive ventilation in do-not-intubate patients in acute respiratory failure. Crit Care Med 2013;41(2):481–8.

23. Schallom M, Cracchiolo L, Falker A, et al. Pressure ulcer incidence in patients wearing nasal-oral versus full-face noninvasive ventilation masks. Am J Crit Care 2015;24(4):349–56 [quiz: 357].

24. Yamaguti WP, Moderno EV, Yamashita SY, et al. Treatment-related risk factors for development of skin breakdown in subjects with acute respiratory failure undergoing noninvasive ventilation or CPAP. Respir Care 2014;59(10):1530–6.

25. Pinto T, Chatwin M, Banfi P, et al. Mouthpiece ventilation and complementary techniques in patients with neuromuscular disease: a brief clinical review and update. Chron Respir Dis 2017;14(2):187–93.

26. Bedard ME, McKim DA. Daytime mouthpiece for continuous noninvasive ventilation in individuals with amyotrophic lateral sclerosis. Respir Care 2016;61(10):1341–8.

27. Nardi J, Leroux K, Orlikowski D, et al. Home monitoring of daytime mouthpiece ventilation effectiveness in patients with neuromuscular disease. Chron Respir Dis 2016;13(1):67–74.

28. Garuti G, Nicolini A, Grecchi B, et al. Open circuit mouthpiece ventilation: concise clinical review. Rev Port Pneumol 2014;20(4):211–8.

29. Czell DC. Daytime mouthpiece ventilation plus nighttime noninvasive ventilation improves quality of life in patients with neuromuscular disease. Respir Care 2014;59(9):1460–1.

30. Benditt JO. Full-time noninvasive ventilation: possible and desirable. Respir Care 2006;51(9): 1005–12 [discussion: 1012–5].

31. Carlucci A, Mattei A, Rossi V, et al. Ventilator settings to avoid nuisance alarms during mouthpiece ventilation. Respir Care 2016;61(4):462–7.

32. Hess DR. Noninvasive ventilation for acute respiratory failure. Respir Care 2013;58(6):950–72.

33. Martinez D, Sancho J, Servera E, et al. Tolerance of volume control noninvasive ventilation in subjects with amyotrophic lateral sclerosis. Respir Care 2015;60(12):1765–71.

34. Hess DR. Ventilator waveforms and the physiology of pressure support ventilation. Respir Care 2005; 50(2):166–86 [discussion: 183–6].

35. Hess D. Noninvasive pressure support ventilation. Minerva Anestesiol 2002;68(5):337–40.

36. Hess DR. Patient-ventilator interaction during noninvasive ventilation. Respir Care 2011;56(2):153–65 [discussion: 165–7].

37. Chadda K, Clair B, Orlikowski D, et al. Pressure support versus assisted controlled noninvasive ventilation in neuromuscular disease. Neurocrit Care 2004;1(4):429–34.

38. Chatburn RL. Intermittent mandatory ventilation will live forever. Respir Care 2016;61(9):1281–2.

39. Johnson KG, Johnson DC. Treatment of sleep-disordered breathing with positive airway pressure devices: technology update. Med Devices (Auckl) 2015;8:425–37.

40. Luján M, Sogo A, Grimau C, et al. Influence of dynamic leaks in volume-targeted pressure support noninvasive ventilation: a bench study. Respir Care 2015;60(2):191–200.

41. Nicholson TT, Smith SB, Siddique T, et al. Respiratory pattern and tidal volumes differ for pressure support and volume-assured pressure support in amyotrophic lateral sclerosis. Ann Am Thorac Soc 2017;14(7):1139–46.

42. Schwartz AR, Kacmarek RM, Hess DR. Factors affecting oxygen delivery with bi-level positive airway pressure. Respir Care 2004;49(3):270–5.

43. Hess DR. Aerosol therapy during noninvasive ventilation or high-flow nasal cannula. Respir Care 2015; 60(6):880–91 [discussion: 891–3].

44. Bach JR, Sinquee DM, Saporito LR, et al. Efficacy of mechanical insufflation-exsufflation in extubating unweanable subjects with restrictive pulmonary disorders. Respir Care 2015;60(4):477–83.

45. Fanfulla F, Delmastro M, Berardinelli A, et al. Effects of different ventilator settings on sleep and inspiratory effort in patients with neuromuscular disease. Am J Respir Crit Care Med 2005;172(5):619–24.

46. Johnson KG, Johnson DC. Bilevel positive airway pressure worsens central apneas during sleep. Chest 2005;128(4):2141–50.

47. Parreira VF, Jounieaux V, Aubert G, et al. Nasal two-level positive-pressure ventilation in normal subjects. Effects of the glottis and ventilation. Am J Respir Crit Care Med 1996;153(5):1616–23.

48. Rabec CA, Reybet-Degat O, Bonniaud P, et al. Leak monitoring in noninvasive ventilation. Arch Bronconeumol 2004;40(11):508–17 [in Spanish].

49. Piquilloud L, Thevoz D, Jolliet P, et al. End-tidal carbon dioxide monitoring using a naso-buccal sensor is not appropriate to monitor capnia during noninvasive ventilation. Ann Intensive Care 2015;5:2.

Swallowing and Secretion Management in Neuromuscular Disease

Deanna Britton, PhD, CCC-SLP, BC-ANCDS[a,b,*],
Chafic Karam, MD[c], Joshua S. Schindler, MD[b]

KEYWORDS

- Neuromuscular disease (NMD) • Dysphagia • Sialorrhea • Amyotrophic lateral sclerosis
- Muscular dystrophy • Myasthenia gravis

KEY POINTS

- Dysphagia associated with neuromuscular diseases reflects underlying disease patterns, such as severity, natural course, progression, and intervention options.
- The clinical swallowing examination provides information regarding underlying neuromuscular function leading to dysphagia symptoms, potential benefit from and timing for further instrumental studies, prognosis for improvements in swallowing function and potential to benefit from intervention.
- Supplemental instrumental assessment is needed when the clinical examination is inadequate to determine aspects of swallowing that will impact outcome.
- Dysphagia intervention aims to reduce risk for medical complications, including pneumonia and respiratory failure, and improve participation with life activities involving intake of food and quality of life.

INTRODUCTION

Neuromuscular disease (NMD) frequently leads to difficulty swallowing (dysphagia) and managing secretions (sialorrhea and/or excessive thick mucus). The act of swallowing is complex and involves at least 3 phases (oral, pharyngeal, and esophageal). Swallowing requires adequate strength and coordination of the bulbar musculature and production of saliva, as well as intact sensory, esophageal, respiratory, and cortical functions. Swallowing function is also important for saliva management, because humans typically generate more than one-half liter of saliva per day[1] and unconsciously swallow approximately every 1 to 3 minutes.[2,3] Bulbar and respiratory muscle weakness, often associated with NMDs, disrupt the ability to swallow safely and efficiently. Dysphagia may lead to deleterious medical complications, such as malnutrition,[4] dehydration,[5] aspiration pneumonia, and other pulmonary sequelae,[6] such as pulmonary

Disclosure Statement: D. Britton receives royalties for prior publications and on-line presentations from Plural Publishing, Pro-Ed, Inc, and Medbridge Education. C. Karam – None. J.S. Schindler – None.
[a] Department of Speech and Hearing Sciences, Portland State University (PSU), PO Box 751, Portland, OR 97207, USA; [b] Department of Otolaryngology–Head & Neck Surgery, Oregon Health & Science University (OHSU), Northwest Clinic for Voice and Swallowing, Physician's Pavilion 250/PV01, 3181 SW Sam Jackson Park Road, Portland, OR 97239, USA; [c] Department of Neurology, Oregon Health & Science University (OHSU), Hatfield Research Center, 12D44A/CH8C, 3181 Southwest Sam Jackson Park Road, Portland, OR 97239, USA
* Corresponding author. Department of Speech and Hearing Sciences, Portland State University (PSU), PO Box 751, Portland, OR 97207.
E-mail address: db23@pdx.edu

Clin Chest Med 39 (2018) 449–457
https://doi.org/10.1016/j.ccm.2018.01.007

fibrosis, localized lung inflammation, or abscess. In many NMDs, the ultimate cause of death is respiratory failure, which is often preceded by aspiration pneumonia.[7–9] Not surprisingly, dysphagia in individuals with NMD is also associated with increased health care costs, and mortality.[10] For many, dysphagia may also interfere with participation in communicative events involving food, such as conversation around the dinner table with family and other social events, and lead to reduced enjoyment of eating and quality of life.[11] This, in turn, may lead to depression and/or social isolation.[12] The identification and management of dysphagia can help to mitigate these complications and consequences. This review provides an overview of dysphagia associated with NMD in adults, along with a concise review of swallowing assessment and intervention options.

DYSPHAGIA ASSOCIATED WITH NEUROMUSCULAR DISEASE: AN OVERVIEW

Specific patterns of dysphagia associated with NMD reflect the underlying disease. Therefore, these patterns vary depending on several factors, including the characteristics of the disorder; the severity, natural course, or stage of progression; and the intervention options. For instance, dysphagia in some NMDs, such as Duchenne muscular dystrophy, progresses relatively slowly, whereas others, such as amyotrophic lateral sclerosis (ALS), often progress rapidly. Furthermore, dysphagia in myasthenic patients tends to fluctuate and is typically reversible with adequate treatment of the disease. In addition, the pattern of swallowing-related impairments reflects the pattern of neuromuscular weakness. For instance, reduced speed,[13] aspiration (including silent aspiration),[14] coughing and choking,[15] upper esophageal sphincter (UES) hypertonicity[16] and laryngospasm[17] in individuals with ALS may be related to the combination of spastic and flaccid weakness associated with ALS. However, in Duchenne muscular dystrophy, a pattern of difficulty with chewing and oropharyngeal transport of solid foods, as well as pharyngeal residue without aspiration is more common,[18] and is likely due to flaccid weakness of jaw, tongue,[19] and pharyngeal constrictor musculature. Many NMDs occur in individuals of advancing age. For instance, peak age of onset is typically between 55 and 75 years for ALS,[20] and 70 years for inclusion body myositis.[21] In these cases, the impact of the NMD is overlaid upon age-related changes to swallowing, such as those caused by the loss of dentition, presbylarynx or presbyesophagus.[22]

For these reasons, the overall prevalence and incidence of dysphagia in individuals with NMD is challenging to determine. **Table 1** outlines the literature describing the prevalence of dysphagia in selected NMDs.

Respiratory muscle weakness is associated with NMDs, leading to restrictive lung disease and impairment of the ability to cough, which contributes to the risk for dysphagia, aspiration pneumonia, and other pulmonary complications. Discoordination of breathing and swallowing may also occur.[30] When respiratory impairments are combined with bulbar impairments, the impact on swallowing and pulmonary defenses may be synergic, even lethal.[31] For instance, because the ability to cough requires the active coordination of respiratory musculature and intrinsic laryngeal muscles, the combination of bulbar and respiratory muscle impairment may render the ability to cough or use compensatory strategies for cough completely ineffective at a time when the protective defense of cough is needed to guard the lungs from aspiration.

Excessive saliva or drooling frequently co-occurs with dysphagia and is a manifestation of swallowing difficulty and clearance of normal secretions, rather than an increase in salivary flow.[32] Indeed, increasing salivary flow is a treatment challenge—even pharmacologically—whereas a decreased frequency of automatic saliva swallowing has been observed in individuals with dysphagia.[3] In addition, individuals with dysphagia owing to

Table 1	
Prevalence of dysphagia in selected neuromuscular diseases	
Examples	**Prevalence**
Inclusion body myositis	65%[23] to ≤80%[24]
Duchenne muscular dystrophy (muscle level)	Unknown; ≤30% report dysphagia[25] >95% based on MBSS findings[26]—greater with advancing age
Myasthenia gravis (neuromuscular junction disease)	30% as an early symptom[27] Up to two-thirds of individuals with myasthenia gravis[28]
Amyotrophic lateral sclerosis (motor neuron disease)	95%–98% bulbar onset[29] 35%–73% spinal onset[29]

Abbreviations: CNS, central nervous system; MBSS, modified barium swallow study.
Data from Refs.[23,26–29]

NMD may have difficulty with management of excessive thick mucus,[33] which may contribute to breathing discomfort.

PATIENT EVALUATION OVERVIEW

Clinical swallowing assessment and intervention are indicated for individuals with symptoms and/ or underlying conditions potentially associated with dysphagia to eliminate or minimize complications of dysphagia. For individuals who are asymptomatic but at risk for dysphagia, a validated dysphagia screening tool may identify the need for swallowing assessment. However, further development of swallowing screening tools for NMD populations is needed. In the United States, speech pathologists evaluate oral and pharyngeal swallowing concerns in adults. Gastroenterologists assess esophageal phase concerns. A clinical swallowing examination, as completed by a speech pathologist, includes 3 components[34]: (1) obtaining a history via medical records, interview with the individual and family or caregivers, (2) oral mechanism examination, including bulbar cranial nerve function, muscle strength and coordination, and observation of intraoral tissues and dentition, and (3) observations during swallowing of food or liquid, depending on patient tolerance. The clinical swallowing examination provides information regarding the underlying neuromuscular function leading to dysphagia symptoms, potential benefit from and timing for further instrumental studies, prognosis for improvements in swallowing function, and the potential to benefit from intervention.[13] For individuals with progressive NMDs, periodic reassessment to monitor for progression of dysphagia and update recommendations is beneficial.

A specific limitation of the clinical swallowing examination is the inability to definitively determine the presence of aspiration and other aspects of pharyngeal phase swallowing.[35] However, certain observations from the clinical swallowing examination may be associated with a higher risk for aspiration, such as a reduced lingual range of motion[36] and a reduced frequency of spontaneous swallowing.[32] In addition, experienced dysphagia clinicians may have an informed sense of potential swallowing impairments based on what is known about patterns of dysphagia related to the underlying condition. Some patients may experience substantial dysphagia without aspiration. For instance, pharyngeal or esophageal phase obstruction to bolus flow may lead to regurgitation without aspiration; however, pharyngeal or esophageal phase residue may increase risk for aspiration of the

residue after swallowing; this sort of delayed postswallow aspiration may go undetected by instrumental studies, such as the modified barium swallow study (MBSS).

The risk for the development of aspiration pneumonia is not determined solely by the presence or absence of aspiration. For instance, Langmore and colleagues[37] found that the presence of dysphagia, including aspiration, was not an independent risk factor for the development of pneumonia in nursing home residents. Instead, factors such as dependency for feeding or oral care, number of decayed teeth, tube feeding, multiple diagnoses ($\geq$1), number of medications, and smoking were independent predictors of aspiration pneumonia.[37] In addition to dysphagia, other factors were associated with the development of aspiration pneumonia, including pulmonary diagnoses, gastrointestinal disease, dental disease, poor oral care, and tube feeding.[37] Many of these independent predictors and other factors may be related to and/or cooccur with 1 or more impairments in pulmonary defenses. The clinical swallowing examination may reveal factors linked with a higher risk for pneumonia, including impairment of fundamental pulmonary defenses, such as impaired protective reflexes, ability to cough, mucociliary clearance, and/or immunologic defenses.[38] Because risk for pneumonia is multifactorial, aspiration is only one of many factors important to determining tolerance for safe oral intake.[37]

Instrumental assessment such as dynamic imaging of the swallowing mechanism via MBSS or fiberoptic endoscopic evaluation of swallowing (FEES), or dynamic assessment of swallowing-related pressures via manometry, may provide additional objective information on aspects of swallowing function. Current guidelines regarding when it is beneficial to recommend dysphagia diagnostic imaging are based largely on expert opinion documented with an American Speech-Language-Hearing Association guideline,[39] and continue to be debated. Imaging is needed when the clinical examination is inconsistent or inadequate, such as suspected inadequacy of UES opening. Similar to guidelines for neuroimaging,[40] key considerations include value or cost effectiveness, risk of harm, and whether or not the imaging findings ultimately make a difference for the intervention outcome.[39] Part of the rationale for selecting instrumental swallowing assessment stems from the specific information provided. **Tables 2 and 3** outline benefits and limits of MBSS versus FEES, respectively. However, other considerations include the availability of instrumentation and the expertise necessary for assessment,

Table 2
Benefits of MBSS versus FEES

MBSS	FEES
MBSS provides assessment of the following:	FEES provides assessment of the following:
• Dynamic swallowing biomechanics across all phases of swallowing: oral, pharyngeal, and esophageal	• Hypopharynx and laryngeal surface anatomy, including adequacy of glottic closure
• Airway protection before, during, and after swallows	• Mucosal abnormalities
• Oropharyngeal residue, as well as underlying patterns and contributing factors to residue and aspiration	• Pooled saliva or secretions
• Adequacy of upper esophageal sphincter opening	• Laryngeal sensation
• Submucosal structural abnormalities, for example, osteophytes	• Adequacy of velopharyngeal closure
• Effectiveness of postural adjustments, maneuvers, texture modification and other intervention strategies on swallowing safety and efficiency	In addition:
	• Portable
	• No adverse complications with repeated or longer examinations (no radiation exposure)
	• Can be used as a means of therapeutic biofeedback

Abbreviations: FEES, fiberoptic endoscopic evaluation of swallowing; MBSS, modified barium swallow studies.
Data from American Speech-Language-Hearing Association (ASHA). Clinical indicators for instrumental assessment of dysphagia [Guidelines]. 2000. Available at: www.asha.org/policy. Accessed September 20, 2017; and Langmore S. Endoscopic evaluation of oral and pharyngeal phases of swallowing. GI Motility Online. 2006. Available at: http://www.nature.com/gimo/contents/pt1/full/gimo28.html. Accessed September 26, 2017.

Table 3
Limitations of MBSS versus FEES

MBSS	FEES
• Constraints on study time and repeated examinations to minimize radiation exposure	• Oral and esophageal phases are not visualized
• Unnatural food (contrast media – barium) and environment	• Limited visualization of the upper esophageal sphincter opening
• Unable to visualize pooled saliva or secretions	• Cannot visualize swallowing biodynamics at the height of the swallow

Abbreviations: FEES, fiberoptic endoscopic evaluation of swallowing; MBSS, modified barium swallow studies.
Data from American Speech-Language-Hearing Association (ASHA). Clinical indicators for instrumental assessment of dysphagia [Guidelines]. 2000. Available at: www.asha.org/policy. Accessed September 20, 2017; and Langmore S. Endoscopic evaluation of oral and pharyngeal phases of swallowing. GI Motility Online. 2006. Available at: http://www.nature.com/gimo/contents/pt1/full/gimo28.html. Accessed September 26, 2017.

instrumental assessment. Finally, it may be challenging to determine the optimal timing of instrumental assessment for individuals with progressive NMDs, because dysphagia continues to progress and change after assessment.

MULTIDISCIPLINARY THERAPEUTIC OPTIONS

A primary goal of dysphagia intervention is to reduce the risk for aspiration pneumonia and other complications of dysphagia. For patients with rapidly progressive neurodegenerative disorders with associated dysphagia, such as ALS, the goal is to maintain swallowing function for as long as possible and to manage symptoms. Intervention goals vary depending on the specific biomechanical aspects of an individual's dysphagia, natural course of the underlying disease, and preferences of the individual. In developing intervention plans for each patient, clinicians combine evidence from clinical research, which is often limited in scope and applicability to patients with unique sets of comorbidities, with pathophysiologic reasoning, clinical experience, consideration of patient and family preferences, and available resources or limits.[41]

Pharmacologic Treatment Options

Pharmacologic treatment options for dysphagia in individuals with NMDs fall into 3 categories: (1) intervention for neurologic disease, (2) symptom

which may differ between institutions and locations, and the individual's ability to adequately participate with various forms of assessment. For instance, many rural clinics, as well as urban nursing facilities, do not have access to MBSS or providers capable of performing FEES. A variety of factors may also preclude the ability to participate with instrumental assessment, such as the need for intensive monitoring in an intensive care unit, mobility issues, and behavioral or cognitive issues impacting the ability to cooperate with management, and (3) management of contributing factors, such as reflux. Because dysphagia occurs secondary to disease, intervention to improve the underlying condition may also lead to an improvement in swallowing. An example of this type of improvement is in myasthenia gravis, an autoimmune disease that causes global weakness that frequently leads to dysphagia. Swallowing typically improves after controlling the disease with medications such as pyridostigmine and/or immunosuppression.[28] In conditions such as ALS, for which there are very few medical or pharmaceutical options for slowing progression, there are also limited options for slowing progression of the underlying dysphagia.

For patients struggling with sialorrhea and/or excessive thick mucus, pharmacologic management may aid the balance between the extremes of excessive dryness or secretions. In addition to behavioral management techniques and/or the use of a suction machine, oral or transdermal medications may offer relief. For sialorrhea, medications with drying side effects are used, such as amitriptyline (Elavil), scopolamine (transdermal hyoscine), atropine, and/or glycopyrrolate (Robinul). For management of excessive thick mucus, medications that thin out saliva (eg, guaifenesin) without additional drying are helpful.

Botulinum toxin (Botox, Myobloc, etc) injections are sometimes used to temporarily alleviate a variety of dysphagia symptoms, including inadequate relaxation of the UES[42] and severe sialorrhea. Botulinum injections to the parotid glands may be helpful for more severe cases of sialorrhea; however, some investigators have reported concern that the botulinum injection may spread and further weaken musculature for swallowing.[43] Salivary gland irradiation is also sometimes considered in severe cases, usually when the aforementioned management techniques are ineffective.[44]

Nonpharmacologic Treatment Options

Nonpharmacologic treatments fall into 2 categories: (1) behavioral management and maintenance strategies that offer an immediate counteractive effect of the neurologic condition on swallowing, and (2) rehabilitative interventions that seek to improve or restore swallowing function. These categories are not entirely exclusive and may overlap. Best intervention plans include both components.

Behavioral management approaches include a variety of compensatory strategies, such as diet modification, sensory stimulation, position or posture adjustments, swallowing maneuvers,

saliva management, respiratory support, cough assistance, and nutritional management. Specific strategies recommended depend on the underlying impairments contributing to the dysphagia. For instance, water thickening agents may be suggested for individuals who aspirate thin liquids owing to spastic weakness and slowness of laryngeal closure, because nectar thick liquids will move down the throat more slowly, thereby reducing risk for aspiration.[45] However, honey thick or thicker liquids are often avoided, owing to the risk for dehydration and pneumonia.[46] Another example is the strategy of an ipsilateral head turn, which may reduce pharyngeal residue for individuals with unilateral pharyngeal and/or laryngeal weakness.[47] In addition, manual cough assist strategies and/or use of mechanical insufflation and exsufflation will aid the key pulmonary defense of an effective cough in individuals with weakened abdominal muscles. Prevention strategies also fall under this rubric. For instance, optimal oral care (including regular mechanical cleaning of the teeth, tongue, and palate), has been linked with a reduced risk for pneumonia.[48] Positional strategies and/or the use of suction may be used to facilitate oral care when there is concern for aspiration.

Rehabilitative interventions for dysphagia include exercises to improve the strength, skill, or biomechanical support needed for swallowing. In accordance with the neural and muscle plasticity principles of specificity and "use it or lose it,"[49,50] swallowing is the best exercise for swallowing. A complete cessation of swallowing can render needed musculature weaker owing to disuse. For these reasons, any effort, compensatory or otherwise, to keep an individual swallowing safely, even if limited, is worthwhile. Per the principle of transference, exercises targeting the strengthening of the underlying musculature beyond the level of normal use may also benefit swallowing function, and functional reserve needed for swallowing endurance.[50] Exercises recommended vary depending on the underlying impairment. For example, the Shaker exercise targets laryngeal elevation and UES patency during swallowing,[51] whereas the Masako maneuver targets pharyngeal constriction and tongue base retraction weakness.[52] Expiratory muscle strength training may benefit cough strength as well as airway protection,[53] because it targets the muscles for expiration and laryngeal elevation.[54] However, very few dysphagia-related exercises have been studied in NMD populations. Theoretically, tolerance and the potential to benefit from exercise differ depending on the type of underlying NMD. For instance, intensive exercises are not typically recommended for individuals with untreated myasthenia gravis owing to the highly fatigable nature of this condition. The benefit of exercise for individuals with ALS is debatable; for instance, Plowman and colleagues[55] (2016) reported that expiratory muscle strength training at a moderate intensity was tolerated by some, but without significant benefit for cough strength or airway protection during swallowing.

Various forms of biofeedback may facilitate rehabilitation of swallowing skills. One example of this is surface electromyography biofeedback to track laryngeal elevation during swallowing efforts.[56] Biofeedback via FEES and high-resolution manometry may also facilitate use of swallowing strategies,[57] and coordination of pharyngeal pressures during swallowing,[58] respectively. Surface electrical stimulation has emerged as an adjunct modality toward the goal of improving swallowing strength and function. However, research findings on this approach have been mixed, and the underlying physiologic rationale for use with NMD populations has not yet been elucidated fully.[59] Currently, neither surface electromyography or surface electrical stimulation have been systematically studied in many NMDs, such as ALS, myasthenia gravis, and Duchenne muscular dystrophy.

Surgical Treatment Options

Surgical options may be appropriate for some individuals with dysphagia and include methods for maintaining nutrition, airway protection, bolus flow, and saliva management. Tracheostomy with an inflated cuff may reduce risk for greater amounts of aspiration. A caveat, however, is that tracheostomy does not fully block aspiration and may increase the risk for pneumonia owing to leakage of aspirated material around the cuff,[60,61] esophageal compression from an overinflated cuff,[62] laryngeal desensitization,[63] reduced subglottic air pressure,[64] and potentially laryngeal disuse atrophy.

Inadequate UES opening during swallowing can occur for different reasons, including reduced or uncoordinated laryngeal elevation leading to delayed or shorter duration of UES opening time, reduced bolus driving pressures, inadequate relaxation of UES musculature, and structural fibrotic UES changes such as a cricopharyngeal hypertonicity with or without an associated Zenker's diverticulum.[65] In the latter scenario, surgical procedures of myotomy or dilation with botulinum toxin may be helpful. For instance, individuals with inclusion body myositis frequently experience fibrotic changes to the UES that can be managed with UES opening.[66]

Depending on the underlying NMD, vocal fold paralysis, weakness, or severe bowing may interfere with airway protection during swallowing. In these instances, restoration of glottic competence through vocal fold augmentation with injection laryngoplasty or medialization thyroplasty may be performed. Medialization for unilateral vocal fold immobility may improve swallowing through valving and improved cough for airway protection.[67]

Patients with NMDs who are unable to adequately meet their hydration and nutrition needs may benefit temporarily or in the long term from the surgical placement of a gastrostomy tube.[68] Gastrostomy support provides stability for nutritional intake, and may also decrease anxiety and time pressure with eating.[13] Guidelines exist for gastrostomy placement for some NMDs, such as ALS,[69] but not for others. For those with neurodegenerative conditions, it is best practice to educate regarding the option of gastrostomy before urgent need arises and significant respiratory impairment occurs. Gastrostomy use does not preclude eating or drinking for those able to tolerate eating transiently or in limited amounts.

Laryngectomy and other chronic aspiration procedures are considered for some individuals with severe bulbar impairments (usually with preserved respiratory and limb musculature).[70] Separating the alimentary and respiratory pathways eliminates aspiration, alleviates the discomfort associated with chronic coughing and choking on secretions, and eliminates the distress of severe laryngospasms. An alternative to total laryngectomy is laryngotracheal separation, where the trachea is routed to an anterior neck stoma without removal of the larynx.[71] This procedure leaves a tracheal stump where food or saliva collects and pools, but clears for most within 24 hours.[72] Laryngotracheal separation has been reported to aid quality of life and tolerance of limited eating in individuals with severe bulbar ALS.[73] However, functional swallowing is not guaranteed, because severe tongue, lip, and/or palate weakness could preclude effective swallowing, despite the elimination of aspiration. In addition, posterior oropharyngeal stasis may lead to gagging, which cannot be easily cleared, because cough efforts would clear material through the stoma only. These procedures also render the individual unable to voice, and it is best to establish communication strategies before the surgery.

EVALUATION OF OUTCOME

Key outcomes of interest for individuals with dysphagia owing to NMD include the ability to tolerate oral intake without pulmonary compromise or discomfort and to maintain adequate nutrition and hydration. For those with greater severity or rapid progression of dysphagia, goals may be adjusted to the maintenance of nutrition fully or partially via alternative means, or tolerating oral intake for as long as possible. Outcomes for therapeutic targets related to swallowing physiology may also be tracked, such as aspiration and bolus clearance. Clinician and patient-reported tools are available as well, such as use of the Eating Assessment Tool to track dysphagia symptoms,[74] Functional Oral Intake Scale to track changes in oral intake,[75] and the swallowing-related quality of life tool.[76]

SUMMARY

NMDs frequently result in dysphagia and sialorrhea. Because dysphagia is a symptom of the underlying disease, the characteristics of swallowing or saliva management impairments vary with the natural course of the underlying NMD. Treatment options depend on the underlying characteristics of the individual's dysphagia, as well as the underlying causal condition, and may include behavioral, pharmacologic, and/or surgical interventions. Dysphagia intervention aims to reduce the risk for the medical complications of dysphagia and to improve participation with life activities involving intake of food and quality of life.

REFERENCES

1. Dawes C, Pedersen AM, Villa A, et al. The functions of human saliva: a review sponsored by the World Workshop on Oral Medicine VI. Arch Oral Biol 2015;60(6):863–74.
2. Tanaka N, Nohara K, Kotani Y, et al. Swallowing frequency in elderly people during daily life. J Oral Rehabil 2013;40(10):744–50.
3. Crary MA, Carnaby GD, Sia I, et al. Spontaneous swallowing frequency has potential to identify dysphagia in acute stroke. Stroke 2013;44(12):3452–7.
4. Serra-Prat M, Palomera M, Gomez C, et al. Oropharyngeal dysphagia as a risk factor for malnutrition and lower respiratory tract infection in independently living older persons: a population-based prospective study. Age Ageing 2012;41(3):376–81.
5. Leibovitz A, Baumoehl Y, Lubart E, et al. Dehydration among long-term care elderly patients with oropharyngeal dysphagia. Gerontology 2007;53(4):179–83.
6. Prather AD, Smith TR, Poletto DM, et al. Aspiration-related lung diseases. J Thorac Imaging 2014;29(5):304–9.
7. Kiernan MC, Vucic S, Cheah BC, et al. Amyotrophic lateral sclerosis. Lancet 2011;377(9769):942–55.
8. Cohen MS, Younger D. Aspects of the natural history of myasthenia gravis: crisis and death. Ann N Y Acad Sci 1981;377:670–7.
9. Baydur A, Gilgoff I, Prentice W, et al. Decline in respiratory function and experience with long-term assisted ventilation in advanced Duchenne's muscular dystrophy. Chest 1990;97(4):884–9.
10. Altman KW, Yu GP, Schaefer SD. Consequence of dysphagia in the hospitalized patient: impact on prognosis and hospital resources. Arch Otolaryngol Head Neck Surg 2010;136(8):784–9.
11. Ekberg O, Feinberg MJ. Altered swallowing function in elderly patients without dysphagia: radiologic findings in 56 cases. AJR Am J Roentgenol 1991;156(6):1181–4.
12. Cichero JA, Altman KW. Definition, prevalence and burden of oropharyngeal dysphagia: a serious problem among older adults worldwide and the impact on prognosis and hospital resources. Nestle Nutr Inst Workshop Ser 2012;72:1–11.
13. Miller RM, Britton D. Dysphagia in neuromuscular diseases. San Diego (CA): Plural Publishing, Inc; 2011.
14. Briani C, Marcon M, Ermani M, et al. Radiological evidence of subclinical dysphagia in motor neuron disease. J Neurol 1998;245(4):211–6.
15. Hadjikoutis S, Eccles R, Wiles CM. Coughing and choking in motor neuron disease. J Neurol Neurosurg Psychiatry 2000;68(5):601–4.
16. Ertekin C, Aydogdu I, Yuceyar N, et al. Pathophysiological mechanisms of oropharyngeal dysphagia in amyotrophic lateral sclerosis. Brain 2000;123:125–40.
17. van der Graaff MM, Grolman W, Westermann EJ, et al. Vocal cord dysfunction in amyotrophic lateral sclerosis: four cases and a review of the literature. Arch Neurol 2009;66(11):1329–33.
18. Aloysius A, Born P, Kinali M, et al. Swallowing difficulties in Duchenne muscular dystrophy: indications for feeding assessment and outcome of videofluoroscopic swallow studies. Eur J Paediatr Neurol 2008;12(3):239–45.
19. van den Engel-Hoek L, Erasmus CE, Hendriks JC, et al. Oral muscles are progressively affected in Duchenne muscular dystrophy: implications for dysphagia treatment. J Neurol 2013;260(5):1295–303.
20. Byrne S, Jordan I, Elamin M, et al. Age at onset of amyotrophic lateral sclerosis is proportional to life expectancy. Amyotroph Lateral Scler Frontotemporal Degener 2013;14(7–8):604–7.
21. Molberg O, Dobloug C. Epidemiology of sporadic inclusion body myositis. Curr Opin Rheumatol 2016;28(6):657–60.
22. Britton D. The impact of aging and progressive neurological disease on swallowing: a concise overview. J Texture Stud 2016;47(4):257–65.

23. Cox FM, Verschuuren JJ, Verbist BM, et al. Detecting dysphagia in inclusion body myositis. J Neurol 2009;256(12):2009–13.

24. Houser SM, Calabrese LH, Strome M. Dysphagia in patients with inclusion body myositis. Laryngoscope 1998;108(7):1001–5.

25. Toussaint M, Davidson Z, Bouvoie V, et al. Dysphagia in Duchenne muscular dystrophy: practical recommendations to guide management. Disabil Rehabil 2016;38(20):2052–62.

26. Hanayama K, Liu M, Higuchi Y, et al. Dysphagia in patients with Duchenne muscular dystrophy evaluated with a questionnaire and videofluorography. Disabil Rehabil 2008;30(7):517–22.

27. Beekman R, Kuks JB, Oosterhuis HJ. Myasthenia gravis: diagnosis and follow-up of 100 consecutive patients. J Neurol 1997;244(2):112–8.

28. Shoesmith C, Nicolle MW. Myasthenia gravis (MG). In: Jones H, Rosenbek J, editors. Dysphagia in rare conditions. San Diego (CA): Plural Publishing, Inc; 2010. p. 393–400.

29. Onesti E, Schettino I, Gori MC, et al. Dysphagia in amyotrophic lateral sclerosis: impact on patient behavior, diet adaptation, and riluzole management. Front Neurol 2017;8:94.

30. Hadjikoutis S, Wiles CM. Respiratory complications related to bulbar dysfunction in motor neuron disease. Acta Neurol Scand 2001;103(4):207–13.

31. Benditt JO. Respiratory complications of amyotrophic lateral sclerosis. Semin Respir Crit Care Med 2002;23(3):239–47.

32. Murray J, Langmore SE, Ginsberg S, et al. The significance of accumulated oropharyngeal secretions and swallowing frequency in predicting aspiration. Dysphagia 1996;11(2):99–103.

33. Raheja D, Stephens HE, Lehman E, et al. Patient-reported problematic symptoms in an ALS treatment trial. Amyotroph Lateral Scler Frontotemporal Degener 2016;17(3–4):198–205.

34. Yorkston KM, Miller RM, Strand EA, et al. Management of speech and swallowing disorders in degenerative diseases. 3rd edition. Austin (TX): Pro-Ed, Inc; 2013.

35. Rangarathnam B, McCullough GH. Utility of a clinical swallowing exam for understanding swallowing physiology. Dysphagia 2016;31(4):491–7.

36. Leder SB, Suiter DM, Murray J, et al. Can an oral mechanism examination contribute to the assessment of odds of aspiration? Dysphagia 2013;28(3):370–4.

37. Langmore SE, Terpenning MS, Schork A, et al. Predictors of aspiration pneumonia: how important is dysphagia? Dysphagia 1998;13:69–81.

38. Happel KI, Bagby GJ, Nelson S. Host defense and bacterial pneumonia. Semin Respir Crit Care Med 2004;25(1):43–52.

39. American Speech-Language-Hearing Association (ASHA). Clinical indicators for instrumental assessment of dysphagia [Guidelines]. 2000. Available at: www.asha.org/policy. Accessed September 20, 2017.

40. Culebras A, Kase CS, Masdeu JC, et al. Practice guidelines for the use of imaging in transient ischemic attacks and acute stroke. A report of the Stroke Council, American Heart Association. Stroke 1997;28(7):1480–97.

41. Tonelli MR, Curtis JR, Guntupalli KK, et al. An official multi-society statement: the role of clinical research results in the practice of critical care medicine. Am J Respir Crit Care Med 2012;185(10):1117–24.

42. Restivo DA, Marchese-Ragona R, Patti F, et al. Botulinum toxin improves dysphagia associated with multiple sclerosis. Eur J Neurol 2011;18(3):486–90.

43. Leigh PN, Abrahams S, Al-Chalabi A, et al. The management of motor neurone disease. J Neurol Neurosurg Psychiatry 2003;74(Suppl 4):iv32–47.

44. Slade A, Stanic S. Managing excessive saliva with salivary gland irradiation in patients with amyotrophic lateral sclerosis. J Neurol Sci 2015;352(1–2):34–6.

45. Rofes L, Arreola V, Mukherjee R, et al. The effects of a xanthan gum-based thickener on the swallowing function of patients with dysphagia. Aliment Pharmacol Ther 2014;39(10):1169–79.

46. Robbins J, Gensler G, Hind J, et al. Comparison of 2 interventions for liquid aspiration on pneumonia incidence: a randomized trial. Ann Intern Med 2008; 148(7):509–18.

47. Logemann J. Evaluation and treatment of swallowing disorders. 2nd edition. Austin (TX): Pro-Ed., Inc; 1998.

48. Pace CC, McCullough GH. The association between oral microorganisms and aspiration pneumonia in the institutionalized elderly: review and recommendations. Dysphagia 2010;25(4):307–22.

49. Kleim JA, Jones TA. Principles of experience-dependent neural plasticity: implications for rehabilitation after brain damage. J Speech Lang Hear Res 2008;51(1):S225–39.

50. Burkhead LM, Sapienza CM, Rosenbek JC. Strength-training exercise in dysphagia rehabilitation: principles, procedures, and directions for future research. Dysphagia 2007;22(3):251–65.

51. Shaker R, Easterling C, Kern M, et al. Rehabilitation of swallowing by exercise in tube-fed patients with pharyngeal dysphagia secondary to abnormal UES opening. Gastroenterology 2002;122(5):1314–21.

52. Fujiu M, Logemann JA. Effect of a tongue-holding maneuver on posterior pharyngeal wall movement during deglutition. Am J Speech Lang Pathol 1996; 5:25–30.

53. Pitts T, Bolser D, Rosenbek J, et al. Impact of expiratory muscle strength training on voluntary cough and swallow function in Parkinson Disease. Chest 2009;135(5):1301–8.

54. Wheeler-Hegland KM, Rosenbek JC, Sapienza CM. Submental sEMG and hyoid movement during Mendelsohn maneuver, effortful swallow, and expiratory muscle strength training. J Speech Lang Hear Res 2008;51(5):1072–87.

55. Plowman EK, Watts SA, Tabor L, et al. Impact of expiratory strength training in amyotrophic lateral sclerosis. Muscle Nerve 2016;54(1):48–53.

56. Athukorala RP, Jones RD, Sella O, et al. Skill training for swallowing rehabilitation in patients with Parkinson's disease. Arch Phys Med Rehabil 2014;95(7): 1374–82.

57. Langmore S. Endoscopic evaluation of oral and pharyngeal phases of swallowing. GI Motility Online; 2006. Available at: http://www.nature.com/gimo/contents/pt1/full/gimo28.html. Accessed September 26, 2017.

58. Walczak CC, Jones CA, McCulloch TM. Pharyngeal pressure and timing during bolus transit. Dysphagia 2017;32(1):104–14.

59. Humbert IA, Michou E, MacRae PR, et al. Electrical stimulation and swallowing: how much do we know? Semin Speech Lang 2012;33(3):203–16.

60. Bailey RL. Tracheostomy and dysphagia: a complex association. Perspectives in Swallowing and Swallowing Disorders; 2005. p. 2–7.

61. Zanella A, Scaravilli V, Isgro S, et al. Fluid leakage across tracheal tube cuff, effect of different cuff material, shape, and positive expiratory pressure: a bench-top study. Intensive Care Med 2011;37(2): 343–7.

62. Nash M. Swallowing problems in the tracheotomized patient. Otolaryngol Clin North Am 1988;21(4): 701–9.

63. Leder SB. Incidence and type of aspiration in acute care patients requiring mechanical ventilation via a new tracheotomy. Chest 2002;122(5):1721–6.

64. Gross RD, Atwood CW Jr, Grayhack JP, et al. Lung volume effects on pharyngeal swallowing physiology. J Appl Physiol (1985) 2003;95(6):2211–7.

65. Cook IJ. Clinical disorders of the upper esophageal sphincter. Edition 2006. GI Motility Online; 2006.

66. Murata KY, Kouda K, Tajima F, et al. Balloon dilation in sporadic inclusion body myositis patients with Dysphagia. Clin Med Insights Case Rep 2013;6:1–7.

67. Cates DJ, Venkatesan NN, Strong B, et al. Effect of vocal fold medialization on dysphagia in patients with unilateral vocal fold immobility. Otolaryngol Head Neck Surg 2016;155(3):454–7.

68. Rahnemai-Azar AA, Rahnemaiazar AA, Naghshizadian R, et al. Percutaneous endoscopic gastrostomy: indications, technique, complications and management. World J Gastroenterol 2014; 20(24):7739–51.

69. Miller RG, Jackson CE, Kasarskis EJ, et al. Practice parameter update: the care of the patient with amyotrophic lateral sclerosis: drug, nutritional, and respiratory therapies (an evidence-based review): report of the Quality Standards Subcommittee of the American Academy of Neurology. Neurology 2009;73(15): 1218–26.

70. Garvey CM, Boylan KB, Salassa JR, et al. Total laryngectomy in patients with advanced bulbar symptoms of amyotrophic lateral sclerosis. Amyotroph Lateral Scler 2009;10(5–6):470–5.

71. Lindeman RC, Yarington CT, Sutton D. Clinical experience with the tracheoesophageal anastomosis for intractable aspiration. Ann Otol Rhinol Laryngol 1976;85:609–12.

72. Suzuki H, Hiraki N, Murakami C, et al. Drainage of the tracheal blind pouch created by laryngotracheal separation. Eur Arch Otorhinolaryngol 2009;266(8): 1279–83.

73. Mita S. Laryngotracheal separation and tracheoesophageal diversion for intractable aspiration in ALS–usefulness and indication. Brain Nerve 2007; 59(10):1149–54 [in Japanese].

74. Belafsky PC, Mouadeb DA, Rees CJ, et al. Validity and reliability of the eating assessment tool (EAT-10). Ann Otol Rhinol Laryngol 2008;117(12):919–24.

75. Crary MA, Mann GD, Groher ME. Initial psychometric assessment of a functional oral intake scale for dysphagia in stroke patients. Arch Phys Med Rehabil 2005;86(8):1516–20.

76. McHorney CA, Robbins J, Lomax K, et al. The SWAL-QOL and SWAL-CARE outcomes tool for oropharyngeal dysphagia in adults: III. Documentation of reliability and validity. Dysphagia 2002;17(2): 97–114.

Diaphragm Pacing

Anthony F. DiMarco, MD

KEYWORDS

- Diaphragm pacing • Spinal cord injury • Ventilatory support • Mechanical ventilation

KEY POINTS

- Diaphragm pacing is a useful and cost-effective alternative to mechanical ventilation.
- Benefits of diaphragm pacing include improved mobility, speech, olfaction, and quality of life.
- Diaphragm pacing is cost-effective, being less expensive compared with long-term mechanical ventilation.
- Diaphragm has few side effects and complications.

INTRODUCTION

Chronic ventilatory support is most commonly required for management of patients with respiratory failure consequent to severe dysfunction of the lungs or respiratory muscles. These patients are typically maintained on either traditional mechanical ventilation (MV) via tracheostomy tube or noninvasive methods. A unique category of patients with chronic respiratory failure, however, are those in whom the lungs, chest wall, and respiratory muscles are fully intact. These patients experience chronic respiratory failure due to lack of neural input from the central nervous system to the major inspiratory muscles. These include patients with central hypoventilation syndrome (CHS)[1,2] in whom there is inadequate drive from the respiratory centers in the medulla and patients with cervical spinal cord injury (SCI) in whom there is interruption of nerve impulses from the respiratory center to the inspiratory muscles.[3–11] Because the respiratory neuromuscular apparatus is otherwise normal, these patients are candidates for an alternative method of ventilatory support involving the application of electrical stimulation to the phrenic nerves, that is, diaphragm pacing (DP).

RESPIRATORY PHYSIOLOGY

The diaphragm, which is a thin dome-shaped sheet of skeletal muscle separating the thoracic and abdominal cavities, is the primary muscle of inspiration (Fig. 1). This is illustrated by patients breathing comfortably at rest with singular function of the diaphragm alone. The muscular fibers of the diaphragm originate from the abdominal wall and lumbar vertebrae posteriorly, the xiphoid process and floating ribs anteriorly, and the lateral rib cage laterally and insert on a central tendon. The diaphragm consists of anteriorly located costal fibers and posteriorly located crural fibers. The vena cava, esophagus, and aorta pass through the diaphragm posteriorly.[12]

Normal inspiration is associated with contraction of both the diaphragm and inspiratory intercostal muscles lasting approximately 1 second, 8 times per minute to 12 times per minute. The inspiratory intercostal muscles are primarily located in the upper 6 interspaces. Contraction of the inspiratory muscles results in the development of a negative intrathoracic pressure causing inhalation of air into the chest. After diaphragm relaxation, exhalation occurs passively due to the positive pressure developed by lung and chest wall recoil pressure. The function of the intercostal muscles is illustrated by the contraction of the diaphragm alone resulting in paradoxic inward movement of the anterior rib cage. This phenomenon is most significant in infants with an immature flexible rib cage but does not interfere with adequate tidal volume generation in adults in whom the rib cage is much less compliant.

Potential Conflict of Interest: Dr A.F. DiMarco is stakeholder in Synapse Biomedical, in Oberlin, Ohio, a manufacturer of diaphragm pacing systems.

Physiology and Biophysics, Case Western Reserve University, MetroHealth Medical Center, 2500 MetroHealth Drive, Cleveland, OH 44109, USA

E-mail address: afd3@case.edu

Clin Chest Med 39 (2018) 459–471
https://doi.org/10.1016/j.ccm.2018.01.008

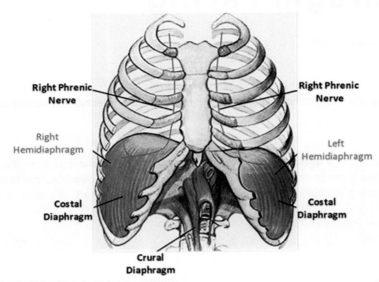

Fig. 1. Schematic drawing of the human diaphragm.

Relevant to the anatomic location of cervical spinal cord lesions, the diaphragm is innervated by a single right phrenic nerve and single left phrenic nerve, each of which is supplied by cervical spinal nerves C3, C4, and C5. The phrenic motoneurons, however, are most plentiful at the C4 level. Each phrenic nerve trifurcates just above the dome of the diaphragm as it enervates this muscle.

With regard to potential candidates for DP, virtually all patients with CHS and secondary chronic respiratory failure are potential candidates for this modality because the phrenic nerve/diaphragm neuromuscular apparatus is fully intact. Patients with cervical SCI, however, need to be carefully evaluated to assess the integrity of the phrenic nerves. Patients with cervical lesions limited to the C3 level and higher are usually excellent candidates for DP. In patients with damage to the phrenic motoneuron pools at the C4/C5 level and/or direct damage to the phrenic nerves, however, DP will not be successful. It is also important to point out that bilateral phrenic nerve integrity is necessary for successful DP.

MECHANICAL VENTILATION VERSUS DIAPHRAGM PACING—CLINICAL CONSIDERATIONS

In the management of acute and chronic respiratory failure, positive-pressure MV is a life-sustaining modality. MV can be applied via tracheostomy tube or less invasive means via nasal/facial mask appliances. In patients with CHS in early childhood, tracheostomy may be preferred due to the potential development of midface hypoplasia with mask ventilation.[13] In addition, these devices can be uncomfortable and poorly tolerated in many individuals. Given that this is life support device, MV via tracheostomy may be preferable.

With regard to SCI and excluding those who die at the scene, there are approximately 17,500 new cases per year, of which more than half occur at the cervical level.[14] Although a majority of tetraplegics require at least temporary MV via tracheostomy, most are successfully weaned from these devices. Nonetheless, as many as 400 to 500 per year new patients require chronic mechanical ventilatory support. Importantly, ventilator dependency is an independent negative prognostic factor for long-term survival. During the first-year postinjury, there is as much as a 40-fold increase in mortality that remains elevated at 2-fold to 3-fold in subsequent years. Compared with a normal 20 year old, life expectancy for patients surviving at least 1 year postinjury is markedly diminished, from 60 years to only 18 years. In high tetraplegics who do not require MV, life expectancy is significantly higher, at 35 years.[14]

In properly selected individuals, DP provides an important alternative to MV with significant advantages (**Box 1**).[4,5,10,15–20] Compared with MV, most patients describe an improved sense of well-being and overall health. This could occur consequent to these patients engaging their own inspiratory muscles and sensing more normal breathing. Patients also describe the benefit of no longer requiring connection to an external machine and attached tubing. Negative-pressure ventilation may reduce the incidence of barotrauma and also have

Box 1
Potential advantages of diaphragm pacing

Increased mobility

   Easier transfers from bed to chair

   Easier transport to occupational and recreational activities outside the home

Restoration of olfactory sensation

Improved speech

Subjective sense of more normal breathing

   Engagement of intrinsic respiratory muscles

   Normal negative-pressure ventilation

Reduced anxiety and embarrassment

   Elimination of ventilator tubing

   Elimination of ventilator noise

   Daytime closure of tracheostomy

Improved level of comfort

   Elimination of fear of ventilator disconnection

   Elimination of the pull of ventilator tubing

   Elimination of the discomfort associated with positive-pressure breathing

Reduction in the incidence of respiratory tract infections

Reduction in overall costs

   Reduction and/or elimination of ventilator supplies

   Reduction in the level of required caregiver support

beneficial cardiovascular effects. Moreover, tension on the tracheostomy tube and fear of disconnection from the ventilator are eliminated. Quality of speech may improve because ventilator noise and interference are not present. Speech can also be improved by use of an abdominal binder.[21] Preserved speech facilitates the use of adaptive communication devices, such as computers and phones. Olfactory sensation is also restored with DP and associated with an improved quality of life.[22]

Patient mobility and ease of transport are also enhanced because attachment to a machine with tubing is restrictive. Daily bed-to-chair transfers and transport outside the home are also easier. Improved mobility may have substantial benefits, including the potential to participate in rehabilitation programs, participate in social events, and even obtain gainful employment. The ability to engage more fully in society can be life changing.[15,18,23–25]

Because DP is virtually indistinguishable from normal breathing, the social stigma and embarrassment of being tethered to a machine are also removed.

There is also some evidence the DP may reduce the incidence of respiratory tract infections.[26] If borne out in additional studies, this argues for a reduction in morbidity and possibly mortality consequent to DP.

MECHANICAL VENTILATION VERSUS DIAPHRAGM PACING—COST CONSIDERATIONS

The initial costs of DP, including the costs of the device and surgical implantation, are high and, depending on the type of device, can range from approximately $30,000 to $100,000. Despite this initial high cost, however, there is compelling evidence that DP is highly cost effective.[17,26–28] The cost of maintenance supplies associated with MV, especially when extrapolated over many years, is substantial and eliminated with DP. In addition, patients can be transferred to less intensive and, therefore, less expensive care settings.[10,11,15,16,29] Perhaps the major driver of cost savings is that the level of caregiver expertise needed to care for these patients is reduced significantly. If proved true that the incidence of respiratory tract infections is reduced, DP also may be associated with reduction in the costs of treatment, including the high costs of hospitalization.

DEVICES

Glenn and colleagues[7–11,30,31] performed the basic science and clinical studies that led to the initial commercial application of DP. The basic design of DP systems are similar. Each device requires stimulation of each phrenic nerve and consists of implanted materials and external components (**Fig. 2**). Currently available devices include the Mark IV Diaphragm Pacing System (Avery Biomedical Devices, Commack, NY). With this device and other radiofrequency devices,[32,33] the internal components include the electrodes, radiofrequency receivers, and connecting wires. The external components include an external power supply radiofrequency transmitter and antenna wires. Surgery is required to attach the electrodes to the phrenic nerves bilaterally either by open thoracotomy or video-assisted thoracoscopic surgery. Wires are tunneled subcutaneously to connect each electrode to a radiofrequency receiver that is positioned over the anterior chest wall. The external battery-powered transmitter generates radiofrequency signals, which are inductively

EXTERNAL
COMPONENTS

INTERNAL
COMPONENTS

Fig. 2. Illustration of the external and internal components of the direct phrenic nerve and intramuscular DP systems.

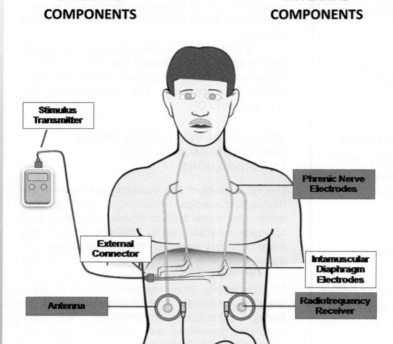

coupled to the receivers via circular rubberized antennas. Each antenna must be positioned directly over each receiver and secured in place to ensure transmission of the signal. The transmitter signal is demodulated by the receivers, converting the radiofrequency signals to electrical signals, which are transmitted to the electrodes.[9,16] Amplitude and frequency can be modulated to adjust tidal volume. Respiratory rate can be adjusted by altering train rate delivery. Inspiratory time and flow rate can also be adjusted. Similar devices are manufactured in Europe including the Atrotech OY (Tampere, Finland) and MedImplant (Vienna, Austria) Biotechnisches Labor devices. These are not available, however, in the United States.

DP can also be achieved by placement of electrodes in the body of the diaphragm via laparoscopic surgery using the NeuRx RA/4 device (Synapse BioMedical, Oberlin, Ohio).[34–39] This technique also represents a form of phrenic nerve pacing and not direct diaphragm muscle pacing. Using a mapping technique,[40,41] 2 intramuscular electrodes are implanted into each hemidiaphragm near the motor points of the phrenic nerves bilaterally (see **Fig. 2**). Full-time ventilator support

can be maintained in ventilator-dependent tetraplegics with success rates similar to systems involving electrodes implanted directly on the phrenic nerves.[40] The advantages of this technique include less invasive surgery and eliminating the small risk of phrenic nerve injury. Another important difference lies in that with the NeurRx RA/4 device, electrode wires penetrate the skin and are connected directly to an external stimulator. Finally, this device is much less expensive compared with the radiofrequency systems.

DIAPHRAGM PACING COMBINED WITH INSPIRATORY INTERCOSTAL PACING

Many patients with tetraplegia and secondary respiratory failure have damage to 1 or both phrenic motoneurons pools and/or phrenic rootlets and, therefore, are not candidates for DP.[8–10,15,31,42] Previous studies, however, have demonstrated that the inspiratory intercostal muscles can be activated by electrodes positioned epidurally and ventrally in the high thoracic region of the spinal cord by stimulating the ventral roots.[43–46] In initial clinical trials in patients with absent diaphragm function, stimulation of the intercostal muscles alone produced inspired volumes similar in magnitude to those resulting from a single hemidiaphragm. Inspired volume generation was not sufficient to maintain ventilation for prolonged periods.[45] In subsequent trials in ventilator-dependent patients with unilateral diaphragm function, however, combined stimulation of intercostal ventral roots with unilateral phrenic nerve stimulation was successful in providing long-term ventilatory support.[46]

Intercostal muscle stimulation resulted in some side effects, including mild flexion of both hands and contraction of the muscles of the upper torso, which was well tolerated. Intercostal pacing, therefore, may be a useful adjunct to enhance tidal volume generation in patients with inadequate phrenic nerve function.[45,46]

This technique is not commercially available but received FDA approval via an investigational device exemption.

MICROSURGICAL INTERCOSTAL TO PHRENIC NERVE TRANSFER

Another potential approach to patients with respiratory failure secondary to tetraplegia and damage to the phrenic motor neuron pools and/or phrenic rootlets is simultaneous bilateral intercostal to phrenic nerve transfers and pacemaker placement. By this method, phrenic nerve integrity is restored resulting in reinnervation of each hemidiaphragm. These nerves are then amenable to DP. Krieger and Krieger[47] first reported on this technique in 10 patients and found that each patient could be successfully weaned from MV.

More recently, Kaufman and colleagues[48] performed bilateral intercostal to phrenic nerve transfers in 14 mechanically dependent tetraplegics with phrenic nerve injury. In this retrospective analysis, recovery of diaphragm electromyographic activity was observed in 13 patients and 8 of these patients achieved at least 1 hour of weaning per day. Mean weaning time was an impressive 10 h/d. These favorable outcomes support consideration of this method for patients without adequate phrenic nerve function and who, therefore, are not candidates for conventional DP.

PATIENT SELECTION

Prospective candidates for DP should be free from significant lung disease or primary muscle disease because these factors preclude successful long-term pacing. As discussed previously, DP has the potential to provide clinical benefit in 2 patient groups: ventilator-dependent tetraplegia with

bilateral intact phrenic nerve function in patients with CHS.[4,5,49] DP has been tried in other patient groups, including chronic obstructive pulmonary disease[50] and amyotrophic lateral sclerosis, without success. There is some evidence that the application of DP in patients with ALS may be harmful.[51]

Ventilator-dependent Tetraplegia

Prior to application of DP, vigorous attempts should be made to wean these patients from MV. Vital capacity measurements of less than 10 mL/kg suggest inadequate inspiratory muscle function to maintain spontaneous ventilation. In some patients with sufficient inspiratory muscle function, noninvasive ventilator support may be a suitable alternative to DP.[52–54]

Psychosocial factors should also be considered prior to DP.[15,18,30,34,55] A high level of motivation and cooperation of the patient and family members are important factors determining outcomes. In home situations in which the family seeks to improve the mobility, social interaction, ability of the patient to function independently, and occupational potential significantly increase the likelihood of success.

Central Hypoventilation Syndromes

CHS can be congenital[1,2] or occur secondary to brainstem dysfunction from mechanical injury, bleeding, tumor or Arnold-Chiari malformation.[3,8,10,11] Most patients are initially managed with MV via tracheostomy. Institution of DP can be performed in infants as young as 9 months old. Patients who are not full-time ventilator dependent and able to undergo tracheal decannulation after pacer placement may later develop obstructive apnea. Because diaphragm activation is not synchronized with upper airway activation, the upper airway may collapse. Some centers, therefore, prefer to offer DP to patients 5 years of age and older with the intention of decannulating soon thereafter, because obstructive apnea is less frequent in older children.[56]

EVALUATION OF PHRENIC NERVE FUNCTION

The technical and clinical success of DP is dependent on adequate phrenic nerve function. Therefore, a thorough evaluation of phrenic nerve function must be performed in each patient.[9,57–59] Function of the phrenic nerves can be assessed via measurements of phrenic nerve conduction times.[58,59] This method involves applying electrical stimulation of the phrenic nerves in the cervical region with surface or monopolar needle electrodes at the posterior border of the sterno-cleidomastoid muscle at the level of the cricoid cartilage. Using surface electrodes, diaphragmatic action potentials are monitored between the 7th and 9th intercostal spaces in the anterior axillary line. Single pulses of gradually increasing intensity are applied until a supramaximal M-wave is observed. Phrenic nerve conduction time can then be calculated as the time interval between the applied stimulus and first appearance of the compound motor action potential (CAP). Stimulation results in outward motion of the abdominal wall. Normal conduction times in adults range between 7 ms and 9 ms.[58,59] Mild prolongation, however, up to 14 ms does not preclude successful DP.[11] In children, mean latencies are shorter, in the range of 2 ms at 6 months and increasing to 4.2 ms between 5 years and 11 years of age.[6,60] The magnitude of the CAP, which reflects the number of stimulated diaphragm motor units in the vicinity of the recording electrode, is a less reliable indicator of phrenic nerve function.[16,58] Low amplitude may reflect a low number of functional phrenic nerve fibers but may also be secondary to technical factors or reversible diaphragm atrophy. Conduction times, therefore, are considered a more reliable indicator of phrenic nerve function.

The assessment of phrenic nerve function should be performed by a physician experienced in the performance of this test. Although considered the gold standard in the assessment of phrenic nerve function, measurements of phrenic nerve conduction times are associated with a small rate of both false-positive results and false-negative results. For this reason, it is useful to observe motion of the diaphragm with fluoroscopy during electrodiagnosis. Visual estimate of diaphragm descent of at least 3 cm in adults[9,15,35] and 2 rib spaces in children[3] during phrenic nerve stimulation is a useful confirmatory test.

If phrenic nerve function is still in doubt, this parameter can also be assessed by measurements of diaphragm force development during phrenic nerve stimulation. This test involves the placement of small balloon-tipped catheters in the esophagus and stomach to measure the pressure difference across the diaphragm, that is, the transdiaphragmatic pressure (Pdi).[27] Unilateral single-shock stimulation typically results in Pdi values of approximately 10 cm H_2O in normal subjects.[61] This value may be lower in ventilator-dependent individuals, however, due to diaphragm atrophy.

INITIATION OF DIAPHRAGM PACING

DP is a life support system and should be initiated under close supervision. Typically, DP is started approximately 2 weeks after surgical implantation to allow for resolution of inflammation and edema at the electrode/nerve interface and healing of surgical wounds.

Assessment of Stimulus-output Parameters

The integrity of the pacing system should be assessed initially and monitored on a regular basis thereafter.[11,16] Important parameters include the minimum stimulus amplitude that results in visible or palpable diaphragm contraction (stimulus threshold) and lowest stimulus parameters that result in maximum inspired volume generation (supramaximal amplitudes and stimulus frequencies). Threshold and supramaximal amplitudes should be determined for each lead or lead combination. Because the diaphragm has most likely developed varying degrees of disuse atrophy, the magnitude of inspired volumes and force generation gradually increase during the conditioning phase. Achievement of a plateau in these values indicates that the conditioning phase is complete.

Determination of Stimulus Parameters for Chronic Use

It is useful to determine P_{CO_2} values either by arterial blood gases or end-tidal values prior to initiation of DP. Many patients are maintained in a hyperventilated state while on MV. Chronic hyperventilation results in a reduction in bicarbonate stores. With initiation of pacing, therefore, which is designed to maintain near normal P_{CO_2} values, an acidosis may develop secondary to the rise in P_{CO_2}. This development can be prevented by adjusting the ventilator to achieve eucapnia prior to initiation of pacing.

Inspired volume generation is initially adjusted by changing stimulus frequency at supramaximal stimulus amplitudes. Using respiratory rates between 8 breaths per minute and 14 breaths per minute (stimulus train rate delivery), stimulus frequency should be adjusted to achieve inspired volumes necessary to maintain P_{CO_2} values in the low normal range (approximately 35 mm Hg). Respiratory rate and tidal volume should be further adjusted for patient comfort. To avoid potential diaphragm injury, stimulus frequency should be maintained at the lowest possible level and not exceed 20 Hz. There is some evidence the chronic stimulation at high frequencies may cause myopathic changes in the diaphragm resulting in reductions in force generation.[7,18,62,63]

During the conditioning phase, stimulus frequencies and respiratory rates should be reduced to the lowest values that maintain adequate ventilation and patient comfort. With the Avery DP system, stimulation frequency can usually be reduced to 7 Hz to 9 Hz with respiratory rates of 6 breaths per minute to 12 breaths per minute.[7] The Atrotech DP system typically requires less adjustment because the initial frequencies are lower. With the Synapse DP system, stimulus frequency can be reduced to 11 Hz.[34] Infants and young children require higher respiratory rates, up to 20 breaths per minute, with lower inspiratory times of 0.6 seconds to 0.9 seconds compared with 1 second to 1.4 seconds in adults.[4,63,64] Conditioning time can vary between a few weeks to several months. For most, conditioning is accomplished within 6 weeks to 10 weeks.

Low-frequency stimulation during the initial phases of DP may result in shaking motion of the abdominal wall. This occurs consequent to diaphragm stimulation below its intrinsic fusion frequency.[65] With continued daily stimulation during the conditioning process, vibrating diaphragm contractions are gradually replaced by smooth coordinated contractions even at very low stimulus frequencies.[7,8] This occurs secondary to the gradual transformation of the diaphragm, which is normally constituted with nearly equal populations of both type I and type II fibers, to one consisting of a uniform population of type I fibers.[7,66] Type I fibers have a lower fusion frequency and are highly oxidative and fatigue resistant. Although a type I muscle has a higher endurance, it is also characterized by reductions in maximum force-generating capacity and, thereby, maximum inspired volume generation. This is not a concern for most patients because generalized muscle paralysis in SCI patients restricts the need for higher levels of ventilation. Nonetheless, this factor may account for reductions in the success rate of DP.

Once full-time pacing is achieved during the day, DP should be provided during sleep while oxygen saturation is continuously monitored, with alarms in place. Patients can typically cap the tracheostomy tube while pacing during the day. The tracheostomy should be maintained open at night, however, to prevent upper airway obstruction. This occurs secondary to asynchronous contraction of the upper airway muscles and diaphragm, a form of sleep apnea.[4,57,63]

Ventilation during DP should be measured in both the supine and upright postures. Higher levels of applied stimulation may be necessary in a sitting posture compared with a supine posture.[67] While upright, the gravitational effects of the abdominal contents on the diaphragm are reduced, resulting in diaphragm shortening. Diaphragm force-generating capacity becomes less and, therefore, inspired volume generation is reduced for a given level of stimulation. Therefore, most patients find it useful to wear a tight-fitting binder while sitting. This serves to compress the abdominal wall and increase diaphragm length, resulting in greater diaphragm force production and larger inspired volumes.[67]

PATIENT OUTCOMES

Clinical studies have clearly demonstrated that DP is an effective and cost-effective method of maintaining ventilatory support in patients with SCI and CHS. In many patients, DP can be used as the sole mode of ventilatory support. There are numerous reports of successful long-term pacing in individual patients for 10 years or longer.[7,10,18,34]

When assessing any technique, the term, success, should be carefully defined. Success should also adhere to each individual patient goals. Some patients may tolerate DP for only very short periods, for instance, 20 minutes. This small degree of independence from MV, however, may allow for easier bed-to-chair transfer, which may have a positive impact on mobility. Most patients, however, have expectations of greater freedom from MV.

In 1 study, the clinical outcome of patients who underwent DP before 1981 were compared with patients implanted between 1981 and 1987.[18] In the latter group, low-frequency stimulation was applied at low respiratory rates and pacing was successful in each of the 12 patients evaluated. In fact, 6 patients continued pacing for a mean duration of approximately 15 years. The other patients did not achieve long-term pacing success due to lack of adequate financial and social support or medical comorbidities.

Based on an analysis of 64 patients with the Atrotech OY device in whom the average duration of pacing was 2 years, approximately 50% were able to maintain full-time DP whereas approximately 80% were able to maintain pacing throughout the day.[68] With this device, involving an analysis of 64 patients, successful pacing was achieved in 95% of pediatric and 86% of adult patients. At the time of the study, however, the average duration of pacing was approximately 2 years. With the Synapse Biomedical intramuscular DP device, approximately 50% of patients also were able to maintain full-time pacing. In patients not using the device full time, the duration of use was as short as 4 hours to 5 hours.[40] High success rates have also been observed in infants and children in whom a more modest goal of part-time pacing (<15 h/d) was achieved.[3]

There are several factors why DP is not more successful in maintaining full-time ventilatory support. Lack of long-term maintenance of inspired volume production may account for many of these factors. First, peripheral nerve electrodes generally do not achieve complete diaphragm activation due to the high thresholds of some axons.[69] As discussed previously, conversion of the diaphragm to a type I muscle increases endurance but reduces maximum force generation and, thereby, inspired volume production. Moreover, the diaphragm accounts for only approximately 60% of the inspiratory capacity and only a portion of the diaphragm is stimulated with DP.[70] Lack of coincident intercostal muscle activation, therefore, may account for insufficient inspired volumes. Another factor that may also play a role includes a greater sense of security with MV, a device equipped with more alarm systems.

The effects of DP on survival is unknown. Complicating any analysis between patients managed with MV versus DP is that there are multiple prognostic factors that have an impact on survival, including age, level and completeness of injury, and time since injury. There is some evidence, however, that DP is associated with a lower incidence of respiratory tract infections,[26] which is a frequent cause of death in SCI, driving a trend toward improved survival.

COMPLICATIONS AND SIDE EFFECTS

Currently the incidence of complications and side effects associated with DP is low due to technical advances and clinical experience garnered over the past several decades. With use of modern-day equipment, proper use of stimulus parameters, and adequate patient monitoring, serious complications are uncommon. Because DP is a life support system and DP may fail to provide adequate ventilatory support, back-up MV or other means of providing respiratory support, for example, use of an Ambu bag, should always be readily available. Potential complications and side effects are shown in **Box 2**.

Surgical Complications

One of the most serious complications is iatrogenic phrenic nerve injury,[10,63,71] which may occur during manipulation of the nerve during initial electrode placement. Damage to the nerve can occur via direct mechanical trauma or compromise of nerve blood supply. Late injury can also occur due to mechanical injury or the development of fibrosis around the nerve. Fortunately, the incidence of this complication is low. This complication is more likely to occur with cervical electrode placement. Because most patients have motor

---

Box 2
Potential complications and side effects of diaphragm pacing

Mechanical injury to the phrenic nerve

  Iatrogenic injury at the time of surgery

  Late injury due to tension on the nerve, loss of nerve blood supply, or fibrosis

Technical malfunction

  External components

    Battery failure

    Breakage of antenna wires

  Implanted components

    Receiver failure

    Breakage of implanted connecting wires

    Electrode malfunction

Infection

Upper airway obstruction after tracheostomy closure

Paradoxic movement of the upper rib cage, particularly in children

---

control of their cervical muscles, excessive neck motion may result in stretching of the nerve/electrode assembly and secondary injury. For this reason, intrathoracic electrode placement is preferred. Improved electrode design, however, has also significantly reduced the occurrence of this complication. The intramuscular electrode system developed by Synapse Biomedical, in which the electrodes are not in direct contact with the nerve, virtually eliminates this small risk.

As with any surgical procedure, there are infection risks. With modern surgical techniques and use of preoperative antibiotics, however, the rate of infection is low.[63,68,71] Infection involving any of the implanted materials, however, usually requires their removal. Placement of intramuscular diaphragm electrodes involves a small risk of pneumothorax and infection at the exit site of the electrode wires. With implantation of intramuscular electrodes, there is a high incidence of capnothorax, that is, tracking of CO_2 above the diaphragm from the pressurized abdomen required for laparoscopy. This could be managed by either observation or simple aspiration and does not result in any hemodynamic or respiratory compromise.

Technical Malfunction

By far the most common cause of mechanical failure is loss of battery power. This is completely avoidable by following the required routine mainte-nance procedures involving regular battery changes and recharging schedules. Low battery alarms are also present. With the radiofrequency devices, the external antenna wires may break at stress points, either near the connection to the transmitter or at the connection to the receivers. With the intramuscular electrode device, wire breakage may occur at the exit point from the body.

With regard to the internal components, the radiofrequency receiver may fail. Due to leakage of body fluids through the epoxy capsule, this was a frequent. problem with older devices, occur-ring within 5 years.[18,64,71] In newer devices with improved housing materials, however, receiver life has been extended significantly and the inci-dence or receiver failure is less common.[68] Elec-trode breakage or malfunction can also occur at variable time periods after implantation. In 1 anal-ysis of the Atrotech OY quadripolar electrode sys-tem in patients who had undergone DP for approximately 2 years, the electrode failure rate was 3.1%.[68] Failure rates were similar in patients with SCI and those with CHS. Failure of 1 or more of the 4 electrode combinations was com-mon but usually did not interfere significantly with the performance of the device.

Upper Airway Obstruction

Although there are reports of successful tracheos-tomy closure after maintenance of ventilation on DP, these are uncommon. As discussed previ-ously, most patients cap their tracheostomy tubes during wakefulness. At night, however, diaphragm contraction may not be synchronized with upper airway contraction.[4,72,73] Contraction of the dia-phragm with a flaccid upper airway would result in intermittent airway collapse and possibly signif-icant hypoxemia during sleep. Maintenance of a patent tracheostomy is also useful in instances when MV is necessary due to pacemaker malfunc-tion or instances of increased respiratory demand, such as atelectasis or respiratory tract infections.

EFFECTS OF MAGNETIC AND RADIOFREQUENCY FIELDS

With the radiofrequency devices, it is possible that the strong magnetic fields associated with MRI scanning can override the electronic circuitry of pacing systems, resulting in significant damage. In addition, the phrenic nerve may be damaged by the potentially high levels of energy transmis-sion to the electrode. Electrotherapeutic devices that generate strong radiofrequency fields may also interfere with the normal function of the DP system.

MAINTENANCE AND TROUBLESHOOTING OF DIAPHRAGM PACING SYSTEMS

The DP system should be monitored on a routine basis and also in situations in which patients are experiencing respiratory distress. In this regard, most patients are able to detect small changes in inspired volume delivered by DP and, therefore, alert caregivers to early signs of DP system malfunction.[74] Diaphragm contraction can be assessed by palpation of the chest wall. Inspira-tion should be accompanied by outward move-ment of the abdominal wall and lateral expansion of the lower rib cage. Reductions in the magnitude of chest wall movement signals reductions in inspired volume. Readily available use of a simple spirometer, which can be attached to the trache-ostomy tube, allows for a direct measurement of inspired volume. The transmitter can also be adjusted to assess separately inspired volume production from each hemidiaphragm. Pulse oximetry and end-tidal CO_2 monitors are also use-ful devices to monitor ventilation. With the onset of inadequate ventilation, MV should be instituted promptly until the specific problems are addressed. The battery power should be first checked followed by replacement of a back-up antenna and transmitter, if available.

Changes in lung mechanics may also have an impact on the function of the DP system. Increases in airway resistance and/or reductions in respira-tory system compliance may result in reductions in inspired volume. For example, retained secre-tions, which are a common occurrence in SCI, may increase airway resistance and cause atelec-tasis, resulting in reductions in lung compliance. Prompt suctioning or use of other means of secre-tion management may quickly address this problem. Respiratory tract infections, such as pneumonia, may also result in abnormalities in lung mechanics. Infections, such as pneumonia, may result in marked increases in airway resis-tance and reductions in lung compliance. When severe alterations occur, DP may become ineffec-tive, necessitating a need to switch to MV.

If inspired volumes remain low despite func-tional external components and there are no obvious signs of alterations in lung mechanics, pa-tients should be referred to specialized centers to evaluate the function of the internal components.

FUTURE DIRECTIONS

DP is usually reserved for patients with chronic SCI that is at least several months after injury. This delay is a prudent approach because the phrenic nerve may recover over a period of several weeks to several months, resulting in successful weaning from MV.[8,15,16,23,75] Moreover, DP is expensive and requires a surgical procedure. Implantation of intramuscular diaphragm electrodes, which is less expensive, requires a minimally invasive procedure and does not require implantation of a receiver but, however, may be an attractive alternative to MV in the acute phase of SCI. With this approach, deconditioning of the diaphragm would be prevented and successful transition to DP would occur more quickly compared with chronic SCI. If a patient is eventually weaned from MV, the electrodes can then be removed. Prior to adoption, however, clinical trials are necessary to assess the risks and benefits of such an approach as well as a cost-benefit analysis.

All DP systems are open-loop in design, that is, the diaphragm is stimulated independent of the spontaneous generation of inspiratory signals in the brainstem. Consequently, the upper airway muscles may not be activated in synchrony with the diaphragm, resulting in upper airway obstruction during sleep. This problem could be solved if diaphragm activation could be triggered by a signal from a functional inspiratory muscle, such as an upper airway muscle.[76] Such a closed loop system would eliminate need for a tracheostomy and also allow for ventilatory adjustments to speech and changes in metabolic demand.

Finally, animal studies suggest that both the diaphragm and the inspiratory intercostal muscles can be activated in synchrony by the application of high-frequency spinal cord applied to the ventral epidural surface of the spinal cord.[77] This technique can be applied with a single electrode with small currents (1–2 mA) and stimulus frequencies of approximately 300 Hz. Near-maximal activation of the inspiratory muscles can be achieved, resulting in inspired volumes approaching the inspiratory capacity. The electromyographic pattern of both the diaphragm and intercostal also resembles normal breathing, with an asynchronous pattern and firing frequencies similar to those occurring during normal breathing. Moreover, ventilation could be maintained on a chronic basis for at least 6 hours without signs of system fatigue. Consequently, this seems to be a more natural and effective means of inspiratory muscle pacing. Clinical trials of this technique are necessary to assess it safety and efficacy in patients with SCI.[77]

SUMMARY

DP is a practical and cost-effective method of providing ventilatory support in patients with respiratory failure secondary to cervical SCI and CHS.

Compared with MV, this method has significant health and lifestyle advantages, including greater mobility, improved speech and olfaction, reduced level of anxiety and embarrassment, and overall sense of well-being. It is important that all patients be screened to determine adequacy of phrenic nerve function, including measurements of phrenic nerve conduction studies. In addition, social factors, including level of patient motivation and caregiver support, should be assessed. Serious coexisting medical conditions, such as significant cardiac or brain disease, may also preclude eligibility. In patients with inadequate phrenic nerve function, emerging technologies, such as intercostal to phrenic nerve transfer to restore phrenic nerve viability and combined intercostal and phrenic nerve pacing, may emerge as standard techniques to increase the number of patients who can be weaned from MV. Finally, early work in animal studies suggests that high-frequency spinal cord stimulation may be a more natural and effective means of weaning patients from MV.

REFERENCES

1. Mellins RB, Balfour HH Jr, Turino GM, et al. Failure of automatic control of ventilation (Odine's curse). Report of an infant born with this syndrome and review of literature. Medicine (Baltimore) 1970;49:487–504.
2. Deonna T, Arczynska W, Torrado A. Congenital failure of automatic ventilation (Odine's curse). A case report. J Pediatr 1974;84:710–4.
3. Weese-Mayer DE, Hunt CE, Brouillette RT, et al. Diaphragm pacing in infants and children. J Pediatr 1992;120:1–8.
4. Hunt CE, Brouillette RT, Weese-Mayer DE, et al. Diaphragm pacing in infants and children. Pacing Clin Electrophysiol 1988;11:2135–41.
5. Ilibawi MN, Idriss FSL, Hunt CE, et al. Diaphragmatic pacing in infants: techniques and results. Ann Thorac Surg 1985;40:323–9.
6. Brouillette RT, Ilbawi MN, Hunt CE. Phrenic nerve pacing in infants and children: a review of experience and report on the usefulness of phrenic nerve stimulation studies. J Pediatr 1983;102:32–9.
7. Glenn WW, Hogan JF, Loke JS, et al. Ventilatory support by pacing of the conditioned diaphragm in quadriplegia. N Engl J Med 1984;310:1150–5.
8. Glenn WW, Hogan JF, Phelps ML. Ventilatory support of the quadriplegic patient with respiratory paralysis by diaphragm pacing. Surg Clin North Am 1980;60:1055–78.
9. Glenn WW, Phelps ML. Diaphragm pacing by electrical stimulation of the phrenic nerve. Neurosurgery 1985;17:974–84.

10. Glenn WW, Phelps ML, Elefteriades JA, et al. Twenty years of experience in phrenic nerve stimulation to pace the diaphragm. Pacing Clin Electrophysiol 1986;9:780–4.

11. Glenn WW, Sairenji H. Diaphragm pacing in the treatment of chronic ventilatory insufficiency. In: Roussos C, Macklem PT, editors. The thorax: lung biology in health and disease, vol. 29. New York: Marcel Dekker; 1985. p. 1407–40.

12. Drake RL, Vogl WA. Gray's anatomy for students. Elsevier/Church Livingstone; 2005. p. 134–5.

13. Weese-Mayer DE, Berry-Kravis EM, Ceccherini I, et al. An official ATS clinical policy statement: congenital central hypoventilation syndrome. Am J Respir Crit Care Med 2010;181:626–44.

14. National Spinal Cord injury statistical Center, University of Alabama at Birmingham. Annual statistical report 2017. Birmingham (United Kingdom): University of Alabama; 2017.

15. DiMarco AF. Diaphragm pacing in patients with spinal cord injury. Top Spinal Cord Inj Rehabil 1999;5:6–20.

16. DiMarco AF. Respiratory muscle stimulation in patients with spinal cord injury. In: Horch KW, Dhillon GS, editors. Neuroprosthetics: theory and practice. River Edge (NJ): World Scientific; 2004. p. 951–78.

17. Dobelle WH, D'Angelo MS, Goetz BF, et al. 200 cases with a new breathing pacemaker dispel myths about diaphragm pacing. ASAIO J 1994;40:M244–52.

18. Elefteriades JA, Quin JA, Hogan JF, et al. Long-term follow-up of pacing of the conditioned diaphragm in quadriplegia. Pacing Clin Electrophysiol 2002;25:897–906.

19. Tibballs J. Diaphragmatic pacing: an alternative to long-term me chanical ventilation. Anaesth Intensive Care 1991;19:597–601.

20. Langou RA, Cohen LS, Sheps D, et al. Odine's curse: hemodynamic response to diaphragm pacing (electrophrenic respiration). Am Heart J 1978;95:295–300.

21. Holt JD, Banzett AB, Brown R. Binding the abdomen can improve speech in men with phrenic nerve pacers. Am J Speech Lang Pathol 2002;11:71–6.

22. Adler D, Gonzalez-Bermejo J, Duguet A, et al. Diaphragm pacing restores olfaction in tetraplegia. Eur Respir J 2009;34(2):365–70.

23. DiMarco AF. Neural prostheses in the respiratory system. J Rehabil Res Dev 2001;38:601–7.

24. Fodstad H. The Swedish experience in phrenic nerve stimulation. Pacing Clin Electrophysiol 1987;10:246–51.

25. Fodstad H. Pacing of the diaphragm to control breathing in patients with paralysis of central nervous system origin. Stereotact Funct Neurosurg 1989;53:209–22.

26. Hirschfeld S, Exner G, Luukkaala T, et al. Mechanical ventilation or phrenic nerve stimulation for treatment of spinal cord injury-induced respiratory insufficiency. Spinal Cord 2008;46:738–42.

27. Moxham J, Shneer JM. Diaphragmatic pacing. Am Rev Respir Dis 1993;148:533–6.

28. Whiteneck GG, Charlifue SW, Frankel HL, et al. Mortality, morbidity, and psychosocial outcomes of persons spinal cord injured more than 20 years ago. Paraplegia 1992;30:617–30.

29. DiMarco AF, Supinski G, Petro J, et al. Artificial respiration via combined intercostal and diaphragm pacing in a quadriplegic patient. Am Rev Respir Dis 1994;149:A135.

30. Glenn WWL, Hageman JH, Mauro A, et al. Electrical stimulation of exciteable tissue by radiofrequency transmission. Ann Surg 1964;160:338–50.

31. Judson JP, Glenn WWL. Radio-frequency electrophrenic respiration: long-term application to a patient with primary hypoventilation. JAMA 1968;203:1033–7.

32. Talonen PP, Baer GA, Hakkinen V, et al. Neurophysiological and technical considerations for the design of an implantable phrenic nerve stimulator. Med Biol Eng Comput 1990;28:31–7.

33. Thoma H, Gerner H, Holle J, et al. The phrenic pacemaker: substitution of paralyzed functions in tetraplegia. ASAIO Trans 1987;33:472–9.

34. DiMarco AF, Onders RP, Ignagni A, et al. Phrenic nerve pacing via intramuscular diaphragm electrodes in tetraplegic subjects. Chest 2005;127:671–8.

35. DiMarco AF, Onders RP, Kowalski KE, et al. Phrenic nerve pacing in a tetraplegic patient via intramuscular diaphragm electrodés. Am J Respir Crit Care Med 2002;166:1604–6.

36. Peterson DK, Nochomovitz M, DiMarco AF, et al. Intramuscular electrical activation of the phrenic nerve. IEEE Trans Biomed Eng 1986;33:342–52.

37. Peterson DK, Nochomovitz ML, Stellato TA, et al. Longterm intramuscular electrical activation of phrenic nerve: safety and reliability. IEEE Trans Biomed Eng 1994;41:1115–26.

38. Peterson DK, Nochomovitz ML, Stellato TA, et al. Longterm intramuscular electrical activation of phrenic nerve: efficacy as a ventilatory prosthesis. IEEE Trans Biomed Eng 1994;41:1127–35.

39. Schmit BD, Stellato TA, Miller ME, et al. Laparoscopic placement of electrodes for diaphragm pacing using stimulation to locate the phrenic nerve motor points. IEEE Trans Rehabil Eng 1998;6:382–90.

40. Onders RP, Elmo MJ, Khansarinia S, et al. Complete worldwide operative experience in laparoscpic diaphragm pacing: results and differences in spinal cord injured patients and amotrophic lateral sclerosis patients. Surg Endosc 2009;23:1433–40.

41. Onders RP, DiMarco AF, Ignagni AR, et al. Mapping the phrenic nerve motor point: the key to a

successful laparoscopic diaphragm pacing system in the first human series. Surgery 2004;136:819–26.

42. Oliven A. Electrical stimulation of the respiratory muscles. In: Cherniack NS, Altose MD, Homma I, editors. Rehabilitation of the patient with respiratory disease. New York: McGraw-Hill; 1999. p. 535–42.

43. DiMarco AF, Altose MD, Cropp A, et al. Activation of intercostäl muscles by electrical stimulation of the spinal cord. Am Rev Respir Dis 1987;136:1385–90.

44. DiMarco AF, Budzinska K, Supinski GS. Artificial ventilation by means of electrical activation of intercostal/accessory muscles alone in anesthetized dogs. Am Rev Respir Dis 1989;139:961–7.

45. DiMarco AF, Supinski GS, Petro J, et al. Evaluation of intercostal pacing to provide artificial ventilation in quadriplegics. Am J Respir Crit Care Med 1994;150:934–40.

46. DiMarco AF, Takaoka Y, Kowalski KE. Combined intercostal and diaphragm pacing to provide artificial ventilation in patients with tetraplegics. Arch Phys Med Rehabil 2005;86:1200–7.

47. Krieger LM, Krieger AJ. The intercostal to phrenic nerve transfer: an effective means of reanimating the diaphragm in patients with high cervical spine injury. Plast Reconstr Surg 2000;105:1255–61.

48. Kaufman MR, Elkwood AI, Aboharb F, et al. Diaphragmatic reinnervation in ventilator-dependent patients with cervical spinal cord injury and concomitant phrenic nerve lesions using simultaneous nerve transfers and implantable neurostimulators. J Reconstr Microsurg 2015;5:391–5.

49. Flageole H. Central hypoventilation and diaphragmatic eventration: diagnosis and management. Semin Pediatr Surg 2003;12:38–45.

50. Glenn WW, Gee JBL, Schachter EN. Diaphragm pacing: application to a patient with chronic obstructive lung disease. J Thorac Cardiovasc Surg 1978;75:273–81.

51. DiPals Study Group Collaborators. Safety and efficacy of diaphragm pacing with respiratory insufficiency due to amyotrophic lateral sclerosis (DiPALS): a multicenter, open-label, randomized controlled trial. Lancet Neurol 2016;14:883–92.

52. Bach JR, Alba AS. Noninvasive options for ventilatory support of the traumatic high level tetraplegic patient. Chest 1990;98:613–9.

53. Bach JR, Alba AS. Management of chronic alveolar hypoventilation by nasal ventilation. Chest 1990;97:52–7.

54. Chae J, Triolo RI, Kilgore KL, et al. Neuromuscular electrical stimulation in spinal cord injury. In: Kirshblum S, Campagnolo DI, DeLisa JA, editors. Spinal cord medicine. Philadelphia: Lippincott Williams & Wilkins; 2002. p. 360–88.

55. Oakes DD, Wilmot CB, Halverson D, et al. Neurogenic respiratory failure: a 5-year experience using implantable phrenic nerve stimulators. Ann Thorac Surg 1980;30:118–21.

56. Nicholson KJ, Nosanov LB, Bowen KA, et al. Thoracoscpic placement of phrenic nerve pacers for diaphragm pacing in congenital central hypoventilation syndrome. J Pediatr Surg 2015;50:78–81.

57. DiMarco AF. Diaphragm pacing. In: Tobin MJ, editor. Principles and practice of mechanical ventilation. New York: McGraw-Hill; 2006. p. 1263–76.

58. MacLean IC, Mattioni TA. Phrenic nerve conduction studies: a new technique and its application in quadriplegic patients. Arch Phys Med Rehabil 1981;62:70–3.

59. Mckenzie DK, Gandevia SC. Phrenic nerve conduction times and twitch pressures of the human diaphragm. J Appl Physiol 1985;58:1496–504.

60. Moosa A. Phrenic nerve conduction in children. Dev Med Child Neurol 1981;23:434–48.

61. Miller JM, Moxham J, Green M. The maximal sniff in the assessment of diaphragm function in man. Clin Sci (Lond) 1985;69:91–6.

62. Ciesielski TE, Fukuda Y, Glenn WW, et al. Response of the diaphragm muscle to electrical stimulation of the phrenic nerve. A histochemical and ultrastructural study. J Neurosurg 1983;58:92–100.

63. Brouillette RT, Ilbawi MN, Klemka-Walden L, et al. Stimulus parameters for phrenic nerve pacing in infants and children. Pediatr Pulmonol 1988;4:33–8.

64. Glenn WW, Brouillette RT, Dentz B, et al. Fundamental considerations in pacing of the diaphragm for chronic ventilatory insufficiency: a multi-center study. Pacing Clin Electrophysiol 1988;11:2121–7.

65. Oda T, Glenn WWL, Fukuda Y, et al. Evaluation of electrical parameters for diaphragm pacing: an experimental study. J Surg Res 1981;30:142–53.

66. Salmons S, Henriksson J. The adaptive response of skeletal muscle to increased use. Muscle Nerve 1981;4:94–105.

67. Brown R, DiMarco AF, Hoit JF, et al. Respiratory dysfunction and mangement in spinal cord injury. Respir Care 2006;51:853–70.

68. Weese-Mayer DE, Silvestri JM, Kenny AS, et al. Diaphragm pacing with a quadripolar phrenic nerve electrode: an international study. Pacing Clin Electrophysiol 1996;19:1311–9.

69. Enoka RM. Activation order of motor axons in electricaly evoked cotractions. Muscle Nerve 2002;25:763–4.

70. Agostoni E, Mognoni P, Torri G, et al. Static features of the passive rib cae and abdomen-diaphragm. J Appl Physiol 1965;20:1187–93.

71. Vanderlinden RG, Epstein SW, Hyland RH, et al. Management of chronic ventilatory insufficiency with electrical diaphragm pacing. Can J Neurol Sci 1988;15:63–7.

72. Weese-Mayer DE, Morrow AS, Brouillette RT, et al. Diaphragm pacing in infants and children.

A life-table analysis of implanted components. Am Rev Respir Dis 1989;139:974–9.

73. Glenn WW, Gee JB, Cole DR, et al. Combined central alveolar hypoventilation and upper airway obstruction. Treatment by tracheostomy and diaphragm pacing. Am J Med 1978;64:50–60.

74. DiMarco AF, Wolfson DA, Gottfried SB, et al. Sensation of inspired volume in normal subjects and quadriplegic patients. J Appl Physiol 1982;53:1481–6.

75. Oo T, Watt JWH, Soni BM, et al. Delayed diaphragm recovery in 12 patients after high cervical spinal cord injury. A retrospective review of the diaphragm status of 107 patients ventilated afteracute spinal cord injury. Spinal Cord 1999;37:117–22.

76. Scharf SM, Feldman NT, Goldman MD, et al. Vocal cord closure. A cause of upper airway obstruction during controlled ventilation. Am Rev Respir Dis 1978;117:391–7.

77. DiMarco AF, Kowalski KE. High frequency spinal cord stimulation of inspiratory muscles in dogs: a new method of inspiratory muscle pacing. J Appl Physiol 2009;107:662–9.

Moving?

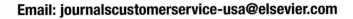

Make sure your subscription moves with you!

To notify us of your new address, find your **Clinics Account Number** (located on your mailing label above your name), and contact customer service at:

Email: journalscustomerservice-usa@elsevier.com

800-654-2452 (subscribers in the U.S. & Canada)
314-447-8871 (subscribers outside of the U.S. & Canada)

Fax number: 314-447-8029

Elsevier Health Sciences Division
Subscription Customer Service
3251 Riverport Lane
Maryland Heights, MO 63043

*To ensure uninterrupted delivery of your subscription, please notify us at least 4 weeks in advance of move.